# Genetic Control
## of Natural Resistance
## to Infection and Malignancy

# Perspectives in Immunology

## A Series of Publications Based on Symposia

# GENETIC CONTROL OF NATURAL RESISTANCE TO INFECTION AND MALIGNANCY

edited by

**EMIL SKAMENE**

*Montreal General Hospital Research Institute*
*Montreal, Quebec, Canada*

**PATRICIA A. L. KONGSHAVN**

*Montreal General Hospital Research Institute*
*and*
*Department of Physiology*
*McGill University*
*Montreal, Quebec, Canada*

**MAURICE LANDY**

*Schweizerisches Forschungsinstitut*
*Davos, Switzerland*

**ACADEMIC PRESS**    **1980**

A Subsidiary of Harcourt Brace Jovanovich, Publishers

New York   London   Toronto   Sydney   San Francisco

Academic Press Rapid Manuscript Reproduction

Proceedings of an International Symposium of the Canadian Society for Immunology held in Montreal, Quebec, March 18–20, 1980.

ACADEMIC PRESS, INC.
111 Fifth Avenue, New York, New York 10003

*United Kingdom Edition published by*
ACADEMIC PRESS, INC. (LONDON) LTD.
24/28 Oval Road, London NW1 7DX

**Library of Congress Cataloging in Publication Data**

International Symposium on the Genetic Control of
    Natural Resistance to Infection and Malignancy,
    Montréal, Québec, 1980.
    Genetic control of natural resistance to infection
and malignancy.

    (Perspectives in immunology)

    Includes index.
    1. Natural immunity—Congresses. 2. Infection—
Immunological aspects—Congresses. 3. Cancer—Immuno-
logical aspects—Congresses. 4. Immunogenetics—
Congresses. I. Skamene, Emil. II. Kongshavn,
Patricia A. L. III. Landy, Maurice. IV. Canadian
Society for Immunology. V. Title. [DNLM: 1. Im-
munity, Natural—Congresses. 2. Immunogenetics—
Congresses. 3. Infection—Immunology—Congresses.
4. Neoplasms—Immunology—Congresses. QW700 G328 1980.]
QR185.2.I57 1980        616.07'9        80-22733
ISBN 0-12-647680-2

PRINTED IN THE UNITED STATES OF AMERICA

80 81 82 83    9 8 7 6 5 4 3 2 1

# CONTENTS

## Section II. Genetic Control of Resistance to Bacterial Infections

## Section III. Genetic Control of Resistance to Virus Infection

**Section IV. Genetic Control of Natural Resistance to Tumor Growth**

**Section V. Genetic Control of Macrophage Differentiation and
Function**

# CONTRIBUTORS

*Numbers in parentheses indicate the pages on which authors' contributions begin.*

M. Alimohammadian, *Department of Pathology, School of Public Health, Tehran University, Tehran, Iran (29)*

E. M. Allen, *Immunology Laboratories, Research Service, Wood VA Medical Center, The Medical College of Wisconsin, Milwaukee, Wisconsin 53193 (191)*

D. B. Amos, *Department of Microbiology and Immunology, Duke University Medical Center, Durham, North Carolina 27710 (381)*

H. Arnheiter, *Division of Experimental Microbiology, Institute for Medical Microbiology, University of Zurich, P. O. Box 8028, Zurich, Switzerland (227)*

P. Baker, *Cellular Immunology Unit of the Tumor Institute, University of Alabama in Birmingham, Birmingham, Alabama 35294 (173)*

G. J. Bancroft, *Department of Microbiology, University of Western Australia, Perth, Western Australia (277)*

F. B. Bang, *Department of Pathobiology. The Johns Hopkins University, School of Hygiene and Public Health, Baltimore, Maryland 21205 (215)*

S. P. Bartlett, *Transplantation Unit, General Surgical Services, Massachusetts General Hospital, Boston, Massachusetts 02114 (413)*

H. G. Bedigian, *The Jackson Laboratory, Bar Harbor, Maine 04609 (461)*

R. G. Bell, *James A. Barker Institute for Animal Health, New York State College of Veterinary Medicine, Cornell University, Ithaca, New York 14853 (67)*

M. Bennett, *Department of Pathology, Boston University, School of Medicine, Boston, Massachusetts 02118 (431)*

P. N. Bhatt, *Section of Comparative Medicine, Yale University, School of Medicine, New Haven, Connecticut 06510 (305)*

B. R. Bloom, *Department of Microbiology and Immunology, Albert Einstein College of Medicine, Bronx, New York 10461 (313)*

D. Boraschi, *Laboratory of Immunobiology, National Cancer Institute, Bethesda, Maryland 20014 (537)*

D. J. Bradley, *Ross Institute of Tropical Hygiene, London School of Hygiene and Tropical Medicine. London, England WC1E 7HT (9)*

D. Briles, *Cellular Immunobiology, Unit of the Tumor Institute, University of Alabama in Birmingham, Birmingham, Alabama 35294 (173)*

M. A. Brinton, *The Wistar Institute, Philadelphia, Pennsylavia 19104 (297)*

W. J. Britt, *Laboratory of Persistent Viral Diseases, National Institute of Allergy and Infectious Diseases, Rocky Mountain Laboratories, Hamilton, Montana 59840 (329)*

J. Brock, *Department of Pathology, University of Cambridge, Cambridge, England (121)*

R. C. Burton, *Transplantation Unit, General Surgical Services, Massachusetts General Hospital, Boston, Massachusetts 02114 (413)*

G. Campbell, *Department of Immunology, University of Alberta, Edmonton, Alberta T6G 2H7, Canada (445)*

G. A. Carlson, *The Jackson Laboratory, Bar Harbor, Main 04609 (445)*

W. S. Ceglowski, *Department of Microbiology and Immunology, Temple University, School of Medicine, Philadelphia, Pennsylvania 19140 (367)*

J. E. Chalmer, *Central Laboratories of Netherlands Red Cross, Blood Transfusion Service, P.O. B. 9190, 1006 AD Amsterdam, The Netherlands (277, 283)*

M. A. Chan, *McMaster University, Hamilton, Ontario L85 4J9, Canada (345)*

Y. Y. Chan, *Department of Microbiology, University of Melbourne, Parkville, Victoria 3052 Australia (141)*

C. Cheers, *Department of Microbiology, University of Melbourne, Parville, Victoria 3052, Australia (141)*

B. Chesebro, *National Institute of Allergy and Infectious Diseases, Laboratory of Persistent Viral Diseases, Rocky Mountain Laboratories, Hamilton, Montana 59840 (329)*

D. A. Chow, *Manitoba Institute of Cell Biology, University of Manitoba, Winnipeg, Manitoba R3E OV9 (455)*

D. A. Clark, *McMaster University, Hamilton, Ontario L85 4J9, Canada (345)*

O. Closs, *University of Oslo, Institute for Experimental Medical Research, Ullevaal Hospital, Oslo 1, Norway (201)*

T. S. Cody, *Department of Pathobiology, The Johns Hopkins University School of Hygiene and Public Health, Baltimore, Maryland 21205 (215)*

E. Cudkowicz, *Immunology Branch, National Cancer Institute, Bethesda, Maryland 20205 (485)*

C. S. David, *Departments of Medicine and Immunology, Mayo Clinic and Foundation, Rochester, Minnesota 55901 (75)*

J. Davie, *National Institute of Allergy and Infectious Diseases, National Institutes of Health, Bethesda, Maryland 20014 (173)*

L. W. Deakins, *Department of Microbiology and Immunology, Temple University School of Medicine, Philadelphia, Pennsylvania 19140 (115)*

L. J. DeTolla, Jr., *Department of Pathobiology, University of Pennsylvania, School of Veterinary Medicine, Philadelphia, Pennsylvania 19104 (39)*

C. L. Diggs, *Walter Reed Army Institute of Research, Washington DC 20012 (89)*

C. Dupuy, *Institut Armand-Frappier, Laval-des-Rapides, Laval, Quebec H7N 4Z3, Canada (241)*

J. M. Dupuy, *Institut Armand-Frappier, Laval-des-Rapides, Laval, Quebec H7N 4Z3, Canada (241)*

M. C. Edelstein, *Laboratory of Immunobiology, National Cancer Institute, Bethesda, Maryland 20014 (537)*

B. M. Eig, *Section of Medical Oncology, Department of Medicine, Northwestern University, Chicago, Illinois 60611 (177)*

T. K. Eisenstein, *Department of Microbiology and Immunology, Temple University School of Medicine, Philadelphia, Pennsylvania 19140 (115)*

H. Engler, *Institute of Virus Research, German Cancer Research Center, 69 Heidelberg 1, Germany (267)*

J. P. Farrell, *Department of Pathobiology, University of Pennsylvania School of Medicine, Philadelphia, Pennsylvania 19104 (39)*

J. A. Frelinger, *Department of Microbiology, University of Southern California School of Medicine, Los Angeles, Californai 90033 (247)*

H. Friedman, *University of South Florida College of Medicine, Tampa, Florida 33612 (83, 367)*

J. S. Gavora, *Animal Research Institute, Research Branch in Agriculture, Ottawa, Ontario K1A OC6, Canada (361)*

S. R. Gee, *McMaster University, Hamilton, Ontario L85 4J9, Canada (345)*

G. J. Gleich, *Departments of Medicine and Immunology, Mayo Clinic and Foundation, Rochester, Minnesota 55901 (75)*

A. A. Glynn, *Bacteriology Department, Wright-Fleming Institute, St. Mary's Hospital Medical School, London, England W2 1PG (133)*

A. H. Greenberg, *Manitoba Institute of Cell Biology, University of Manitoba, Winnipeg, Manitoba R3E OV9, (455)*

H. C. Greenblatt, *Albert Einstein College of Medicine, Bronx, New York 10461 (89)*

M. G. Groves, *Department of Rickettsial Diseases, Walter Reed Army Institute of Research, Washington, D.C. 20012 (165)*

T. Haliotis, *Department of Microbiology and Immunology, Queen's University, Kingston, Ontario K7L 3N6, Canada, (419)*

O. Haller, *Division of Experimental Microbiology, Institute for Medical Microbiology, University of Zurich, P.O. Box 8028, Zurich, Switzerland (227)*

N. Haran-Ghera, *Department of Chemical Immunology, The Weizmann Institute of Science, Rehovot, Israel (321)*

C. E. Hormaeche, *Department of Pathology, University of Cambridge, Cambridge, England (121)*

E. Israel, *Lady Davis Institute for Medical Research, Sir Mortimer B. Davis Jewish General Hospital, Montreal, Quebec H3T 1E2, Canada (373)*

R. O. Jacoby, *Section of Comparative Medicine, Yale University School of Medicine, New Haven, Connecticut 06510 (305)*

D. A. Johnson, *The Jackson Laboratory, Bar Harbor, Maine 04609 (461)*

G. Ju, *Department of Cell Biology, Roche Institute of Molecular Biology, Nutley, New Jersey 07110 (313)*

M. Kamali, *Department of Pathobiology, School of Public Health, Tehran University, Tehran, Iran (29)*

K. Kärre, *Department of Tumor Biology, Karolinska Institutet, S-104 01 Stockholm 60, Sweden (389)*

E. Katz, *Department of Chemical Immunology, The Weizmann Institute of Science, Rehovot, Israel (321)*

A. Khamesipour, *Department of Pathobiology, School of Public Health, Tehran University, Tehran, Iran (29)*

R. Kiessling, *Department of Tumor Biology, Karolinska Institutet, S-104 01 Stockholm, Sweden (389, 467)*

H. Kirchner, *Institut for Virus Research, German Research Center, 69 Heidelberg 1, Germany (267)*

G. Klein, *Department of Tumor Biology, Karolinska Institutet, S-104 01 Stockholm 60, Sweden (467)*

G. O. Klein, *Department of Tumor Biology, Karolinska Institutet, S-104 01 Stockholm 60, Sweden (389, 467)*

T. W. Klein, *University of South Florida College of Medicine, Tampa, Florida 33612 (83)*

P. A. L. Kongshavn, *Department of Physiology, McGill University, Montreal General Hospital, Research Institute, Montreal, Quebec H3G 1A4, Canada (149, 499, 565)*

V. Kumar, *Department of Pathology, Boston University School of Medicine, Boston, Massachusetts 02118 (431)*

F. Labrador, *I.V.I.C. Centro de Microbiologia y Biologia Celular, Apartado 1827, Caracas 1010 A, Venezuela (47)*

D. Laforrêt-Cresteil, *Inserum U. 56 Hôpital, Bichêtre, France (241)*

E. Ledezma, *I.V.I.C. Centro de Microbiologia y Biologia Celular, Caracas 1010 A, Venezuela (47)*

J. R. Leininger, *University of Iowa, Iowa City, Iowa 52242 (353)*

E. Levy, *Department of Pathology and Microbiology, Boston University School of Medicine, Boston, Massachusetts 02118 (431)*

F. Lilly, *Department of Genetics, Albert Einstein College of Medicine, Bronx, New York 10461 (337)*

J. Lindenmann, *Division of Experimental Microbiology, Institute for Medical Microbiology, University of Zurich, P.O. Box 8028, Zurich, Switzerland (227)*

P. Lonai, *Department of Chemical Immunology, The Weizmann Institute of Science, Rehovot, Israel (321)*

C. Lopez, *Sloan-Kettering Institute for Cancer Research, New York, New York 10021 (253)*

M. Lovik, *University of Oslo, Institute for Experimental Medical Research, Ullevaal Hospital Oslo 1, Norway (201)*

T. J. MacVittie, *Experimental Hematology Department, Armed Forces Radiobiology Research Institute, Bethesda, Maryland 20014 (511)*

K. H. Mahoney, *Department of Microbiology, Medical College of Virginia, Virginia Commonwealth University, Richmond, Virginia 23298 (575)*

T. E. Mandel, *The Walter and Eliza Hall Institute, University of Melbourne, Parkville, Victoria 3052, Australia (141)*

D. N. Mannel, *Laboratory of Immunobiology, National Cancer Institute, Bethesda, Maryland 20014 (537)*

R. M. Massanari, *University of Iowa, Iowa City, Iowa 52242 (353)*

D. D. McGregor, *James A. Baker Institute for Animal Health, New York State College of Veterinary Medicine, Cornell University, Ithaca, New York 14853 (67)*

I. F. C. McKenzie, *Department of Medicine, University of Melbourne, Austin Hospital, Heidelberg, Victoria, Australia (141)*

H. Meier, *The Jackson Laboratory, Bar Harbor, Maine 04609 (461)*

R. Melvold, *Section of Medical Oncology, Department of Medicine, Northwestern University, Chicago, Illinois 60611 (425)*

M. S. Meltzer, *Laboratory of Immunobiology, National Cancer Institute, Bethesda, Maryland 20014 (537, 555)*

E. S. Metcalf, *Department of Microbiology, Uniformed Services, University of the Health Sciences, Bethesda, Maryland 20014 (101)*

M. W. Miller, *Immunology Branch, National Cancer Institute, Bethesda, Maryland 20205 (485)*

F. Z. Modabber, *Institut Pasteur, 28 rue du Dr. Roux, 75724 Paris cedex 15, France (29)*

S. C. Mogensen, *Institut of Medical Microbiology, University of Aarhus, Aarhus, Denmark (291)*

M. A. S. Moore, *Sloan-Kettering Institute for Cancer Research, Rye, New York 10580 (519)*

V. L. Moore, *Immunology Laboratories, Research Service, Wood VA Medical Center, The Medical College of Wisconsin, Milwaukee, Wisconsin 53193 (191)*

P. S. Morahan, *Department of Microbiology, Medical College of Virginia, Virginia Commonwealth University, Richmond, Virginia 23298 (575)*

S. S. Morse, *Department of Microbiology, Medical College of Virginia, Virginia Commonwalth University, Richmond, Virginia 23298 (575)*

C. A. Nacy, *Division of Communicable Diseasers and Immunology, Walter Reed Army Institute of Research, Washington, D.C. 20012 (555)*

M. Nahm, *Cellular Immunobiology Unit of the Tumor Institute, University of Alabama in Birmingham, Birmingham, Alabama 35294 (173)*

R. M. Nakamura, *Department of Tuberculosis, National Institute of Health, Shinagawa-ku, Tokyo 141, Japan (185)*

I. Nakoinz, *Sloan-Kettering Institute for Cancer Research, Rye, New York 10580 (519)*

M. Nasseri, *Department of Microbiology and Immunology, Center for Health Sciences, University of California, Los Angeles, California 90024 (29)*

P. A. Neighbour, *Department of Microbiology and Immunology, Albert Einstein College of Medicine, Bronx, New York 10461 (313)*

A. J. Norin, *Montefiore Hospital and Medical Center, New York, New York 10467 (531)*

A. D. O'Brien, *Department of Microbiology, Uniformed Services, University of the Health Sciences, Bethesda, Maryland 20014 (101)*

J. J. Oppenheim, *Laboratory of Microbiology and Immunology, National Institute of Dental Research, Bethesda, Maryland 20014 (583)*

J. V. Osterman, *Department of Rickettsial Diseases, Walter Reed Army Institute of Research, Washington, D.C. 20012 (165)*

H. Pérez, *I.V.I.C., Centro de Microbiologia y Biologia Celular, Apartado 1827 Caracas 1010 A, Venezuela (47)*

R. Pettifor, *Department of Pathology, University of Cambridge, Cambridge, England (121)*

J. E. Plant, *Bacteriology Department, Wright-Fleming Institute, St. Mary's Hospital Medical School, London, England W2 1PG (133)*

R. P. Polisson, *Immunology Branch, National Cancer Institute, Bethesda, Maryland 20014 (485)*

J. E. R. Potter, *The Jackson Laboratory, Bar Harbor, Maine 04609 (519)*

M. H. Pourmand, *Department of Pathobiology, School of Public Health, Tehran University, Tehran, Iran (29)*

G. Radlick, *Division of Communicable Diseases and Immunology, Walter Reed Army Institute of Research, Washington, D.C. 20012 (555)*

B. Rager-Zisman, *Department of Microbiology and Immunology, Albert Einstein College of Medicine, Bronx, New York 10461 (313)*

P. Ralph, *Sloan-Kettering Institute for Cancer Research, Rye, New York 10580 (519, 591)*

W. E. Rawls, *McMaster University, Hamilton, Ontario L85 4J0 Canada (345)*

J. C. Roder, *Department of Microbiology and Immunology, Queen's University, Kingston, Ontario K7L 3N6 Canada (405, 419)*

P. Rodday, *Departments of Pathology and Microbiology, Boston University School of Medicine, Boston, Massachusetts 02118 (431)*

D. L. Rosenstreich, *Albert Einstein College of Medicine, Bronx, New York 10461 (89, 97, 101, 165, 583)*

L. P. Ruco, *Laboratory of Immunobiology, National Cancer Institute, Bethesda, Maryland 20014 (537)*

C. Sadarangani, *Montreal General Hospital Research Institute, Montreal Quebec H3G 1A4 Canada (149)*

I. Scher, *Department of Immunology, Naval Medical Research Institute, Bethesda, Maryland 20014 (101)*

D. J. Schrier, *Immunology Laboratories, Research Service, Wood VA Medical Center, The Medical College of Wisconsin, Milwaukee, Wisconsin, 53193 (191)*

C. H. Schroder, *Institute of Virus Research, German Cancer Research Center, 69 Heidelberg 1, Germany (267)*

K. Schroer, *Cellular Immunobiology Unit of the Tumor Institute, University of Alabama in Birmingham, Birmingham, Alabama 35294 (173)*

P. A. Scott, *Department of Pathobiology, University of Pennsylvania School of Veterinary Medicine, Philadelphia, Pennsylvania 19104 (39)*

G. M. Shearer, *Immunology Branch, National Cancer Institute, Bethesda, Maryland 20014 (485)*

G. F. Shellam, *Department of Microbiology, University of Western Australia, Perth, Western Australia (277)*

D. E. Singer, *Department of Medicine, Massachusetts General Hospital, Boston, Massachusetts 02114 (477)*

E. Skamene, *Montreal General Hospital Research Institute, Montreal, Quebec H3G 1A4 Canada (149, 209, 499, 565)*

A. L. Smith, *Section of Comparative Medicine, Yale University School of Medicine, New Haven, Connecticut 06510 (305)*

S. Specter, *Department of Medical Microbiology, University of South Florida, College of Medicine, Tampa, Florida 33612 (367)*

J. L. Spencer, *Animal Diseases Research Institute, Agriculture, Canada, Nepean Ontario K2H 8P9 (361)*

R. Steeves, *Department of Genetics, Albert Einstein College of Medicine, Bronx, New York 10461 (337)*

J. L. Sternick, *Immunology Laboratories, Research Service, Wood VA Medical Center, The Medical College of Wisconsin, Milwaukee, Wisconsin, 53193 (191)*

M. M. Stevenson, *Montreal General Hospital Research Institute, Montreal, Quebec H3G 1A4 Canada (565)*

C. C. Stewart, *Section of Cancer Biology, Mallincrodt Institute of Radiology, Washington University School of Medicine, St. Louis, Missouri 63110 (499)*

S. A. Stohlman, *Department of Neurology, University of Southern California School of Medicine, Los Angeles, California 90033 (247)*

B. M. Sultzer, *Department of Microbiology and Immunology, State University of New York, Downstate Medical Center, Brooklyn, New York 11203 (115)*

B. A. Taylor, *The Jackson Laboratory, Bar Harbor, Maine 04609 (1, 191)*

T. Tokunaga, *Department of Tuberculosis, National Institute of Health, Shinagawa-ku, Tokyo 141, Japan (185)*

A. C. Vickery, *University of South Florida College of Medicine, Tampa, Florida 33612 (83)*

S. N. Vogel, *Laboratory of Microbiology and Immunology, National Institute of Dental Research, Bethesda, Maryland 20014 (583)*

M. A. Wainberg, *Lady Davis Institute for Medical Research, Sir Mortimer B. Davis Jewish General Hospital, Montreal, Quebec H3T 1E2 (373)*

A. Wake, *First Department of Bacteriology, National Institute of Health, Tokyo 141, Japan (179)*

D. Wakelin, *Wellcome Laboratories for Experimental Parasitology, University of Glasgow, Bearsden Road, Bearsden, Glasgow, Scotland (55)*

Wassom, D. L., *Allergic Diseases Research, Mayo Clinic, Rochester, Minnesota 55901 (75)*

L. L. Weedon, *Laboratory of Microbiology and Immunology, National Institute of Dental Research, Bethesda, Maryland 20014 (583)*

S. R. Weinberg, *Experimental Hematology Department, Armed Forces Radiobiology Research Institute, Bethesda, Maryland 20014 (511)*

R. M. Williams, *Section of Medical Oncology, Department of Medicine, Northwestern University, Chicago, Illinois 60611 (425, 477)*

M. L. Wilson, *University of Iowa, Iowa City, Iowa 52242 (353)*

H. J. Winn, *Transplantation Unit, General Surgical Services, Massachusetts General Hospital, Boston, Massachusetts 02114 (413, 495)*

L. B. Wolosin, *Manitoba Institute of Cell Biology, University of Manitoba, Winnipeg, Manitoba R3E OV9 (455)*

C. Yoosook, *Department of Microbiology, Faculty of Science, Mahidol University, Bangkok 4, Thailand (337)*

R. Zawatzky, *Institute of Virus Research, German Cancer Research Center, 69 Heidelberg 1, Germany (267)*

# PREFACE

History provides numerous examples of variable susceptibility of human populations to viral, bacterial, and parasitic infections both during epidemics and in the endemic areas of the world. Although the influence of environmental factors must be considered in any explanation of such variability, it has recently become clear, mainly on the basis of studying experimental infections in inbred animals, that genetic factors play the decisive role in individual susceptibility. Similarly, most tumor biologists believe that there are multiple mechanisms that influence the growth and spread of cells transformed to the neoplastic state and that most of them are, in a broad sense, genetically influenced.

In principle, the entire basis of susceptibility or resistance to infection and malignancy is genetically determined but, because of the immense variety of offenders and the complexities of host defenses, few common patterns of resistance are discernible. Thus, we are compelled to study step-wise processes affecting individual organisms and cancer cell types with the hope of extending the studies to other infections and malignancies and to other hosts.

Genetic studies have, in the last few years, proved to be a most valuable tool for analysis of host resistance processes This volume provides a review and discussion of a large body of information on various models of genetic resistance that have recently been discovered. Interaction of geneticists with investigators studying mechanisms of host defense to infection and malignancy, such as occurred at the symposium, that formed the basis for this volume, proves mutually beneficial. Thus, several polymorphic systems controlling genetic resistance among populations of inbred animals were defined by formal genetic analysis and located on the chromosomal map. Similarly, well-defined defects in host defenses in certain animal sublines were traced to single mutations in the genome of such strains. Another, perhaps more important, aspect of this interaction is an understanding of the action of genes controlling host resistance. In this case, genetic analysis is not the aim but serves to probe the processes that lead to successful host defense. As yet, there is not a single case in which the phenotypic expression of a host resistance gene has been identified at the molecular level. However, the cellular mechanisms of their action are clearly different from adaptive, specific immune responses and they mostly seem to fit into the category of natural or noninduced resistance.

It is apparent from this volume that systems of genetic resistance are all-important, not only in the first-line surveillance of infections and tumors, but also by their strong influence on the success of chemotherapy and immunotherapy. Thus, it is hoped that further analysis of these systems will lead to their more successful manipulation in favor of the host.

*Emil Skamene*
*Patricia A. L. Kongshavn*

# ACKNOWLEDGMENTS

The Symposium on Genetic Control of Natural Resistance to Infection and Malignancy, which formed the basis of this volume, was held under the auspices of the Montreal General Hospital Research Institute. We are greatly indebted to the Institute's Executive Director, Mr. L. G. Elliott, for his help, support, and constant encouragement in preparation of the symposium. Miss Pat Valois provided invaluable assistance in looking after the management of the symposium with great efficiency and attention to detail. We gratefully acknowledge the superb secretarial assistance of Mrs. Mary Bergin and her hard work, patience, and understanding in both the organization of the symposium and in preparation of the manuscript of this volume for publication.

# RECOMBINANT INBRED STRAINS OF MICE: USE IN GENETIC ANALYSIS OF DISEASE RESISTANCE

Benjamin A. Taylor
The Jackson Laboratory
Bar Harbor
Maine 04609

Recombinant inbred (RI) strains are derived by systematic inbreeding beginning with the $F_2$ generation of the cross of two preexisting inbred (progenitor) strains (1). From random pairings of $F_2$ mice, multiple independent strains are derived without selection (usually by brother-sister inbreeding). Once inbred, such a set of RI strains can be thought of as a stable segregant population. It is intuitively clear that each RI strain is expected to have received one-half of its autosomal genes from each of the progenitor strains. Thus, in a set of RI strains, half are expected to become fixed for each of the two alleles at every differential locus. Unlinked genes are randomized in the $F_2$ generation and are therefore equally likely to be fixed in parental or recombinant phases. However, linked genes will tend to become fixed in the same (parental) combinations as they entered the cross. These properties of RI strains permit several strong predictions: (a) for a phenotype under the control of a single locus only the two parental phenotypes are expected among the RI strains, and these are expected in equal frequencies; (b) linked loci will exhibit an excess of parental combinations, and the extent of the excess will be a function of the recombination frequency between the two loci in question; (c) different phenotypes under the control of a single locus (pleiotropic effects) will exhibit identical patterns of inheritance among the RI strains. Thus sets of RI strains can be used to test whether a particular trait is under the control of a single locus, to establish linkage (or independence), to estimate recombination frequency, to determine gene order, and to detect or test for possible pleiotropic effects of genes.

The strategy then is to develop a set of RI strains from the cross of two unrelated progenitors, and then to type them for as many genetic markers as feasible. When new genetic differences are discovered that distinguish between the progenitor strains, the RI strains are typed to determine whether the inheritance is simple or complex, and to evaluate potential linkage or pleiotropic relationships with previously typed loci. The enormous advantage of this approach is that the data are cumulative. Each RI strain needs to be typed only once for a particular locus. Therefore the

GENETIC CONTROL OF NATURAL RESISTANCE
TO INFECTION AND MALIGNANCY

1

discoverer of a new variant needs only to type the RI
strains for that variant. The investigator can immediately
determine whether the "new" locus is independent of, closely
linked to, or possibly a pleiotropic manifestation of, any
previously typed locus.

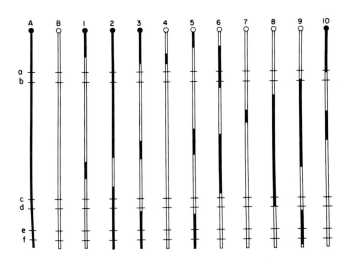

**Fig. 1.** Genetic consequences of RI strain formation, showing the result of a simulated example of ten RI strains derived from hypothetical progenitor strains A and B. Solid
and open lines are used to depict chromosomal material inherited from the A and B progenitor chromosome (shown at
left), respectively.

Figure 1 illustrates the genetic consequences of RI
strain formation using results obtained by computer simula-
tion. It shows the segregation and recombination of a single autosome 100 centimorgans in length for ten RI strains.
Genetic material from the A and B hypothetical progenitors
is represented by solid and open lines, respectively, in
both the progenitors' chromosomes (shown at left) and ten RI
strain chromosomes. The traces of six loci are shown to
illustrate the fact that short chromosomal segments are usually inherited intact, but that one or more genetic inter-
changes frequently separate more distantly linked loci. The
example also shows that it is not unusual for an RI strain

chromosome to be derived principally from one of the progenitor strains. The same processes of segregation and recombination would occur independently for other chromosomes.
The length of the chromosome in this example is approximately equal to the longest mouse chromosome, Chromosome 1.

Since there may be multiple opportunities for genetic
recombination between linked genes during the inbreeding
process, an equation is needed that expresses the probability of fixing a recombinant genotype in an RI strain ($\underline{R}$) as a
function of the recombination frequency ($\underline{r}$) in a single
meiosis. For the case of brother-sister inbreeding, $\underline{R} = 4\underline{r}$-
$/(1+6\underline{r})$ (3). By solving for $\underline{r}$, we obtain an equation which
can be used to calculate an estimate of the recombination
frequency ($\hat{\underline{r}}$) in terms of the observed frequency of RI stra-
ins with recombinant gentotypes ($\hat{\underline{R}}$), $\hat{\underline{r}} = \hat{\underline{R}}/(4-6\hat{\underline{R}})$ (7). A detailed exposition of the uses of RI strains for linkage ana-
lysis is published elsewhere (5).

The use of RI strains for linkage detection is best
illustrated by an example. Mishkin, et al. (4) found significant interstrain differences in the mean level of the enzyme galactokinase in erythrocytes. Differences were noted
between the progenitors of two sets of RI strains: the AKXL
RI strains, derived from AKR/J and C57L/J; and the BXH RI
strains, derived from C57BL/6J and C3H/HeJ. The RI strains
were tested and found to separate cleanly into the two parental classes. The results are shown in Table 1. In tab-
ulating genotypic data for RI strains, we follow the convention of using a generic symbol to indicate the source of any
allele. Thus A, L, B, and H are used to designate alleles
inherited from AKR/J, C57L/J, C57BL/6J, and C3H/HeJ, respectively. This convention facilitates the search for similar
patterns of inheritance. Such a search revealed a high degree of concordance between the patterns for the galacto-
kinase locus ($\underline{Glk}$) and esterase-3 ($\underline{Es-3}$), a kidney esterase
electrophoretic variant previously mapped to Chromosome 11
(Table 1). Only two recombinants were found among the 20
AKXL strains, and only one among the 14 BXH strains, for a
total of three recombinants among 34 RI strains. Substitut-
ing 3/34 for $\hat{R}$ in the previous equation $\hat{\underline{r}} = \hat{\underline{R}}/(4-6\hat{\underline{R}})$, we
obtain $\hat{\underline{r}} = 0.0254$. An estimate of the variance of $\hat{\underline{r}}$ is
given by the equation $\underline{V}(\hat{\underline{r}}) = \hat{\underline{r}}(1+2\hat{\underline{r}})(1+6\underline{r})^2/4\underline{n}$, where $\underline{n}$ is
the number of RI strains used in estimating $\underline{r}$ (Taylor et al.
1975). $\underline{V}(\hat{\underline{r}}) = .000254$. The standard error of $\hat{\underline{r}}$ is the
square root of $\underline{V}(\hat{\underline{r}})$, or 0.0160. Therefore the estimated
recombination frequency is 0.025 ± 0.016.

Table 2 lists some well established sets of RI strains
that are available at the Jackson Laboratory. These RI
strains have been typed for numerous genetic loci, the ma-

Table 1. Strain distribution patterns of Glk and ES-3 in the AKXL and BXH RI strains*

AKXL

| Locus | 4 | 6 | 8 | 11 | 12 | 13 | 14 | 16 | 17 | 18 | 19 | 21 | 23 | 24 | 25 | 28 | 29 | 36 | 37 | 38 |
|---|---|---|---|---|---|---|---|---|---|---|---|---|---|---|---|---|---|---|---|---|
| Glk | A | L | A | L | L | A | L | L | A | A | A | L | A | L | L | L | L | L | A | L |
|  |  |  |  |  |  | x |  |  |  |  |  |  |  |  |  |  |  |  |  | x |
| Es-3 | A | L | A | L | L | L | L | L | A | A | A | L | A | L | L | L | L | L | A | A |

BXH

| Locus | 2 | 3 | 4 | 5 | 6 | 7 | 8 | 9 | 10 | 11 | 12 | 14 | 18 | 19 |
|---|---|---|---|---|---|---|---|---|---|---|---|---|---|---|
| Glk | B | B | H | H | B | H | H | B | B | H | B | H | B | B |
| Es-3 | B | B | H | H | B | H | H | B | B | H | B | B | B | B |
|  |  |  |  |  |  |  |  |  |  |  |  | x |  |  |

*An x is used to denote the location of crossovers.

4

Table 2. Several sets of RI strains maintained at the Jackson Laboratory

| Progenitor | RI strain designation | Number of strains | Generations of inbreeding | Number of loci typed | Number of chromosomes * |
|---|---|---|---|---|---|
| BALB/cBy x C57BL/6By | CXB | 7 | 60-69 | 89 | 15 |
| AKR/J x C57L/J | AKXL | 18[†] | 19-47 | 80 | 15 |
| SWR/J x C57L/J | SWXL | 7 | 24-47 | 68 | 13 |
| C57BL/6J x DBA/2J | BXD | 26 | 34-49 | 100 | 15 |
| C57BL/6J x C3H/HeJ | BXH | 12 | 39-47 | 77 | 16 |

*The number of chromosomes known to bear at least one of the loci typed in the various RI strains.
†Two sublines of six strains were established after ten generations of brother-sister inbreeding.

jority of which have been mapped. They have been used in a
wide variety of studies to define new genetic loci, to map
these loci, and in some cases to try to establish the nature
of the genetic difference. I have summarized the published
genetic information on these strains elsewhere (6). The
numerous other sets of RI strains which exist or are under
development are listed in the same reference.

There are several advantages of the RI strain approach
over conventional genetic analysis. Some of these are particularly relevant to the analysis of complex traits such as
disease resistance. The major advantage, as previously
mentioned, is that the data are cumulative. This not only
makes linkage analysis practical, but it also permits the
detection of pleiotropy. Thus evidence may be obtained to
suggest that resistance to two or more organisms are under
the control of a single locus, even though the different
tests are conducted at different places and times, by independent investigators. Another situation in which RI strains are convenient, is that of genetic control by two loci,
one known (and typed already), and the other unknown. In a
hypothetical example resistance may be controlled by a major
gene, but modified by another gene, such as H-2. Previous
knowledge of the H-2 types of the RI strains would permit
the effects of the major gene to be seen in clearer focus.
Since RI strains are homozygous, genetic differences are
maximized, and the recessive genes of both progenitor strains can be expressed. A major advantage is that genotypes
do not need to be inferred from the phenotypes of individual
mice. Thus it is possible to work with statistical phenotypes, where the terms resistant and susceptible may be relative, not absolute. Unusual genotypes, such as rare recombinants, when detected in RI material, are immediately
available for confirmation and further characterization.

The major limitation of the RI approach is that
the strains are useful only if the progenitors of a set of
RI strains differ with respect to the trait of interest.
Another limitation is that the number of RI strains available in a particular set may be insufficient to discriminate
among different genetic hypotheses. Availability may be a
problem, particularly if large numbers of contemporary, age-
matched mice are needed. This problem is heightened by the
fact that some RI strains are poor breeders. Despite these
limitations, RI strains are being used to good advantage in
a wide variety of studies, including studies of disease resistance.

## ACKNOWLEDGEMENT

This work was supported by NIH Research Grant GM-18684 from the National Institute of General Medical Sciences. The Jackson Laboratory is fully accredited by the American Association for Accreditation of Laboratory Animal Care.

## REFERENCES

1.  Bailey, D.W.  Transplantation 11:325, 1971.
2.  Bradley, D.J., Taylor, B.A., Blackwell, J., Evans, E.P. and Freeman, J.  Clin.Exp.Immunol. 37:7, 1979.
3.  Haldane, J.B.S., and Waddington, C.H.  Genetics 16:357, 1931.
4.  Mishkin, J.D., Taylor, B.A., and Mellman, W.J. Biochem. Genet. 14:635, 1976.
5.  Taylor, B.A.  "Origins of Inbred Mice".  H. Morse (ed.). Academic Press, New York, p.423, 1978.
6.  Taylor, B.A.  "Genetic Variants and Strains of the Laboratory Mouse".  M.C. Green (ed).  Gustav Fischer Verlag, Stuttgart, 1980 (in press).
7.  Taylor, B.A., Bailey, D.W., Cherry, M., Riblet, R., and Weigert, M.  Nature 256:644, 1975.

## DISCUSSION

Taylor:  The recombinant inbred strains that I decribed (in Table 2) are available on order from Jackson Laboratory. Breeding pairs can also be obtained on those five sets.  A number of other sets of strains are also being reared at Jackson and elsewhere and these are summarized in ref. 6.

# GENETIC CONTROL OF RESISTANCE TO PROTOZOAL INFECTIONS

David J. Bradley
Ross Institute of Tropical Hygiene
London School of Hygiene and Tropical Medicine
Keppel Street
London, England WC1E 7HT

An epidemiologist in a meeting of laboratory scientists must tread warily if he is not to be considered the idiot of the family, and one may also wonder why the protozoa were selected to be the first group of infections to be considered at this meeting. But there is a logic to selecting them and having an epidemiologist with primarily African experience to introduce them. The research funds that are used to breed and feed our rats and mice are usually given with the dual objects of promoting scientific understanding and human welfare. Human disease has provided two large questions in the genetics of resistance and both concern protozoa. First, what enables the sickling gene, so deleterious to survival in its homozygous form, to be so abundant in many parts of Africa? Secondly, why is it that the indigenous inhabitants of West Africa are relatively untroubled by malaria due to Plasmodium vivax? Both questions involve protozoal parasites in man, both involve single genes, and in each case there is considerable understanding at levels from the human population down to molecular mechanisms.

It is therefore my intention to review briefly the range of our knowledge of genetically determined mammalian resistance to protozoan infections (with a glance also at avian hosts) before discussing in greater detail the resistance of mice to Leishmania donovani which has particularly interested the Ross Institute group comprising particularly Jennie Blackwell, Orysia Ulczak, Jacki Channon and Malcolm Guy at present, and earlier involving Joan Freeman, Joseph El-On, Wendy Smith, Jean Kirkley and Ann Zuill at various times. Few things would get completed without them, especially Jennie and a good number would not get started either!

The whole topic of genetics of resistance to parasites was reviewed by Wakelin (1), and recently Blackwell (2) has summarized data on patterns of mouse strain susceptibility to infections, including the protozoan parasites.

There are many protozoa, comprising six main groups, of which all the sporozoa, opalinates and cnidosporidia, and some of the rhizopods, ciliates and flagellates are parasitic. Something is known of the genetic control of susceptibility of invertebrates such as the mosquito vectors of malaria, but I shall consider only the homoiothermic verte-

brates. Data is available on at least eight protozoan genera. These include the malaria parasites of mammals, genus
Plasmodium, and another red cell parasitic group, Babesia.
Toxoplasma which has a stage in the intestine and a tissue
phase has been studied as has the intestinal parasite
Eimeria, the latter chiefly in chickens. Brief attention
has been paid to Entamoeba and much more to the three genera
of flagellates Trypanosoma, Schizotrypanum and Leishmania.

More precision has been obtained for the intracellular
than extracellular parasites. This may be a matter of
chance, but possibly there are fewer genes having a major
effect on the successful intracellular parasites - or to put
it conversely, perhaps a single gene change is more often
enough to produce a large effect on an intracellular than on
an extracellular species. More definitely, it is easier to
do tidy experiments with the intracellular parasites as the
milieu interieur of the cell is better regulated and buffered from environmental changes than is the extracellular
habitat, whether blood, tissue fluid or gut lumen.


                             MALARIA


It is convenient to start with the malaria parasites
and proceed through the other red cell parasites, other sporozoa, and miscellaneous groups, to the flagellates.

The distribution of the sickling gene (S) in human population along with the sub-lethal character of the SS genotype strongly suggested a selective advantage to the AS
heterozygous form and Allison (3) first marshalled substantial evidence that falciparum malaria was the selecting
factor. Subsequent extensive epidemiological data has been
consistent with this. It was early shown that the protection was not against infection as such but against the consequences of infection and very heavy, life-threatening,
infections.

Two main concepts exist for the mode of action of the
gene. One suggests that the parasitised AS red cell is
caused to sickle by being parasitized and is therefore
selectively destroyed in the spleen along with its contained
parasites. An alternative explanation, which has the advantage of explaining why protection is confined to P. falciparum, and does not extend to the other malaria parasites of
man, has been put forward by Pasvol and Weatherall (4) and
Friedman et al. (5) independently. Both show that whereas
P. falciparium grows well in SS, AA and AS red cells under
relatively aerobic conditions, a drop in the oxygen tension
stops growth of the parasite in AS and SS cells, whilst

leaving growth in AA cells at the aerobic rate. Since the
later stages of trophozoite growth and schizogony only in
P. falciparum take place in the deep tissues where oxygen
tension is relatively low, these observations explain both
the occurrence and specificity of the protection afforded by
the AS genotype.

At the clinical level there is also strong evidence of
the relation of malaria to the AS polymorphism. Among children severely ill from falciparum malaria, or with very high
parasitaemias, there are very few with the AS genotype even
where the S gene is present in many of the population, so
that Martin et al. (6) found only one AS and 29 AA genotypes
among severe malaria cases in Nigeria while a control group
gave 8 AS, 1 SS, 2 AC and 27 AA genotypes.

West Africans very rarely suffer from P. vivax malaria,
nor do North Americans of West African pure descent.  The
key to understanding this remarkable phenomenon was the observation (7) that P. knowlesi had a similar host specificity when red cells were tested for invasion in vitro and
the correlation of this resistance with the Duffy negative,
Fy(a-b-), blood group determinants. This suggested that the
Duffy antigens acted as receptors for the P. knowlesi, and
susceptibility was removed by chemotrypsin treatment of
these cells prior to testing.  However, the situation is
more complex than this in that trypsin treatment of the
Duffy negative cells renders them susceptible but does not
make them Duffy positive.  In particular, P. knowlesi
attaches to Duffy negative red cells but does not make an
invagination of the red cell surface.  Further evidence of
the Duffy-specific nature of the phenomenon was obtained
from volunteer experiments in which only the Duffy-negative
exposed people escaped infection (8) and from the unsuccessful invasion in vitro of red cells obtained from three of
the very rare Duffy-negative people of non-African descent
(two Cree Indians and a white Australian woman) (9).  P.
falciparum on the other hand infects all human red cells except for a proportion of those En(a-). The proteolytic
enzymes also affect sensitivity to P. vivax and P. falciparium differently (10).

What is known for the sickling gene has been asserted
for several other haemoglobins, and it is tempting to apply
similar reasoning to other red cell genes which are mainly
prevalent in areas of Africa holoendemic for Plasmodium falciparum.  In the case of HbC and $N_{BALT}$, Friedman et al(5)
have shown experimentally that the red cells do not support
trophozoite growth, but for other genes the malaria hypothesis may not apply.  Martin et al (6) have re-examined
the relation of glucose-6-phosphate dehydrogenase deficiency

to severe malaria and found, among severe clinical cases in
Nigeria, no fewer cases of G-6-P-D deficiency than in a control group from the local population. One earlier study was
consistent with this finding (both were somewhat short of
B-heterozygotes) and they point out that another had an excess of G-6-P-D controls rather than a scarcity of this
genotype among cases. The counter-evidence of Luzzatto,
Usang and Reddy (11) from observations on which cells are
attacked can be explained in part by the red cell age-pref-
erence of P. falciparum but this still leaves the elegant
correlations between malaria endemicity and G-6-P-D deficiency frequencies in Sardinian villages (12) unexplained.

With the exception of the Duffy blood category, red
cell surface antigens have not been shown to relate to
malarial infections. In particular, among 209 children with
heavy parasitaemia, with or without convulsions, who were
seen at two Nigerian hospitals, there was no difference of
antigen frequencies for the M,N,S,s,U system as compared
with controls (13) and the genotypes cDe and $S^uS^u$, particularly seen in Africans, were not missing from the severely ill.

The responses to human malaria have been related to the
HLA complex in a study (14) of three villages in NE Tanzania
where 116 people were typed for HLA-A and B and the malaria
antibody level determined by indirect immunofluorescence.
There was a large excess of the A2, AW30 combination among
those with high antibody titres. Among those with a titre
above 1:2560 an observed gene frequency of 20.4% contrasted
with the expected 11.4%. The combinations A2,BW17 and AW30,
BW17 were also observed more frequently than expected. No
HLA gene taken singly was significantly related to the antibody titre. The finding is remarkable: possible mechanisms
are numerous and could include HLA determined antigen responsiveness, genetically controlled variation in responsiveness to the malaria B-cell mitogen (15) or B-cell levels,
but all are speculative, and data on the haemoglobin types
are not available.

Malaria susceptibility in mice may now be considered
with several principles in mind. The situations with sickling and with P. vivax above make sharp the distinction
between resistance to infection and resistance to disease,
to the consequences of infection. Often the distinction is
much less sharp so that neither can be ignored, but if simple genetic control is being sought then each step in the
natural history of infection and in pathogenesis should be
examined separately where feasible.

Again the broad distinction between innate or natural
resistance and acquired specific immune responses is clear,

but many genes other than specific immune response genes may have a non-specific effect on the induction of immunity or on the effector processes by which immune responses affect parasite populations.

In the case of, for example, intracellular parasites of macrophages, it is possible that a single genetic character may affect innate resistance, induction of immune responses, and acquired effector mechanisms as well. Often the diversity of possible genetic effects is so great and our knowledge so rudimentary that a review must look like stamp collecting by beginners - but this is only the first stage in genetic and biochemical analysis of the variation found in different mouse strains.

The rodent plasmodia, particularly because of their use in drug screening, have been investigated in inbred mice from an early date (16), though some early work gave difficulties due to the dependence of P. berghei on the nutrition of the host, particularly its para-aminobenzoic acid intake. The species P. berghei has subsequently been subdivided and the strains vary in their pathogenicity for mice, while P. chabaudi is increasingly also used in experimental work.

A rather confusing picture emerges. In the early studies parasitaemia and mortality from infection were considered under separate genetic control. However, parasitaemia was shown to be polygenically determined and was not analysed in detail. A comparative table of the relevant papers showing the relation between mouse strains and susceptibility shows great variation, reflecting both the changes in methodology and genetic complexity (17,18). The Biozzi mice of varying antibody responsiveness were more recently studied and the Ab/H and Ab/L strains found to be of comparable innate response but the Ab/H strain was much more responsive to vaccination, both in terms of antibody production and survival of challenge. Over three loci were considered involved (19).

Recently, Eugui and Allison (20) showed that A/HeCre mice were by far the most sensitive of five strains tested with infections of Plasmodium chabaudi or with Babesia microti. They suggested that this resulted from the very low levels of natural killer (NK) cells in the A strain. A better genetically defined difference is the X-linked recessive immunological defect of the CBA/N mouse which reduced immunity to P. yoelii and B. microti (21). Babesia has been shown to have a variable fate in other mouse strains by Ruebush and Hanson (22).

## TOXOPLASMOSIS AND AMOEBIASIS

The response of mice to Toxoplasma gondii has been shown to vary with the mouse strain used (23) as assessed by

time interval between infection and death. At low intraperitoneal inocula the DBA/2 mice were largely dead before any
mortality occurred in other mouse strains, with BALB/c,
C57BL/6J and SW the most resistant and B10.D2, DBA/1 and C3H
occupying intermediate positions. However, a 20x increase
in the inoculum not only raised mortality but also made
BALB/c the most susceptible strain. This finding is reminiscent of some findings in rickettsial disease reported by
Groves at this meeting. Further observations on Toxoplasma
(24) showed survival differences in the B10. congenic resistant series at low challenge doses. All B10.BR and B10.D2
mice survived while B10.Sr were most vulnerable and B10.A
less so. Evidence was obtained of H-2 linked resistance and
also of resistance possibly linked to H-13, with some phenotypic complementarity between these loci.

The search for an experimental model for human amoebi-
asis had led Gold and Kegan (25) to attempt hepatic infections of 8 strains of mice and earlier workers to examine a
few strains. Results have been essentially negative so that
strain susceptibility has not been adequately detected.
However, when usual routes of infection were used, Neal and
Harris (26) had found C3H/mg and CBA/Ca mice susceptible by
intracardiac injection. Most work with amoebae involves
larger mammals. However, Entamoeba histolytica can also be
grown in the chick egg and there are clear strain differences in suitability for this purpose (27).


TRYPANOSOMIASES


The trypanosomiases affecting man fall into two groups:
the African parasites of the genus Trypanosoma which give
rise to sleeping sickness, with related species causing
cattle trypanosomiasis or nagana, and affecting other
animals; and the American genus Schizotrypanum which give
rise to Chagas' disease. The African trypanosomes are primarily extracellular parasites of the blood and tissue fluids while S. cruzi has both aflagellate (amastigote) intracellular and trypanosomal extracellular phases in mammals.

In Africa, several examples of what began as "epidemiological anecdotes" have in recent years been put on a
firmer physioloical and sometimes genetic basis. The resistance of N'dama and Muturu breeds of cattle to trypanosomiasis has been known for many years. It has been confirmed
in experimental infections (28) and the mechanism of resistance asserted to be an increased immune response to infection in early life. These cattle are small, and the

resistant breeds of sheep and goats to trypanosomiasis are
also small (29). Pigs from endemic areas are also relatively resistant (30). The genetics have not been elucidated.

Morrison and his colleagues (31) have gone on to look
at variation in the course of T. congolense, a cattle trypanosome, in mice. Their elegant work demonstrates the complexity of the genetically controlled processes and the de-
cisions needed in selecting the variables for genetic analysis, though with this system as with other blood parasites
repeated sampling from individual mice is possible. Among
the eight strains tested, AKR/A was by far the most resistant when the height of the peak initial parasitaemia was
studied. But the polymorphic trypanosomes - T. brucei, T.
congolense and T. vivax - show a remittent parasitaemia due
to antigenic variation allowing escape from successive
immune responses, and on the third peak AKR/A was more
susceptible than most strains were at that stage, or
initially. Susceptibility corresponded to high levels of B
and null cells in the spleen.

In genetic studies Morrison and Murray (32) showed that
the H-2 complex played little role, as determined by early
parasite counts in congenic resistant strains of the B10.
series. In terms of time to death the b haplotype was of
longest survival. In crosses of the most resistant C57BL/6
with the highly susceptible A strain, the F1 mice were resistant, even more so than the parents, as assessed by time
to death, and were of intermediate susceptibility as judged
by the height of the first peak. The backcrosses were again
spread over the range of the parents. The separation of
parental counts was inadequate for assessment of segregation
while time to death in the backcrosses had a high variance.
An equally diffuse F1 and backcross pattern was seen in C3H
crosses with A and C57BL.

Other work on trypanosomes in mice has shown that the
relative resistance of strains is unaffected by the specific
T. congolense isolate used. Nude mice were always susceptible. Earlier, Olisa and Herson (33) had found no appreciable difference in susceptibility of BALB/c and C57BL mice
at low T. brucei gambiense inocula. Clayton (34) found strain differences in T. brucei responses of different strains,
with C3H the most susceptible. Clarkson (35), comparing the
IgM response in 6 mouse strains found an early rise in
C57BL, intermediate values in 4 strains, and almost no rise
in C3H/mg which was also the first strain to die of the infection.

The true mouse trypanosome T. musculi shows a similar
strain response in that C3H/Bi is more susceptible than mice
of the B10. series as measured by the peak parasitaemia,

though both recover. Interestingly, the peak parasitaemia recorded by Jarvinen and Dalmasso (36) is slightly higher at 54,000 cu mm in the complement C4 deficient B10.D2/old strain than in the congenic B10.D2/new strain where the count was 40,000 at day 12.

Schizotrypanum cruzi combines the biological features of the African trypanosomes and Leishmania, having both blood and intracellular tissue phases. The ranking of 9 mouse strains by degree of resistance to this parasite closely resembles that seen in the polymorphic trypanosomes, while congenic resistant strains demonstrate little effect of the H-2 complex (37). Splenectomy, X-irradiation and silica loading render the C57BL mice susceptible, and the nu/nu mutant alleles in the BALB/c strain, usually of moderate resistance, always lead to death. Cunningham et al (38) found that the susceptible C3H and relatively resistant C57BL/6 strains both developed comparable immunosuppression to heterologous antigens during infection and this was transferable using serum. In studies of the different Biozzi series of mouse strains with varying antibody responsiveness, Kierszenbaum and Howard (39) found the Ab/L strain were more susceptible than the Ab/H strain.

## LEISHMANIASIS

The situation for most major protozoan parasites that will infect mice is becoming comparable. A range of mouse strains has been screened: usually a few in detail and a much larger number perfunctorily, for obvious reasons. Where the assay of infection used requires some time delay from inoculation, either to allow for parasite population growth or because interest is focused on recovery, different workers tend to obtain comparable but not identical results. The choice of the time between infection and assay is often crucial. Then later in the infection, the more complex the genetic control, so that time to death is a particularly difficult phenomenon to analyse. Experience with Leishmania shows the advantage of genetic analysis of the early stages of infection first, so that these genes can be standardized in the study of subsequent more chronic phases. The value of mouse strains differing at a very limited number of loci is apparent, not only for studies of the MHC - controlled response.

In most of the above mouse studies the initial step has been a screening of mouse strains. I do not know what prompted this, except in the case of our own studies on Leishmania donovani which will now be discussed. Here genetic screening was a last despairing resort rather than a planned beginning.

Leishmania donovani, a trypanosomatid flagellate, is an intracellular parasite of the mononuclear phagocytes of man, giving rise to visceral lesihmaniasis or kala-azar which is usually fatal in a year or so if untreated. The liver and spleen are greatly enlarged by parasite-stuffed macrophages, so that the spleen may weight 3 kg. The infection is transmitted by sandflies and may occur as high epidemics (especially in India) or as a sporadic zoonosis with dogs, foxes and sometimes rodents as reservoirs of infection. A similar progressive fatal infection is produced in hamsters, in which the parasite is maintained in the laboratory.

Although infections in mice were documented in 1912 (40,41) and even then a variable response was noted, systematic studies using liver imprints for quantitative assessment of the course of infection are due to Stauber (42) who showed a rise in parasite numbers following intravenous infection of mice, then a fall which levelled off to a prolonged plateau level for some months before final recovery. It was to investigate this apparent partial immunity that our studies began. Although several hypothetical mechanisms involved in this process were individually verified, great difficulty was encountered over 2 years in either getting reproducible experiments or observing the course of infection described by Stauber. Only when concomitant infection with Eperythrozoon, variables of amastigote preparation, and host age and nutrition had been eliminated was strain variation in the mice investigated (43,44), with striking results in that within one month there was a 1600-fold difference in liver parasite burden between the most and least susceptible strains. The mouse strain parasite counts at two weeks after infection feel into two rather sharply separate categories and using the counts at this point as an assay some 25 strains were typed and still formed two discrete groups (45). F1 hybrids were closer in counts to the resistant strains and F2 and backcross generations showed Mendelian ratios of resistant to susceptible mice indicative of single gene, or tight linkage group, control.

In analysis of natural resistance to leishmaniasis, the crucial role of the congenic resistant and recombinant inbred strains discussed by Taylor (this volume) is clear. At the stage of a suggested linkage, the use of Robertsonian translocations both excluded one hypothesis and strongly supported the chromosome 1 location.

Lsh was mapped (46) chiefly using the recombinant inbred strains BXD, BXH, and BRX58N, with smaller numbers of four other RI strain series. It lies near Idh-1 on chromosome 1 and the precise site has recently become of great

interest in relation to <u>Ity</u> which determines susceptibility
to <u>Salmonella typhimurium</u> and maps nearby. The location on
chromosome 1 was confirmed by linkage between <u>Lsh</u> and the
Robertsonian translocation <u>Rb1-Bnr</u> which bears the <u>Lsh</u>
allele. A three-point backcross with typing of <u>Lsh</u>, <u>Idh-1</u>
and <u>Pep-3</u> (the same as <u>Dip-1</u>) favoured that gene order with
<u>Lsh</u> nearest to the centromere. This gave one double cross-
over as compared with three if the gene order were <u>Idh-1</u>,
<u>Lsh</u>, <u>Pep-3</u>, though the single recombination frequencies from
the RI strains were more consistent with that order.

The most interesting outcome of the mapping is its con-
vergence with similar activities by Plant and Glynn (47) who
showed that <u>Ity</u> determining susceptibility to <u>Salmonella</u>
<u>typhimurium</u> also lay on chromosome 1 fairly near to <u>Lsh</u>.
This strengthened the earlier suggestion (48), based on the
strain similarities in response to each parasite, that they
might be determined by the same gene. It is still not certain and some evidence has been accumulated suggesting that
<u>Ity</u> and <u>Lsh</u> are not identical. On the other hand, if they
are separate this does not explain the concordant susceptibilities of mouse strains not closely related. There would
be clear advantages to being able to test the same mouse
simultaneously for susceptibility to both organisms rather
than relying on different individuals of inbred strains.
Jenefer Blackwell and Janet Plant undertook to try this and
in their control initial experiments uncovered modified responses. The genetics of combined infections (polyparasi-
tism: 49) is a new field that may be experimentally confusing yet shed light on the evolutionary processes acting on
the genetic control of natural resistance.

The <u>Lsh</u> gene is present in roughly half the laboratory
mouse strains tested (45); it is not a rare mutant. Since
these strains have a varied origin, the expectation is that
both alleles would be prevalent in wild <u>Mus musculus</u> populations. We have sought them in populations from parts of the
UK, Iraq and elsewhere, both by direct testing of wild mice
and by testing the offspring of crosses with susceptible
laboratory stocks. So far we have not detected the <u>Lsh</u>[S]
allele in a wild mouse, though the UK lacks the sandfly vectors of <u>L. donovani</u>. If the gene also affects <u>Salmonella</u>
resistance this provisional finding is easier to explain.

The objective of genetic analysis may vary, and knowledge at any level may be utilised. For the geneticist it
is an end in itself, and mapping may also allow conclusions
about similarity of mechanisms for different parasite species. For the biochemist genetic analysis is a step towards
the molecular basis of innate resistance, and his findings
in turn may allow the biologist to cross the host species

barrier and explain why some species may act as reservoirs and others not.

The mechanism of action of Lsh is not known, though its functions have been localised to certain cell populations, and some possibilities disproved. Parasite uptake and initial counts do not differ between resistant and susceptible strains, but within 3 days the tritiated thymidine labelling indices differ, being <5% in two resistant strains and >12% in susceptibles (50). T-cell deprivation does not modify the parasite growth rate in resistant mice during the first two weeks of infection. Treatment of the amastigotes with serum from the resistant homozygous form prior to injection into susceptible mice allows the growth rate to remain high, and conversely, so that serum factors do not seem involved.

In the mouse, the Lsh gene effect is expressed both by the Kupffer cells of the liver and by the splenic macrophages, but not in the peritoneal macrophages. In cell cultures also the peritoneal macrophages of resistant and susceptible strains do not show differing parasite multiplication rates but, in spite of the difficulty of producing satisfactory Kupffer cell cultures, these show differences between the susceptible and resistant strains.

Mouse strains that were Lsh$\underline{^S}$ Lsh$\underline{^S}$ differed markedly in the course of infection after two weeks. Some recovered completely, with massive parasite destruction, extensive lymphocyte infiltration, and areas of hepatic necrosis. Others continued with increasing amastigote loads, extensive plasma cell infiltration of the portal tracts, mononuclear phagocytes distended with parasites, and a progressive anaemia with bone marrow infiltration by parasitised macrophages (44). Initially, congenic resistant strains on the C57BL/10 susceptible background with diverse H-2 alleles were infected and clear differences found, with the progenitor strain healing more rapidly even than NMRI (cure) and the B10.D2/new strain carrying heavy parasite loads beyond 130 days (non-cure) (51).

When the C57BL/10 bearing H-2$^{b/b}$ and B10.D2/new bearing H-2$^{d/d}$ were crossed, the F1 generation also failed to cure, while in the F2 and backcross generations the recovery pattern depended on the H-2 haplotypes which were individually determined using two NIH private specificity antisera for each end of H-2. The d/d and b/d haplotypes failed to cure while the b/b mice recovered: parasite counts were approximately 500-fold greater in the non-cure mice by day 130.

Other congenic resistant strains of the B10 series gave a range of responses, (Table 1) with q non-cure and f almost similar, and r and s both curing even more rapidly than the C57BL/10 ancestral strain. When the experiment was carried out using congenic resistant strains on a BALB background the b haplotype BALB/B cured whilst the BALB/c with haplotype d failed to cure (51).

TABLE 1

Recovery of CR strains from L. donovani

| Ancestral Strain | CR Strain | H-2 Haplotype | Recovery |
|---|---|---|---|
| C57BL/10 | C57BL/10 | b | cure +++ |
|  | B10.D2/new | d | non-cure |
|  | B10.G/ola | q | non-cure |
|  | B10.M/Ola | f | cure ++ |
|  | B10.R III(7INS)/Ola | r | cure ++++ |
|  | B10.S/Ola | s | cure ++++ |
| BALB | BALB/B | b | cure ++ |
|  | BALB/C | d | non-cure |
| C57BL/10      x | B10.D2/new | b/d | non-cure |

Thus the H-2 complex or a closely linked gene is a major determinant of recovery from mouse visceral leishmaniasis. Non-cure is unexpectedly dominant, which would tend to favour the hypothesis of an immune suppressor gene. The pattern of apparent recessive immune responsiveness observed differs in its haplotype distribution from other published results, suggesting an undescribed gene which is named Rld-1. Such evidence as is available favours a gene towards the k end of the H-2 complex.

The early findings of varying recovery rates in congenic resistant strains on the C57BL/10 ScSn background suggested that the MHC could act as a marker for genes inaccessible to direct measurement that might affect the prevalence of infection. Much leishmaniasis research has been undertaken as a model of leprosy. It was already clear that HLA-A, B, C did not determine who would have leprosy in the community and therefore family studies were carried out in South India. Before they were completed De Vries and colleagues had published their early results from Surinam (52), and elegant method of analysis which we followed (53). This interplay between experimental work and human field studies, which characterizes the Plasmodium vivax work also, is needed also in leishmaniasis and the other infections being considered at this meeting.

Observations on the early healing phase of L. donovani in mice (54) have suggested that other genes linked to Ir-2 and H-11 may be involved.

Analysis of the genetic basis of resistance has been made more difficult by confounding of the effects of innate susceptibility (narrowly defined), specific acquired immunity, and non-specific factors affecting the latter, which occurs in many acute bacterial and viral infections.  In general, protozoa have a less rapid replication rate than bacteria in vivo, and Leishmania amastigotes are among the slower multiplying parasitic protozoa.  The consequent prolonged course of infection and the slow effects of the acquired specific responses lead to a temporal separation of immediate and acquired responses, which facilitates their separate analysis.  Features of experimental leishmaniasis such as the 3-5 month course of an experiment, which render it unacceptable to many workers are those which make genetic analysis of host resistance tractable, without the need for ablation of the acquired responses experimentally.

Our understanding of genetic control of mouse susceptibility to Leishmania donovani and L. tropica (senulato) may be usefully compared.  More is known about the genetics buy less about the immunology of the former in precise terms than about L. tropica although the latter has been more extensively studied by a larger number of competent workers. This show the importance of a parasite assay, to measure the number of amastigotes, and of also a parasite growth rate assay, using thymidine labelling.  In L. tropica until recently one has been restricted to measuring the size of a lump, which comprises largely host response, and thus at a loss to dissect out the component processes constituting resistance to infection and the disease processes, and also to measuring immunological responses without being able to control for parasite mass or activity.

Nevertheless comparative studies using L. tropica showed a spectrum in 12 mouse strains of lesion size and healing which related to the degree of delayed hypersensitivity developed to leishmanial antigen (55).  Susceptible mice either failed to become hypersensitive or lost their reactivity.  Observations by other workers have given similar though not completely identical results (56,57,58) and all have concurred in finding BALB/c by far the most susceptible strain.  It is also completely clear (Table 2) that the sensitivity patterns of mouse strains to L. tropica and L. donovani differ.  Susceptibility to, and recovery from, closely related parasites may not be under the same genetic control.

Recent L. tropica work has made great progress and James Howard has kindly encouraged me to refer to some of his work which has yet to be published.  This demonstrates, firstly, that in L. tropica, mice of the B10 series of congenic resistants do recover regardless of their H-2 haplotype. Second, and again in contrast to L. donovani, L. tropica in the BALB/B or BALB/C mouse pursues an inexorable course with severe non-healing lesions. BALB/K does not heal either, but its course is very slow. In general, the notable susceptibility of the BALB/series of mice appears to be under single dominant gene control and is associated with the production of immune suppressor cells.

TABLE 2

### Relative susceptibility of mouse strains to Leishmania species

| Mouse Strain | A | B | C | D | E | F | G |
|---|---|---|---|---|---|---|---|
| A/Crc | R | | | | | | |
| A/Jax | | S | | R | | | |
| A | | | | | | R | |
| AKR | | | RR | R | | R | |
| CBA | R | R | | R | R | R | |
| C3H/He | | R | | R | R | R | |
| C57BR | | | | | R | R | |
| C57L | | | | | | R | |
| A2G | | | | | I | R | |
| DBA/2 | S | S | R | | I | R | |
| ASW | I | | | | | | |
| C57BL | R | I | R | R | I | S | |
| C57BL/10 | | | | | | S | Cure |
| DBA/1 | S | | | | | S | |
| NMRI | | | RR | | I | S | Cure |
| B10.D2 | | | | | | S | Not |
| BALB/c | SS | S | SS | SS | S | S | Not |
| BALB/B | SS | | | | | | |

R  resistance I intermediate, S susceptible
Terms broadly interpreted from the papers.

| A | L. tropica | Howard, Hale and Chan-Liew, personal communication |
|---|---|---|
| B | L. tropica | Behlin, Mauel and Sordat (57) |
| C | L. mexicana | Perez, Labrador and Torrealba (58) |
| D | L. tropica | Nasseri and Modabber (56) |
| E | L. tropica | Preston, Bebehani and Dumonde (55) |
| F | L. donovani | Bradley (45) |
| G | L. donovani (chronic) | Blackwell, Freeman and Bradley (51) |

It is clear that the detailed analysis of particular parasite systems is now proving very fruitful and that close interaction between studies of the genetics and the mechanisms of resistance is specially important, while it is necessary for those wishing to understand acquired resistance to do so in strains controlled for innate resistance if confusion is not to result.

Even the 'stamp collecting' is now rewarding since there is a spectrum of host strain responses for each parasite studied so far, and new studies can be matched against these. Thus the similarities and differences in the response spectra of mice to L. donovani, L. tropica and S. typhimurium raise numerous questions susceptible to precise and almost certainly interesting analysis, while the accumulated and unanalysed results of strain-typing of hosts against parasites provide ample material for the immunologist, biochemist and geneticist to study in collaboration.

This paper may have strayed from the more focused interests of many present at this meeting. An obituary of a psychologist of the older school described him as someone, who 'could never settle down with a nice cozy rat' - this, if meant as praise, was overdoing it. The present vigour of our subject is largely due to settling down with some cozy mice of good pedigree, and thus being even more dependent on those who, like Dr. Taylor, have looked after the welfare of inbred mice for so many years. But we should also balance that work with an occasional glance towards the outbred world outside.

## REFERENCES

1. Wakelin, D. Adv. Parasitol. 16:219, 1978.
2. Blackwell, J.F. "Biology of the House Mouse". Symp.Zool.Soc.Lond., 1980 (in press).
3. Allison, A.C. Brit.Med.J. 1:320, 1954.
4. Pasvol, G., and Weatherall, D.J. Nature (Lond). 274:701, 1978.
5. Friedman, M.J., Roth, E.F., Nagel, R.L., and Trager, W. Amer.J.Trop.Med.&Hyg. 28:777, 1979.
6. Martin, S.K., Miller, L.H., Alling, L.H.,, Okoye, V.C., Esan, G.J.F., Osunkoya, B.O., and Deane, M. The Lancet, i:524, 1979.
7. Miller, L.H., Mason, S.J., Dvorak, J.A., McGinniss, M.H., and Rothman, I. Science, 189:561, 1975.
8. Miller, L.H., and Carter, R. Exp.Parasit. 40:132, 1976.
9. Mason, S.J., Miller, L.H., Shiroishi, T., Dvorak, J.A., and McGinniss, M.H. Brit.J.Haematol., 36:327, 1977.

10.  Miller, L.H., McAuliffe, F.M., and Mason, S.J. Amer.J.-
     Trop.Med.& Hlth., 26:204, 1977.
11.  Luzzatto, L., Usanga, E.A., and Reddy, S.  Science,
     164:839, 1969.
12.  Siniscalco, M., Bernini, L., Latte, B. and Motulsky,
     A.G. Nature, 190:1179, 1961.
13.  Martin, S.K., Miller, L.H., Hicks, C.V., David-West, A.
     Ugbode, C., and Deane, M.  Trans.Roy.Soc.Trop.Med.Hyg.,
     73:216, 1979.
14.  Osoba, D., Dick, H.M., Voller, A., Goosen, T.J.,
     Goosen, T., Draper, C.C. and de The, G.
     Immunogenetics, 8:323, 1979.
15.  Greenwood, B.M., Oduloju, A.J., and Platts-Mill, T.A.E.
     Trans.Roy.Soc.Trop.Med.Hyg. 73:178, 1979.
16.  Greenberg, J., and Kendrick, L.P.  J.Parasitol. 43:413,
     1957.
17.  Greenberg, J., and Kendrick, L.P.  J.Parasitol. 44:492,
     1958.
18.  Most, H., Nussenzweig, R.S., Vanderberg, J., Herman, R.
     and Yoeli, M.  Military Med. 131:915, 1966.
19.  Heumann, A.-M., Stiffel, C., Monjour, L., Bucci, A.,
     and Biozzi, G. Infect. Immun. 24:829, 1979.
20.  Eugui, E.M., and Allison, A.C.  Bull.Wld.Hlth.Org.,
     57:231, 1979.
21.  Jayawardena, A.N., and Kemp, J.D. Bull.Wld.Hlth.Org.,
     57:255, 1979.
22.  Rubush, N.J., and Hanson, W.L.  J. Parasitol. 65:    ,
     1979.
23.  Araujo, F.G., Williams, D.M., Grumet, F.C., and
     Remington, J.S. Infect. Immun. 13:1528, 1976.
24.  Williams, D.M., Grumet, F.C.,and Remington, J.S.
     Infect.Immun. 19:416, 1978.
25.  Gold, D., and Kagan, I.G.  J. Parasit. 64:937, 1978.
26.  Neal, R.A., and Harris, W.G.  Protozool. 3:197, 1977.
27.  Jaouni, K.C.  Exp.Parasit., 47:54, 1979.
28.  Murray, P.K., Murray, M., Morrison, W.I., and McIntyre,
     W.I.M. Vet. Parasitol., 1978.
29.  Maclennan, K.J.R. "The African Trypanosomiases". H.W.
     Mulligan, ed., pp751, 1970.
30.  Birkett, J.D. CCTA publication. 45:32, 1958.
31.  Morrison, W.I., Roelants, G.E., Mayor-Withey, K.S., and
     Murray, M. Clin.Exp.Immunol., 32:25, 1978.
32.  Morrison, W.I., and Murray, M. Exp.Parasit., 48:364,
     1979.
33.  Olisa, E.G., and Herson, J. Exp.Parasit., 41:307, 1977.
34.  Clayton, C.E. Exp.Parasitol., 44:202, 1978.
35.  Clarkson, M.J. Parasitol., 73:R8, 1976.
36.  Jarvinen, J.A., and Dalmasso, A.P. Exp.Parasit.,43:

203, 1977.

37. Trischmann, T., Tanowitz, H., Wittner, M., and Bloom, B. Exp.Parasit., 45:160, 1978.

38. Cunningham, D.S., Kuhn, R.E., and Rowland, E.C. Infect. Immun. 22:155, 1978.

39. Kierszenbaum, F., and Howard, J.G. J.Immunol. 116:1208, 1976.

40. Yakimoff, W.L., and Yakimoff, N.K. Bull.Soc.Path.Exot. 5:218, 1912.

41. Laveran, A. Bull.Soc.Path.Exot., 5:715, 1912.

42. Stauber, L.A. Rice Institute Pamphlet 45:80, 1958.

43. Bradley, D.J., and Kirkley, J. Trans.R.Soc.trop.Med.-Hyg. 66:527, 1972.

44. Bradley, D.J., and Kirkley, J. Clin.exp.Immunol. 30:119, 1977.

45. Bradley, D.J. Clin.exp.Immunol. 30:130, 1977.

46. Bradley, D.J., Taylor, B.A., Blackwell, J., Evans, E.P. and Freeman, J. Clin.exp.Immunol. 37:7, 1979.

47. Plant, J., and Glynn, A.A. Clin.exp.Immunol. 37:1, 1979.

48. Bradley, D.J. Nature (Lond.) 250:353, 1974.

49. Buck,A.A., Anderson, R.I., and MacRae, A.A. Trop.med.Parasitol. 29: 253, 1978.

50. Bradley, D.J. Acta Tropica 36:171, 1979.

51. Blackwell, J., Freeman, J., and Bradley, D.J. Nature (Lond.) 283:72, 1980.

52. De Vries, R.R.P., Lai A., Fat, R.F.M., Nijenhuis, L.E., and van Rood, J.J.A. Lancet 2:1328, 1976.

53. Fine, P.E.M., Wolf, E., Pritchard, J., Watson, B., Bradley, D.J., Festenstein, H., and Chacko, C.J.G. J.Infect.Dis. 140:152, 1979.

54. DeTolla, L.J., Semprevivo, L.H., Palczuk, N.C., and Passmore, H.C. 1980 (in press).

55. Preston, P., Bebehani, K., and Dumonde, D.C. J.clin.lab.Immunol. 1:207, 1978.

56. Nasseri, M., and Modabber, F.Z. Infect.Immun. 26:611, 1979.

57. Behin, R., Mauel, J., and Sordat, B. Exper.Parasit. 48:81, 1979.

58. Perez, H., Labrador, F., Torrealba, J.W. Int.J.Parasit. 9:27, 1979.

## DISCUSSION

Poulter: Would Bradley give us his views on some of the possibilities raised by his overview? One can forsee that genetic control of natural defenses would eventually affect

the character and magnitude of specific immune responses.
Following the phase of natural resistance, prior to the
mounting of immune response, there would be rather considerable variations in the number of surviving parasites and
their distribution in various host sites, thus presenting a
variable antigenic load for triggering immune responses.
Could, therefore, the interpretation of Howard's data
(genetic control of resistance to L. tropica is expressed at
the level of suppressor T cells), discussed by Bradley, be
that different levels of suppressor T cell activity in
various mouse strains infected with L. tropica are simply a
reflection of variations in parasite load and distribution,
resulting from operation of natural resitance mechanisms,
rather than being an expression of differences in genetic
control of immune response?

Bradley: Although you are correct in stating that the level
of natural resistance would affect the quality and quantity
of specific immune response by virtue of the differences in
parasite load and presentation, it is equally obvious that
there are distinct genetic systems which control specific T
cell responses to parasites. Our approach was to study acquired responses to L. donovani in mouse strains selected to
express comparable levels of their Lsh gene-controlled
natural resistance. In that situation H-2 linked genetic
systems, presumably influencing T cell responses, were shown
to play a major role in recovery from visceral leishmaniasis.

Poulter: It is unlikely that identification of genes controlling resistance to parasitic infection in inbred mice
would be terribly relevant to the human situation until you
pinpoint the factors controlled by such genes. That being
the case, what can be said about our present knowledge of
any of these?

Bradley: We think these factors are in the area of macrophage biochemistry. I agree entirely with your view that,
only when one finds the biochemical mechanism responsible
for natural resistance, can one cross species barriers. The
Lsh gene is expressed primarily in Kupffer cells and their
equivalent in spleen. Presently the insuperable problem is
that these cells cannot be isolated, cultured and appropriately studied. Analogous work on peritoneal macrophages
as counterpart cells is not acceptable, for, even though
they do belong to the mononuclear phagocytic system, they do
not express the Lsh gene. The other possibility is that the
genetic factor controlled by the Lsh gene acts on the envir-

onment in which macrophages operate. They could well lose
their resistance upon removal from such an environment.

Poulter's comment on the limited value of inbred mice
as a model for the study of genetic control of resistance in
outbred populations is pertinent. Wild mice, which we have
studied extensively, all appear to be resistant to Leishmania although one would expect that the overall population
should include a proportion that is genetically susceptible*.

Skamene: I was intrigued by your statement that the genetic
resistance to malaria in the case of P. chabaudi may be
caused by the high level of NK cell activity. How would you
visualize the NK cell dealing with malaria?

Bradley: I do not visualize it at all. I was only trying
to cover what had been published. I was referring to recent
work (20) stating that one strain of five studied was susceptible and also manifested very low NK cell activity.
Just how NK cells would do this, I do not know. One needs
to look at a lot more strains before getting beyond "stamp
collecting" in that particular situation. It was not a
formal linkage study.

Wyler: For the record, there are observations suggesting
that certain Indian tribes that are highly inbred populations, living in endemic areas, are resistant to Leishmania
tropica. The point is that even within human populations
some patterns are being discerned.

Perez: Bradley's overview emphasized strongly the importance of the genetic contribution of the host in the final
result of host-parasite encounter. However, Leishmania
parasites are very complex organisms, and one could also
conceive a role for the genetic constitution of the parasite
population.

Bradley: This is true; the parasite variations in different forms of leishmaniasis are enormous. We have restrict-

---

*Editor's Comment (E.S.): This may well reflect a high
degree of preselection in nature where only the resistant
ones survive. This may be especially pertinent vis-a-vis
the finding of the possible identity of the Lsh gene and of
the Ity gene controlling natural resistance to Salmonella.
One can visualize that resitance to many other infections
may well be controlled by this locus on the 1st chromosome.

ed ourselves to the study of a single type of parasite only,
thus keeping one part of the equation constant and varying
only the genotype of the host.

# STUDIES ON THE GENETIC CONTROL OF VISCERAL LEISHMANIASIS IN BALB/c MICE BY L.TROPICA

F.Z. Modabber[1], M. Alimohammadian, A. Khamesipour,
M.H. Pourmand, M. Kamali and M. Nasseri[2]
Department of Pathobiology, School of Public Health,
Tehran University,
Tehran, Iran
and Department of Microbiology,
Harvard School of Public Health
Boston, Mass.

[1] Present address (for all communications): Experimental
Immunotherapy, Institut Pasteur, 28 rue du Dr. Roux, 75724
Paris cedex 15, France.
[2] Present address: Dept. of Microbiology and Immunology
Center for Health Sciences, U.C.L.A., Calif. 90024.

## INTRODUCTION

Injection of an infective dose of <u>Leishmania tropica</u> to
different strains of mice produces various forms of leishmaniasis (1). Some strains recover from the infection
(healers) and others retain a persistent lesion (nonheal-
ers). Healer strains may become nonhealer when injected
with higher doses of the organism (2,10). We observed that
the injection of $1-2 \times 10^6$ promastigotes of <u>L.tropica</u> major
produced a visceral and lethal infection with metastatic
lesions in BALB/c mice (9). Weintraub and Weinbaum (15),
Smrkovski and Larson (13), and Bjorvatn and Neva (3) have
also reported the same in BALB/c mice. The visceral disease
in the BALB/c seems to be independent of the infective dose
and the mice can not produce a strong DH reaction to leishmanin ($2 \times 10^5$ phenolized organisms) during the course of infection. Other strains of mice (A/J, C57BL/6, C3H, CBA,
AKR/Cu) similarly infected recovered from the infection and
mounted a DH reaction (8). It therefore seemed that DH and
susceptibility to visceral leishmaniasis in mice are interrelated and genetically controlled.

Bradley and colleagues have analyzed the genetics of
innate susceptibility of mice to <u>L.donovani</u> (4,5,6, this
volume). In this system, the line between "susceptible" and
"resistant" traits is very clear. The gene responsible for
the susceptibility was shown to be located on chromosome 1
and was designated "Lsh".

Handman et al. (7) and Behin et al. (2) have shown a
correlation between the growth of <u>L.tropica</u> in macrophages

GENETIC CONTROL OF NATURAL RESISTANCE
TO INFECTION AND MALIGNANCY

of different mouse strains and their relative susceptibilities to cutaneous leishmaniasis (healing and nonhealing).
Preston et al. (10) also observed a range of susceptibility
in various strains and similar to Behin et al. (2) described
a spectrum of different forms of the cutaneous disease with
increasing doses.

To evade some of the complications of genetic analysis
of a spectral disease, which undoubtedly involves many phenomena, we chose to study the genetic susceptibility of
visceral leishmaniasis in the BALB/c model.

In this paper we report the form of infection in $F_1$ and
their backcrosses to BALB/c (S) and A/J (R) parental strains
the relationship of DH reaction to resistance, and attempts
to modify the immune response by levamisole (lev) and cyclophosphamide (CY) in order to study the mechanisms res- pon-
sible for the generalization of L.tropica infection in BALB-
/c mice. All procedures were the same as described before
(8).

## SUSCEPTIBILITY IN $F_1$ AND BACKCROSSES

All $F_1$ hybrids of BALB/cxA/J (males and females) were
susceptible and had < 1.0 mm 48 hr DH reaction similar to
that of BALB/c. Susceptibility is defined as a generalized
infection with metastatic lesion leading to death. Death is
independent of the dose of inoculum provided an initial
lesion is produced. (Note: Nonhealing localized lesion,
i.e. in DBA/2 mice infected with $1-2 \times 10^6$ L.tropica does not
fit this description and must be considered separately). A
dose of $1-2 \times 10^6$ promastigotes (used routinely) killed 70-80%
of BALB/c, A/JxBALB/c and $F_1$xBALB/c in 4 months. in the resistant backcross ($F_1$xA/J), 13 out of 65 survived beyond 6
months after infection at a time when 100% of BALB/c, A/Jx-
BALB/c and $F_1$xBALB/c were dead with signs of generalization
(Fig. 1). Of the surviving 13, 4 seemed to have controlled
the disease and had signs of recovery. Hence the susceptibility seems to be dominant and under a multigenic control
system.

## DH REACTION IN BACKCROSSES

The DH reaction of $F_1$xA/J and $F_1$xBALB/c 70-80 days post
infection is shown in Table 1. Fifty one percent of the
backcross-resistant mice showed a positive reaction (> 1.0)
in contrast to 21% of the backcross-sensitive mice. The
extent of DH reactions in backcrosses in relation to the
time of death is shown in Fig. 2.

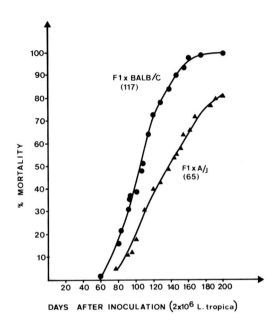

**Fig. 1.** Mortality rates of backcross strains.

**Table 1.** 48 hr DH reaction to leishmanin in infected backcross hybrids.

| Strain | No. of mice giving reactions | | Total | % ≥ 1 |
|---|---|---|---|---|
| | < 0.9 mm | ≥ 1.0 mm | | |
| $F_1$xA/J | 68 | 72 | 140 | 51 |
| $F_1$xBALB/c | 88 | 24 | 112 | 21 |

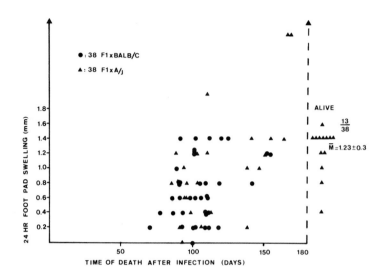

**Fig. 2.**   Relationship of DH and time of death.

Generally, the animals with a positive DH reaction (> 1.0mm) had a longer survival time.   However, there were animals of both backcrosses with positive DH reactions (> 1.4) which died in 6 months and animals with low or negative reactions which survived longer (4 surviving $F_1$xA/J mice had: 0.4, 0.8, 1.4 and 1.6 mm reactions).   The mean DH reaction for $F_1$xA/J mice which survived > 6 months was 1.23±0.3, and for those that died was 1.03±0.71 and hence not significantly different.

Levamisole (Lev) considerably reduced the rate of infection in A/J mice and prolonged the incubation period of BALB/c (Table 2).   However, it did not prevent a visceral disease in BALB/c in spite of enhancement of DH reaction on day 30 (Table 3).

### THE EFFECT OF CY (200 mg/kg BODY WEIGHT)

In a preliminary experiment, an injection of 200 mg/kg body weight (IP) at the time of inoculation delayed the onset of antibody production of both BALB/c and A/J.   However, the rate of infection in A/J mice was increased (from 53 to 100%) but that of BALB/c was reduced (from 100 to 83%).

Table 2.   Effect of Levamisole (25 mg/kg monthly) on the
           rate of infection in A/J and BALB/c mice

| Days after infection | A/J | | BALB/c | |
|---|---|---|---|---|
| | Treated | Control | Treated | Control |
| 20 | 5 | 5 | 20 | 32 |
| 40 | 5 | 36 | 62 | 90 |
| 60 | 5 | 47 | 80 | 100 |
| 80 | 16 | 57 | 90 | 100 |
| 125 | 26 | 78 | 100 | 100 |
| 167 | 31 | 78 | 100 | 100 |

Mice received the first injection of Lev. (IP) at the time
of infection.   Numbers are % of mice with lesion.

Table 3.   Effect of levamisole (25 mg/kg monthly) on 48 hr
           DH reaction

| Days after inoculation | Foot pad swelling (mm) | | | |
|---|---|---|---|---|
| | BALB/c | | A/J | |
| | treated (20) | untreated (10) | treated (19) | untreated (11) |
| 15* | 0.5 ± 1 | 0.3 ± 0.1 | 0.4 ± 0.1 | 0.5 ± 0.1 |
| 30 | 1.4 ± 0.2 | 0.6 ± 0.2 | 1.7 ± 0.1 | 2.4 |
| 48 | 1.2 ± 0.2 | 1.0 ± 0.2 | 1.4 ± 0.2 | 2.0 ± 0.4 |
| 119* | 0.7 ± 0.1** | † | 1.6 ± 0.2 | 1.4 ± 0.4 |

*Leishmanin$_5$ = $1.2 \times 10^5$ phenolized organisms, the rest tested
with $2.4 \times 10^5$.
** Only 15 surviving mice were tested.

Of interest was the observation that 2 out of 12 CY-treated
BALB/c recovered from the infection.   One of them only produced a nodule but the other had a small lesion.   Both had
low antibody titres on day 120 (1:80 and 1:160).   This preliminary experiment indicates that manipulation of the
immune response may prevent the visceral disease.

## DISCUSSION

Murine leishmaniasis produced by L.tropica is a "spectral" disease (10,11) as is leprosy and human leishmaniasis (14); and the immune responses are regulating the course of infection. Therefore genes regulating various immune reactions play a role in the control of this disease. On the other hand the Lsh locus which regulates the acute rate of growth of L.donovani must play a role in the L.tropica infection, since both organisms grow primarily in the macrophages. The isolation of parasites from the spleen of various strains of mice (R and S) injected subcutaneously with L.tropica supports this notion (Leclerc et al., unpublished). Hence, it is understandable to find mouse strains which are either resistant (i.e. C3H), or susceptible (i.e. BALB/c) to both parasites. These mice do not give a spectral disease with different doses of organisms. On the other hand there exist strains of mice (i.e. C57BL/6) which lack $Lsh^r$ gene but are relatively resistant (7,8), however, can give rise to nonhealing lesions in some of the animals with higher doses (2). In these animals another set of genes responsible for acquired immune responses regulate the form of infection. At low parasite load they recover and at high doses they are unable to control the infection. Suppression of in vitro stimulation of lymphocytes by L.-tropica (12) supports this notion.

Although there are contradictory reports from different labs (generalized infection in BALB/c, dose effect in CBA), and this may be a reflection of differences in parasite strains, there is a general agreement that the susceptibility of mice to L.tropica is under a multigenic control system. Our data of $F_1$ and backcrosses support this notion.

Although delayed hypersensitivity per se was shown not to be sufficient to confer resistance, in its absence, the host is highly susceptible. It is therefore not surprising to find that many genes are involved in the regulation of a given form of the disease. The Lsh gene regulates the innate immunity but a host of other genes regulating various macrophage functions, the antibody response and the response of various T-cells interplay in the overall outcome of the infection.

## ACKNOWLEDGEMENT

We thank Drs. A. Nadim and L. Chedid for their support, C. Leclerc for discussion, E. Bourgeois for redaction and B. Cosmao Dumanoir for preparing the manuscript. This work was supported by Grants from the Research Council (Leprosy Fund) and School of Public Health, Tehran University.

## REFERENCES

1.   Behin, R., Mauel, J., Biroum-Noerjasin, and Row, D.S. In "Ecologie des Leishmanioses", Paris:CNRS,p77, 1977.
2.   Behin, R., Mauel, J., and Sordat, B.   Exp.Parasit. 48:81, 1979.
3.   Bjorvatn, B., and Neva, F.A.   Am.J.Trop.Med.Hyg. 28:472, 1979.
4.   Bradley, D.J.   Clin.Exp.Immunol. 30:130, 1977.
5.   Bradley, D.J., and Kirkley, J.   Clin.Exp.Immunol. 30:119, 1977.
6.   Bradley, D.J.,Taylor, B.A., Blackwell, J.,Evans, E.P., and Freeman, J.   Clin.Exp.Immunol. 37:7, 1979.
7.   Handman, E., Ceredig, R., and Mitchell, G.F. Aust.J.Exp.Biol.Med.Sci. 57:9, 1979.
8.   Nasseri, M., and Modabber, F.Z.   Infect.Immun. 26:611, 1979.
9.   Nasseri, M., and Modabber, F.   Proceedings of 8th Pahlavi Medical Congress, Pahlavi Med.J. 8:27, 1977.
10.  Preston, P.M., Behbehani, K., and Dumonde, D.C. J.Clin.Lab.Immunol. 1:207, 1979.
11.  Preston, P.M., and Dumonde, D.C. "Immunology of Parasitic Infection". S. Cohen, E. Sadun (eds). Blackwell Sci.Publications, Oxford. p167, 1976.
12.  Sharma, M.K., Anaraki, F., and Ala, F. Clin.Exp.Immunol. 32:477, 1978.
13.  Smrkovski, L.L., and Larson, C.L.   Infect.Immun. 16:249, 1977.
14.  Turk, J.L., and Bryceson, A.B.M.   Adv.Immunol. 13:209, 1971.
15.  Weintraub, J., and Weinbaum, F.I.   J.Immunol. 118:2288, 1977.

## DISCUSSION

Nacy: Two points deserve comment in discussing mechanisms responsible for genetic resistance to leishmaniasis in implicating macrophages as the effector cells. First of all, a mouse strain with a recognized macrophage defect (P/J) initially manifests no lesions after infection with L. tropica. Later, however, enormous lesions develop progressively and do not resolve with time, as do lesions in other mouse strains mounting effective macrophage responses. The second point deals with the age-dependence of genetic resistance to L. tropica which resembles other age-dependent systems of natural resistance. For instance, C57BL/6 mice infected at 6 weeks of age do not develop lesions, whereas

animals infected at 12-16 weeks of age manifest enormous
lesions which subsequently resolve*.

Kirchner: I would like to ask Modabber about the details of
the cyclophosphamide protocol? I was concerned that he may
have used too high a dose of cyclophosphamide which would
not be selective for suppressor T cells.

Modabber: The data that Kirchner refers to was obtained
with 200 mg/kg body weight and was essentially designed to
suppress the antibody response. It was given either prior
to, or at the time of, the infection, more or less in the
fashion that Turk used cyclophosphamide to suppress the
antibody response. However, we have also used lower doses,
up to a maximum of 20 mg/kg body weight where we sought to
block the suppressor T cells. Here the lesions displayed by
the animals were much smaller, but this study is not yet
completed. In the high dose cyclophosphamide group, it is
noteworthy that these animals do develop delayed hypersensitivity responses, but whether that is related to the
lack of antibody or to elimination of suppressor cells is
not established.

Kirchner: Could it be that one is simply destroying the
target cells of initial parasite replication?

Modabber: The parasites seem to replicate in macrophages.
We all know that. In practical terms it is impossible to
eliminate macrophages or even to substantially reduce their
number. Cyclophosphamide-treated mice eventually develop
lesions and, since the parasite cannot live and replicate
outside the macrophage, it is thus inconceivable that macrophages have been eliminated, but it is possible that they

---

*Editor's comment (E.S.): The formal evidence for macro-
phages expressing the phenotype of genetic resistance to
Leishmania was recently provided by Handman et al. (Aust.J.-
Exp.Biol.Med.Sci. 57:9, 1979) and by Behin et al. (Exp.-
Parasitol. 48:81, 1979). Non-specifically induced peritoneal macrophages from a Leishmania-resistant mouse strain
destroyed ingested parasites in vitro while analogous macrophages from a sensitive strain were unable to kill the intracellular parasites. They did so only after sustained
activation by lymphokines in vitro. These results suggest
the threshold of activation necessary to kill Leishmania is
higher in macrophages of genetically susceptible mice than
in those of resistant mice.

have been biochemically compromised.   It is noteworthy that there have been reports of macrophage activation with cyclophosphamide at dose levels of 200 - 300 mg/kg body weight.

Wyler:   In any of these experiments, I would emphasize that when one inoculates parasites, be it promastigotes or amastigotes, one is dealing with heterogeneous populations.   One can certainly manipulate in vitro, promastigotes at least, in terms of altering their susceptibility.   For example, L. tropica does not grow at 37°C, but if one passages them and adapts them, very often they can be gotten to grow very nicely at 37°C.   Presumably what happens is that one is simply selecting out subpopulations that have different temperature limits.   I cannot help wondering whether some of these susceptibility studies may also relate to selecting out, from the heterogeneous population inoculated, parasites that can survive or cannot survive within that milieu, but it immunologic or biochemical.   So one experiment that would be interesting and important would be to backcross the parasite, in the sense that parasites would be isolated from the resistant host for infection of the sensitive animal and vice versa.   Has Modabber done that?

Modabber:   Yes, it was done, by taking the isolates from Balb/c sensitive host, and injecting them into A/J and various other resistant strains.   The course of infection has not been altered by this procedure, i.e., the animals continue to behave as resistant.   Therefore, I do not see this as involving a selection of organisms.

Wyler:   But, I would expect that the organisms from the resistant animal would be more revealing, in as much as the Balb/c mouse is so permissive for the growth of parasites that one may have effected very little selection.

# INFECTION WITH LEISHMANIA TROPICA MAJOR: GENETIC CONTROL IN INBRED MOUSE STRAINS

Louis J. DeTolla,Jr., Phillip A. Scott, and Jay P. Farrell

Department of Pathobiology
University of Pennsylvania,
School of Veterinary Medicine
Philadelphia, Pennsylvania 19104

Leishmania tropica major is a causative agent of cutaneous leishmaniasis in man and certain wild rodents. The parasites are obligate intracellular parasites of macrophages and usually produce self-limiting, ulcerating cutaneous lesions in a susceptible host. Previous reports (5) suggest that infections in mice with L. tropica show certain similarities to data reported on murine infections with Leishmania donovani (2,3,4). Further data generated on genetic control of cutaneous leishmaniasis, when compared with that on visceral leishmaniasis, should prove to be most interesting.

A series of inbred mouse strains were injected intradermally at the base of the tail with $10^6$ promastigotes of Leishmania tropica. Infected mice were examined on a weekly basis for the development of ulcers and metastatic lesions. The criteria of lesion size, ulceration and persistence of cutaneous lesions were used to divide the mice into two groups: a highly susceptible group including BALB/cJ and SWR/J, and a relatively resistant group that included all of the other strains studied (Table 1). Of all the strains studied, only BALB/cJ and SWR/J developed extensive ulcerous lesions that failed to show signs of resolution. Approximately 50% of the mice of each of these two strains had died within 16 weeks, often with lesions of over 20 mm in diameter. This SWR/J mouse appeared to develop a deeper ulcer than BALB/cJ, but only the BALB/cJ mice developed metastatic lesions.

Within the resistant group, the NZB/BINJ mice appeared to be the most refractory but nevertheless developed small distinct ulcers by 7 weeks with resolution and healing by 11 weeks post infection. Highly significant differences in the time of appearance or extent of ulcers and time of resolution were not noted among most of the other strains studied. It should be noted, however, that the strains A/J and DBA/2J have been previously shown to be somewhat more susceptible to very high parasite doses (1). All of the strains in the resistant group resolved their infections by week 16.

Table 1. Mean diameter (mm) of primary cutaneous lesions in inbred and congenic resistant mouse strains infected intradermally with $10^6$ L. tropica promastigotes.

Time (weeks)

| Mouse Strain | 3 | $7\frac{1}{2}$ | 11 | 16 |
|---|---|---|---|---|
| SWR/J | 4.4 | 14.0 | 15.8 | 19.0 |
| BALB/cJ | 3.8 | 10.2 | 13.9 | 18.1 |
| A/J | 2.1 | 4.8 | 3.8 | 1.0 |
| DBA/1J | 1.2 | 4.5 | 3.0 | 0 |
| DBA/2J | 0 | 2.7 | 0 | 0 |
| AKR/J | 0 | 1.5 | 0 | 0 |
| CBA/J | 2.3 | 4.0 | 0 | 0 |
| C3H/HeJ | 2.5 | 5.6 | 2.5 | 0 |
| NZB/BINJ | 3.0 | 5.0 | 3.2 | 0 |
| C57BL/6J | 0 | 3.2 | 2.1 | 0 |
| C57BL/10Sn | 1.6 | 4.6 | 2.4 | .4 |
| B10.D2 | 1.3 | 4.5 | 1.1 | 0 |
| B10.129(10M) | 3.9 | 5.0 | 2.0 | 0 |
| B10.CE(30NX) | 2.2 | 5.1 | 1.5 | .5 |

From the data it should be apparent that all mouse strains could be considered innately or acutely susceptible to L. tropica since all strains developed a cutaneous ulcer within a few weeks. Since resolution occurs anywhere from 2 to 3 months post infection, it is likely that healing is immunologically mediated. Along these lines, it is interesting to note that only BALB/cJ and SWR/J fail to develop a delayed hypersensitivity to L. tropica antigens (Table 2). All other strains resolved their lesions and developed positive delayed hypersensitivity reactions.

Table 2. Delayed hypersensitivity response[1] of inbred and congenic resistant mouse strains 15 weeks after intradermal infection with $10^6$ L. tropica promastigotes

| Mouse strain | 24 hours | 48 hours |
|---|---|---|
| SWR/J | 0.09 ± 0.10 | 0.00 ± 0.06 |
| BALB/cJ | — | — |
| A/J | 0.33 ± 0.12 | 0.41 ± 0.01 |
| DBA/1J | 0.31 ± 0.10 | 0.19 ± 0.09 |
| DBA/2J | 0.30 ± 0.07 | 0.50 ± 0.28 |
| AKR/J | 0.48 ± 0.03 | 0.33 ± 0.10 |
| CBA/J | 0.45 ± 0.06 | 0.51 ± 0.03 |
| C3H/HeJ | 0.25 ± 0.14 | 0.15 ± 0.10 |
| NZB/BINJ | 0.45 ± 0.15 | 0.50 ± 0.13 |
| C57BL/6J | 0.24 ± 0.10 | 0.35 ± 0.14 |
| C57BL/10Sn | 0.38 ± 0.14 | 0.51 ± 0.21 |
| B10.D2 | 0.33 ± 0.17 | 0.51 ± 0.08 |
| B10.129(10M) | 0.16 ± 0.10 | 0.23 ± 0.19 |
| CB6F$_1$/J | 0.29 ± 0.22 | 0.21 ± 0.19 |

[1] Responses were measured as increased footpad thickness in comparison to saline injected controls in mm (mean ± S.D.) 24 and 48 hrs after injection of 0.025 ml leishmanin.

Because of the probability of immune response gene control over the developed resistance, the possibility of H-2 haplotype influence should be considered. However, BALB/cJ, which is highly susceptible, and NZB/BINJ, which is highly resistant, are both H-2$^d$. In addition, SWR/J, also highly susceptible, and DBA/1, which is resistant, are both H-2$^q$.

Analysis of the course of infection in the $F_1$ hybrid of
BALB/cJ♀ x C57BL/6J♂ (synonym CB6F$_1$/J) indicated the hybrid
to be less resistant than the C57BL/6J (synonym B6) parent
but with a tendency toward resolution of the lesion at or
beyond 16 weeks (Figure 1).

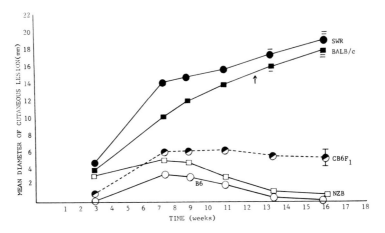

**Figure 1.** Mean diameter of primary cutaneous lesions in
inbred mouse strains infected intradermally with 10 million
L. tropica promastigotes. ( □————□ ) NZB, ( O————O)$^{B6}$,
(●————●)SWR, (■————■)BALB/c, (◐————◐)CB6F$_1$; (↑) time of
appearance of metastatic lesions; (-) time of death of individual mice; 6 mice per group.

The $F_1$ hybrid also showed positive delayed hypersensitivity
to L. tropica antigen (Table 2). If a single gene were
found to control resistance, the trait in the $F_1$ hybrid
would simply be considered one of incomplete or partial
dominance.

An $F_2$ generation of 54 animals was also infected with
L. tropica. As early as 8 weeks post infection the mice
could be divided into three groups. Twenty-eight percent
developed ulcers over 6 mm in diameter with depressed centers and raised borders similar to corresponding BALB/c control mice while 17% were highly resistant and pinpoint
lesions similar to the B6 controls. The remaining 55% showed ulcerous lesions between 3 and 5 mm in diameter resembling the appearance of the lesion in the CB6F$_1$/J hybrids.
Chi-square analysis indicates the data to be in conformity
with a 1:2:1 ratio ($\chi^2$=2.0, P>.30) indicating that resistance may be under control of a single gene.

ACKNOWLEDGEMENT


Support by Grant AI-12663 from the National Institutes of Health and by Grant T16/181/L3/21 from the World Health Organization.


REFERENCES



1. Behin, R., Mavel, J., and Sordat, B. Exp.parasit. 48:81, 1979.
2. Bradley, D.J. Clin.exp.Immunol. 30:130, 1977.
3. Bradley, D.J., and Kirkley, J. Clin.exp.Immunol. 30:119, 1977.
4. DeTolla, L.J., Sempreviro, L.H., Palczuk, N.C., and Passmore, H.C. Immunogenetics, 1980 (in press).
5. Handman, E., Ceredig, R., and Mitchell, G.F. AJEBAK 57:9, 1979.



DISCUSSION


Ali-Khan: We know that Balb mice are high producers of gamma $G_1$ but that all the other strains used in this work are low producers of gamma $G_1$ antibody. I would like to know if De Tolla has any data on the humoral immune response with respect to these antibodies.

DeTolla: We have begun to use the data on antibody levels but we really have not tabulated it. However, there are reasons for coming to the general conclusion at this time that antibody does not seem to play any notable role in acquired resistance to this parasitic disease. This conclusion is based on the work of many investigators whose findings show clearly that cell-mediated immunity is the principle mode of acquired immunity to leishmaniasis.

Ali-Khan: The point that I was seeking to make is the modulating effect of high producers of gamma $G_1$ antibody on the cell-mediated immune response*.

Cudkowicz:   There seems to be a presumption in the communications given by the speakers on this topic that resistance is based on the absence or presence of a certain form
of immune response.   Has anyone tested this in nude mice or
in mice having the genetic B cell defect?

DeTolla:   Studies have indeed been made on nude mice.   It
was found that, whereas normal CBA mice were resistant to
L. tropica, the CBA-nude manifests continually expanding
lesions and dies of the infection.

Cudkowicz:   Then the CBA-nude is as susceptible as the
Balb/c?

DeTolla:   Yes, it seems to be.

Cudkowicz:   Again, referring to the nude mouse, from what I
understood during this session, the susceptibility of Balb/c
mice should be attributed to the lack of delayed hypersensitivity response;  in that case the results on nude mice
would be supportive.   But it was also said that the Balb/c
mice may be susceptible because they generate suppressor T
cells.   However, in that case, the data with the nude mice
would not be supportive - the nude mouse would not have the
source of suppressor cells.

---

*Editor's Comment (E.S.):  Acquired immunity has not been a
principle issue of this conference except for situations
where it might reflect variations originating at the level
of genetically controlled resistance.  As far as the role of
Leishmania antibodies in resistance to this parasite is concerned, it is common knowledge that specific antibodies can
routinely be found in hosts infected with Leishmania:  moreover, the development of immediate hypersensitivity often
coincides with the onset of healing.  Critical experiments,
however, have yielded mixed results;  although specific
antibody can clearly inhibit the growth of Leishmania promastigotes in vitro, the transfer of such antibody (conva-
lescent serum) does not confer protection in normal animals.
The antibody may not be effective in vivo in a host whose
final effector mechanisms of resistance (macrophages, presumably) are genetically unable to handle even well-opsoniz-
ed parasites.

Howard:   It is particularly interesting that if you use a
conventional thymectomized, irradiated and marrow-repopulat-
ed Balb/c mouse, it actually heals its lesions, not all of
them, but all will show a retardation of progression of the
lesions and some of them heal.  You can also see this with
sublethal iradiation prior to the infection.  All these
animals will show a restoration of delayed hypersensitivity
and also have some antibody.  So I think this is a differential effect.  If you try to use nudes they all die anyway
because of the problem of keeping them alive long enough to
do the experiments.

Perez:   I would point out that in leishmaniasis, the ability
to develop delayed hypersensitivity reactions and the ability of the host to resist and eliminate infection are probably two quite separate, unrelated, events.  We should remember, for example, the muco-cutaneous form of American
leishmaniasis, where we may see delayed type hypersensitivity responses and still have a chronic infection.  In our
experimental system, the DBA/2 mice infected with L. mexicana develop persistent infections (non-healing) even with a
low dose of parasites.  However, they develop pronounced delayed type hypersensitivity responses to the parasite and
also protective immunity.  Accordingly, I wonder whether the
delayed type hypersensitivity is not related more to protective immunity than to host ability to eliminate infection.

DeTolla:   That is a possibility;  one has to look at all
sides of the issue in deciding what are proper conclusions.
We do not have any examples of mouse strains, however, that
heal their lesions but fail to develop delayed hypersensitivity reactions.  Nor do we have any correlation from
human data that positive delayed hypersensitive skin test is
present, but lesions are not healing*.

---

*Editor's Comment (E.S.):  Genetic analysis provides a use-
ful means for resolving this issue.  It has been shown by
Modabber et al. (this volume) that there may be a dissociation of resistance to Leishmania (measured as survival) and
DTH (footpad reaction) to Leishmania antigens among the segregating population of $F_1$ (A/J x Balb/c) x A/J backcross
mice.  Several individual mice were sensitive (died) while
having strong DTH, whereas others survived despite insignif-
icant DTH.  DTH and resistance should, therefore, be viewed
as two phenomena which, in the natural course of infection,
are temporally and quantitatively associated;  but there is
possibly no cause-effect relationship between DTH and resistance.

# THE RESPONSE TO THERAPEUTICAL TREATMENT OF RESISTANT AND SUSCEPTIBLE MICE INFECTED WITH LEISHMANIA MEXICANA

Hilda Pérez, Fanny Labrador
and Eliades Ledezma

I.V.I.C. Centro de Microbiologia y Biologia Celular
Apartado 1827
Caracas 1010 A, Venezuela

American cutaneous leishmaniasis (ACL) displays a diverse range of clinical manifestations. These have been related to variations in the host's response (3,13) to a diversity in the pathogenicity and infectivity of Leishmania parasites (5). Different strains of mice show dissimilar patterns of infection after the inoculation of $10^4$ amastigotes of L. mexicana. C3H, CBA, AKR and C57BL/6 are resistant whereas DBA/2 and BALB/c are susceptible (9 and Pérez unpublished data). Hybrids from the cross between resistant and susceptible mice showed a level of resistance similar to that of the more resistant parents (9). These results have suggested that in the mouse susceptibility to L. mexica is under genetic control. Moreover, comparison between the courses of infection with two strains of Leishmania, one isolated from a case of diffuse cutaneous leishmaniasis (DCL) and the other from a non-complicated case of ACL, in C57BL/6 and BALB/c mice revealed that patterns of infection were largely determined by the host (8). However, other factors such as the host's nutritional status and the number of infecting parasites, profoundly modify the response of resistant mice to L. mexicana (10,12).

As a safe vaccine for ACL has not yet been developed, therapeutical treatment remains as the most effective available mean to control the infection. Glucantime (N-methylglucamine antimoniate) is one of the drug of choice for the treatment of ACL. It is usually very effective for the non-complicated form of ACL, it is unsatisfactory for the treatment of mucocutaneos leishmaniasis and it is totally ineffective for DCL.

The lack of efficacy of glucantime in DCL, where specific immune responses are depressed (2,3), has opened the question of whether the activity of the drug is related to cooperation between the drug and the host's immune response to the parasite. It was attractive, therefore, to explore the response of resistant and susceptible mice infected with L. mexicana to therapeutical treatment with glucantime. Drug was administered subcutaneously between the shoulder-

47

blades at the dose of 250 mg/kg/day. Infected mice received
20 injections within 7–34 days after the inoculation of $10^4$
amastigotes of L. mexicana. The results from these experiments made it evident that glucantime at the dose schedule
used was not sufficient to eliminate the parasite. However,
in resistant C57BL/6 mice which are capable to develop cellular and humoral responses to leishmanial antigen and protective immunity to a challenge infection with L. mexicana
(9,11), early chemotherapy markedly diminished the severity
of lesions. However, time of healing was about the same for
both treated and untreated C57BL/6 mice (Fig. 1).

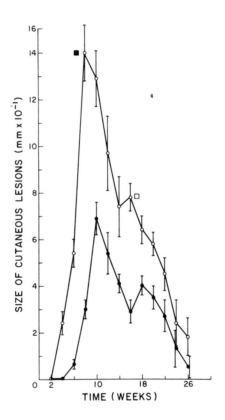

**Figure 1.** Course of infection, as measured by lesion size,
in control, (O) and treated (●) C57BL/6 mice infected with
$10^4$ amastigotes of L. mexicana. Drug treatment administered
within 7–34 days of inoculation of parasites. (■) Ulceration
and (□) cicatrization of lesions. Mean ± SD.

In contrast, in BALB/c mice which show impairment of both <u>in vivo</u> delayed hypersensitivity (DHR) and <u>in vitro</u> lymphocyte reactivity to leishmanial antigen (1,9) early treatment with glucantime although inhibiting the initial development of lesions it did not significantly affect the course of the infection. At 16 weeks of infection lesions of treated and untreated BALB/c mice showed similar sizes (Fig. 2).

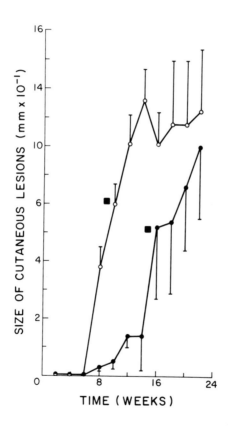

**Figure 2.** Course of infection in control (O) and treated (●) BALB/c mice infected with $10^4$ amastigotes of <u>L. mexicana</u>. Drug treatment administered within 7-34 days of inoculation of parasites. (■) Ulceration of lesions. Mean ± SD.

C57BL/6 mice infected with $10^6$ - $10^7$ amastigotes of L. mexicana develop a chronic infection (12). A further series of experiments were designed to study the effect of glucantime in chronically infected C57BL/6 ($10^6$ amastigotes) and BALB/c ($10^4$ amastigotes) mice. At 20 weeks of infection mice were given 20 daily injections of glucantime at the dose of 250 mg/kg/day. In chronically infected BALB/c mice therapeutical treatment only had a marginal effect and at 26 weeks of infection (3 weeks after the last injection of glucantime) treated and untreated BALB/c mice did not show significant difference in the size of their cutaneous lesions (Fig. 3).

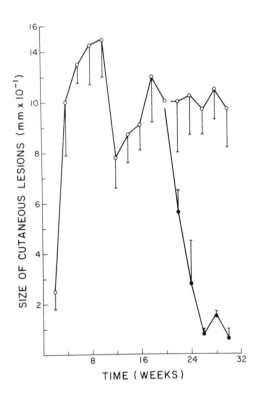

**Figure 3.** Effect of treatment with glucantime in C57BL/6 mice infected with $10^6$ amastigotes of L. mexicana. Drug treatment administered within 20-23 weeks of inoculation of parasites. Control (O) and treated (●) mice. Mean ± SD.

In chronically infected C57BL/6 mice treatment with glucantime had a marked effect, treated mice showed a rapid reduction in the size of their cutaneous lesions and at 26
weeks of infection (3 weeks after the last injection of
drug) mice showed resolved lesions (Fig. 4).

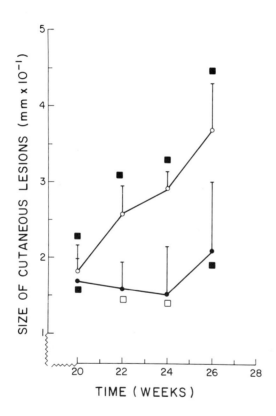

Figure 4.    Effect of treatment with glucantime in BALB/c
mice infected with $10^4$ amastigotes of <u>L. mexicana</u>.   Drug
treatment administered within 20-23 weeks of inoculation of
parasites.   Control (O) and treated (●) mice.   (■) Ulceration and (□) cicatrization of lesions.   Mean ± SD.

Interestingly, chronically infected BALB/c mice which failed to respond to treatment showed suppressed specific and non-specific immune responses and evidence suggested the activation of suppressor cells in the spleen of these mice (1,8).

The effect of glucantime in chronically infected C57BL-/6 mice could be related to a reduction in the parasite load which allowed these animals to recover their capability to control the infection. This is suggested by the fact that at 26 weeks of infection (3 weeks after the last treatment) treated mice showed intensive DHR to parasites antigens whereas untreated C57BL/6 mice showed depressed DHR (data not shown).

Our experiments suggest that the efficacy of glucantime in the tretment of experimental cutaneous leishmaniasis may require cooperation between the drug and the host's immune response.

In vitro evidence suggest that immune mechanisms and in particular intracellular destruction in macrophages are involved in resistance to cutaneous leishmaniasis (6,7). A successful response to therapeutical treatment may result from a two-step mechanism. In the first step parasites are affected by the drug and in the second step damaged parasites are easily destroyed by the host immune response. In the absence of the immune mediated step (in non-responder hosts) the infection persists.

An alternative explanation is that in susceptible mice drug is not properly metabolized. Further work is required to elucidate the relationship between the immune response and the activity of leishmanicidal drugs.

## REFERENCES

1. Arredondo, B., and Pérez, H. Infect.Immun. 25:16, 1979.
2. Bryceson, A.D.M. Trans.R.Soc.Trop.Med.Hyg. 64:380, 1970.
3. Convit, J., Kerdel-Vegas, F. Arch.Dermatol. 91:439, 1965.
4. Convit, J., Pinardi, M.E., and Rondon, A.J. Trans.R.-Soc.Trop.Med.Hyg. 60:526, 1972.
5. Chang, K.P. Am.J.Trop.Med.Hyg. 27:1084, 1978.
6. Handman, E., and Spira, D.T. Z.Parasitenkd. 53:75, 1978.
7. Mauel, J., Buchmuller, Y., and Behin, R. J.Exp.Med. 148:393, 1978.

8.  Pérez, H., Arredondo, B., and Gonzalez, M.   Infect.-
    Immun. 22:301, 1978.
9.  Pérez, H., Labrador, F., and Torrealba, J.W.   Int.J.-
    Parasitol. 9:27, 1979.
10. Pérez, H., Malavé, I., and Arredondo, B.   Clin.exp.-
    Immunol. 38:453, 1979.
11. Pérez, H., Arredondo, B., and Machado, R.   Exp.-
    Parasitol. 47:9, 1979.
12. Pérez, H.   Acta Cient.Venz. 31:1980 (in press).
13. Walton, V. Ann.Trop.Med.Parasit. 73:23, 1979.

# GENETIC CONTROL OF IMMUNOLOGICALLY MEDIATED RESISTANCE TO HELMINTHIC INFECTIONS

DEREK WAKELIN

Wellcome Laboratories for Experimental Parasitology
University of Glasgow
Bearsden Road
Bearsden, Glasgow, Scotland

## INTRODUCTION

The fact that individuals or strains of a species may show variation in the degree of which they are infected by worm parasites, or to which they suffer from the effects of infection, has been known for a comparatively long time. The first well-documented reports concerned parasites of domestic stock (1,9,24,37) where the recognition of variation was facilitated by the existence of defined breeds of host. These early reports not only described the phenomenon but demonstrated the heritability of resistance and confirmed its genetic control. Analysis of the basis of such variation has been limited, until recently, by the paucity of information about the mechanisms which underlie host resistance. However, advanced in this field (28), coupled with a realization that understanding variation in resistance would have important applications in disease management and control, have led to greatly increased research activity and in the last few years significant progress has been made with a number of experimental and field systems.

It is understandable that workers in this area should look to comparable studies with other infectious organisms. Indeed, there are rewarding parallels to be drawn, but helminths, and the host responses they elicit, have characteristics which may necessitate rather different approaches. Not only, as metazoans, are worms antigenically complex in themselves, but during their life cycles they pass through a series of developmental stages which may differ antigenically from one another. These stages may occur within different sites in the host and quite different mechanisms of resistance may operate against them. The size of helminths renders them less susceptible to the cellular mechanisms of natural resistance which protect against smaller organisms, thus in the majority of cases resistance is mediated through both specific (immune) and non-specific effector mechanisms.

ANALYSIS IN EXPERIMENTAL SYSTEMS

1. General Considerations
   Variations in host resistance have been described for a
number of the helminths that can be maintained in the laboratory. However, for many there are limitations which restrict their usefulness as models for detailed analysis. The
most obvious of these is species of host, as such analysis
involves the use of well-defined and readily available strains. At present only the mouse satisfies both requirements.
A further limitation is the extent to which the mechanisms
of resistance operating within a system have been analysed.
In only a few cases have these mechanisms been sufficiently
well defined to permit genetic analysis. A less obvious
limitation may be the status of the host-parasite relationship concerned. Although a number of experimental systems
represent natural relationships, in that the parasite is
maintained in a host in which it occurs in nature, many are
unnatural and the laboratory host is merely a convenient
species in which development is possible. Though generalization is difficult, it may well be that the range of
variation in resistance necessary for analytical work will
be most often encountered in natural relationships. For
example, mouse strains show a wide spectrum of immune-mediated resistance to primary infections with Trichuris muris,
a natural parasite (26). Much less variation, in terms of
worm recovery and survival, is seen in mice infected with
Schistosoma mansoni (7,23), although, intriguingly, wide
variation is apparent after stimulation of the host with BCG
(6).

2. Heritability of Variations in Resistance
   Resistance, as assessed by the time taken to expel
worms from the intestine (e.g. Trichinella spiralis, T.
muris, Trichostrongylus colubriformis, Hymenolepis citelli)
or by the prevention of establishment of larval stages
(e.g. Taenia taeniaeformis), appears most often to be inherited as a dominant characteristic and one controlled by relatively few genes (14,22,26,30,35). In two systems, T.
muris in the mouse (27) and T. colubriformis in the guinea
pig (22) selective breeding from outbred stock has allowed
the separation of distinct resistant and susceptible lines
within a few generations.

3. Expression of Genetic Control in Resistance
   In relatively few cases is resistance to helminths
mediated solely through the immune system. One such case
concerns the cestode T. taeniaeformis, whose larval stages
occur in mice. Resistance is associated with the production

of IgG anti-worm antibody, and particularly of complement-fixing isotypes (13,14,16), and passive transfer confers high levels of protection. Susceptible and resistant strains of mice differ primarily in the rate at which protective antibody is produced (14); in the former adequate titres do not appear until after the larvae have acquired an anticomplementary activity (10) which renders them insusceptible to antibody activity.

Although it is probable that such direct, immunologically-mediated resistance occurs in all helminth infections, the more obvious expressions of resistance appear to derive from the activity of non-specific effectors, such as myeloid cells, which are brought into play by immune mechanisms. This type of response is seen in the antibody-and complement-mediated destruction of larval schistosomes (5) and larval nematodes (11,12), in which granulocytes, and particularly eosinophils, play a major role. Non-specifically acting immune-mediated effector mechanisms are also implicated in the expulsion of intestinal nematodes from the host (28) and the remainder of this paper will be concerned with one such nematode, Trichinella spiralis.

CONTROL OF RESISTANCE MEDIATED THROUGH NON-SPECIFIC EFFECTOR
MECHANISMS

Trichinella spiralis has a life cycle unique among nematodes in that all stages occur within the body of one host organism (Fig. 1). Moderate to heavy infections are pathogenic, and pathogenicity is associated primarily with migration of new-born larvae and their establishment within muscles. Resistance to infection is expressed a) by reduction of adult worm size and fecundity, b) by expulsion of worms from the intestine, c) by parenteral destruction of migrating larvae and is manifest both during primary infection and after challenge.

Much is now known about resistance operating against intestinal stages and it is clear that there is a complex interplay between a variety of specific and non-specific effectors (Fig. 2). Recent evidence suggests that, although related, the expressions of resistance derive from two distinct mechanisms, one a T-cell mediated, intestinal inflammatory response, which results in worm expulsion, the other a T-cell dependent and probably antibody-mediated response which affects growth and reproduction (30,31,32). Any or all of the components involved in these responses may show genetically controlled variation, but it is possible to measure the expression of this variation only by the limited parameters of worm expulsion, reduced growth and fecundity.

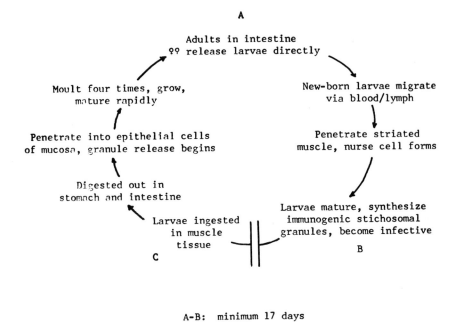

A

Adults in intestine
♀♀ release larvae directly

Moult four times, grow,
mature rapidly

New-born larvae migrate
via blood/lymph

Penetrate into epithelial cells
of mucosa, granule release begins

Penetrate striated
muscle, nurse cell forms

Digested out in
stomach and intestine

Larvae ingested
in muscle
tissue

Larvae mature, synthesize
immunogenic stichosomal
granules, become infective

C                                                      B

A-B:   minimum 17 days

C-A:   minimum  5 days

Figure 1.   Life Cycle of Trichinella Spiralis.

Inbred mice differ markedly in the degree of resistance
they express during a primary infection.   For convenience
strains can be divided into rapid and slow responders, using
the arbitrary criteria of whether worm expulsion is completed before or after day 12 of infection and whether fecundity
is maintained beyond the 8th day.   The status of a number of
strains is shown in Table 1, from which it is apparent that
rapidity of response is not associated with H-2 haplotype,
despite the fact that all the rapid-responder strains in-

cluded are H-2$^q$.  The data from B10 congenic mice indicates that slow response is a non H-2 characeristic;  all B10
background mice had a slow expulsion pattern, although detailed analysis suggests some H-2 influence on other para-
ˇeters of resistance.

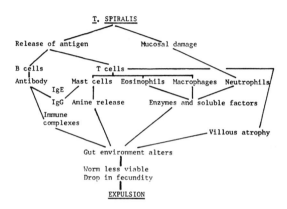

Figure 2.  Summary of responses in intestine associated with
resistance to Trichinella Spiralis

TABLE 1

Response of inbred strains of mice to infection with
Trichinella spiralis (Data from Wakelin, 1980)

| Rapid Response | | | Slow Response | |
|---|---|---|---|---|
| NIH | H-2$^q$ | | B10 (C57BL/10) | H-2$^b$ |
| DBA$_1$ | H-2$^q$ | | B10.G | H-2$^q$ |
| SWR | H-2$^q$ | | B10.BR | H-2$^k$ |
| | | | B10.D2 | H-2$^d$ |

     Non H-2 control of the speed of worm expulsion could be
exerted through the immunologically-specific component of
the response, through the intestinal inflammatory component,
or both.  Reciprocal adoptive transfer experiments, using

the histocompatible NIH and B10.G strains were performed and
the results are summarized in Table 2.

## TABLE 2

Trichinella spiralis in inbred mice:  adoptive transfer of
       immunity with mesenteric lymph node cells[1] in the
   histocompatible rapid- and slow-responder NIH and B10.G
                            strains

| | | Expression of immunity against challenge worms in recipients[2] | |
| | | Lowered | Accelerated |
| Strains of mice | | fecundity of | expulsion |
| Donor | Recipient | female worms | of worms |
| None | NIH | - | - [3] |
| None | B10.G | - | - |
| NIH | NIH | + | + |
| B10.G | B10.G | + | - [3] |
| B10.G | NIH | + | + |
| NIH | B10.G | + | - [3] |

[1] Cells taken from donors infected with 300 larvae 8 days
previously.  Recipients given 2-4 x $10^7$ cells and challenged
with 300 larvae on the same day.

[2] Recipients killed 8 days after challenge.

[3] Expulsion of worms had occurred by day 12.


It is clear that the slow response of B10.G mice is not determined by the rate of development of the immunologically
specific component, as day 8 B10.G cells transferred immunity to NIH mice as effectively as did NIH cells.  (Other experiments showed B10.G mice had competent cells as early as
4 days after infection).  In contrast, NIH cells failed to
bring about significant expulsion of worms from B10.G mice
within the time - 8 days - that they were able to do so in
NIH mice.  This result implies that the rate-limiting factor
in the slow expulsion from B10.G mice and thus the point of
non H-2 genetic control, is the development of the intesti-
inal inflammatory changes in response to the specific immune
component.  This is supported by the fact that when NIH mice
are reconstituted with B10.G bone marrow after lethal irradiation, their response to adoptive transfer of NIH immune

cells resembles that of B10.G mice (Table 3).

## TABLE 3

<u>Trichinella</u> <u>spiralis</u> in inbred mice: adoptive transfer of immunity with mesenteric lymph node cells (MLNC) from rapid-responder NIH mice[1] into NIH mice reconstituted with syngeneic bone mrrow (BM), or BM from histocompatible slow-responder B10.G mice, after 850 rad irradiation[2]

| Group of mice | | | Worm recoveries 8 days after challenge | | |
|---|---|---|---|---|---|
| | | | | | Fecundity |
| | BM | MLNC | Mean | S.D. | larvae/female/h |
| 1 | - | - | - | 102.3 | 30.2 | 2.8 |
| 2 | - | - | + | 46.0 | 26.9 | 0.8 |
| 3 | + | NIH | + | 40.1 | 26.8 | not done |
| 4 | + | B10.G | + | 118.9 | 18.0 | 1.4 |

[1]Cells taken from donors infected with 300 larvae 8 days previously. Recipients given $3 \times 10^7$ cells and challenged with 300 larvae on the same day.

[2]Mice irradiated and given $1 \times 10^7$ BM 90 days before infection.

At present it is not possible to identify which component of the inflammatory response is under non H-2 control. An attractive possibility centres around the involvement of mast cells and reaginic antibody as a central initiating effector mechanism. Although this concept has been current in immunoparasitology for several years, with experimental data both for and against (19), the recent ideas of Askenase (2) on the involvement of amine-containing cells in inflammatory responses has once more focussed attention on this mechanism. Certainly in rapidly-responding mice such as NIH, there is a dramatic rise in intestinal mast cells during a primary infection (Alizadeh and Wakelin, unpublished) and it is also known that inbred mice do vary in their capacity to form IgE and $IgG_1$ antibodies during infection with T. spiralis (20). Recent work with <u>Nippostrongylus</u> <u>brasiliensis</u> (3,18) has shown that the rise in mast cells during infection can be accelerated by transferring immune lymphocytes and there is preliminary evidence that this is true also in the case of <u>T</u>. <u>spiralis</u> in mice. A working hypothesis, therefore, is that non H-2 genes control the production of a lymphocyte-mediated intestinal mastocytosis and/or the production of the reaginic antibody necessary to mediate amine release. Whereas much is presently known about genetic control of reagin production, little or nothing is known about that of mast cell responses. However, it is interesting to note that marked strain differences occur in the mast cell responses of rats infected with N. brasiliensis and in the increased gut permeability that accompanies infection (17,18).

Although it appears that the overall speed of response to T. spiralis is under non H-2 control, it remains to be shown whether H-2 linked genes also play a major role. It is sugestive that the rapidly-responding inbred strains so far studied, using ($^{125}$I) UDR to label mesenteric node blast cells, do show that mice carrying this haplotype have a more rapid cellular response to infection. This is true both of rapid-responders (NIH) and of slow-responders (B10.G); B10 mice, in contrast. show a slower cellular response (Wakelin, unpublished). Wassom et al (35) have shown a clear influence of H-2 linked genes on overall resistance and have confirmed that haplotype H2$^q$ confers greater resistance to T. spiralis.

There is no doubt that present concepts of the genetic control of resistance to T. spiralis are oversimplified and incomplete. The work of Bell and his colleagues (4) has shown that in rats the different stages of infection elicit specific responses in the host; in complete infections the overall characteristics of resistance therefore represent the summation of several component parts. It is not impossible that each could be under independent genetic control. Some support for this view is given by Despommier et al. (8) who reported that in certain rat strains expression of resistance against the intestinal phase of infection included both reduction of fecundity and worm expulsion; in others expulsion occurred without prior effects against reproduction.

In addition, little is yet understood, either at the level of mechanisms or control, of factors operating against the parenteral stages of infection. Recent work has shown that new-born larvae can be killed in vitro by antibody-mediated eosinophil activity (11,12); other studies suggest that a similar mechanism may operate in vivo (15). No systematic study has yet been carried out to test whether there is strain variation in ability to express resistance against parenteral stages. Some workers (25) have assessed strain variation by comparing the numbers of muscle larvae recovered after a standard infection, but such data do not take into account the fact that differences may occur in reproductive output from adult worms, because of variation in a) establishment, b) level of fecundity attained, c) duration of fecundity and d) survival. These difficulties can be overcome by the expedient of direct, intravenous injection of new-born larvae. Not only would this approach provide useful information about host resistance to this stage of T. spiralis, but such information may well prove relevant to understanding the nature of responses to the parenteral stages of nematodes, such as filariids, that are of much greater medical significance.

## CONCLUSION

Despite the complexity of the responses elicited by helminths, genetic control of resistance may still be exerted in a simple and direct manner. This is because, within the complexity, there are relatively few responses that contribute to protection and of these even fewer may act as rate-limiting factors. This fact gives some optimism for the application of genetic studies to the problems of chronic helminth infections, particularly those of domestic animals. If it can be shown that parallels exist between experimental models and field infections then there is scope for the application of controlled vaccination procedures to boost deficient components of the response (discussed by Mitchell et al. 14). there is also the prospect of selecting for resistance within existing stock or of hybridising with native stock to introduce resistance genes into the gene pool. Several workers have demonstrated breed differences in sheep in their responses to intestinal nematode parasites (reviewed in 29) and research into selective breeding for resistance is actively being pursued. Similarly, differences in resistance to infection have been demonstrated between imported and native strains of sheep in areas where nematode infection is endemic (21). As far as parasites of medical significance are concerned application of genetic studies is at present a remote prospect, though there is undoubtedly an urgent need to identify the factors responsible for the apparent failure of resistance in many human helminth infections. Perhaps in the short term it may be more profitable to concentrate on genetic factors relevant to pathological processes in infections. As Class and Deelder (7) have shown, mice of similar susceptibility to infection with Schistosoma mansoni may show very different patterns of morbidity and mortality. If genetic studies could contribute towards a means of reducing pathology in this and similar infections in man, substantial benefits would accrue.

REFERENCES

1.   Ackert, J.E.   J.Paasitol. 28:1, 1942.
2.   Askenase, P.W.   Progr.Allergy 23:199, 1977.
3.   Befus, A.D., and Bienenstock, J.   Immunology 38:95, 1979.
4.   Bell, R.G., McGregor, D.D., and Despommier, D.D. Exp.Parasitol. 47:140, 1979.
5.   Butterworth, A.E.   Amer.J.Trop.Med.Hyg. 26:29, 1977.
6.   Civil, R.H., and Mahmoud, A.A.F.   J.Immunol. 120:1070, 1978.
7.   Class, F.H.J., and Deelder, A.M.   J.Immunogenet. 6:167, 1979.
8.   Despommier, D.D., McGregor, D.D., Crum, E.D., and Carter, P.B.   Immunology 33:7979, 1977.
9.   Gregory P.W., Miller, R.F., and Stewart, M.A.   J.Genet. 39:391, 1940.
10.  Hammerberg, B., and Williams, J.F.   J.Immunol. 120:1033, 1978.
11.  Kazura, J.W., and Grove, D.I.   Nature (Lond.) 274:588, 1978.
12.  Mackenzie, C.D., Preston, P.M., and Ogilvie, B.M. Nature (Lond.) 276:826, 1978.
13.  Mitchell, G.F., Goding, J.W., and Rickard, M.D. Aust.J.Exp.Biol.Med.Sci. 55:165, 1977.
14.  Mitchell, G.F., Rajasekariah, G.R., and Rickard, M.D. Immunology, 1980 (in press).
15.  Moloney, A., and Denham, D.A.   Parasite Immunol. 1:3, 1979.
16.  Musoke, A.J., and Williams, J.F.   Immunology 28:97, 1975.
17.  Nawa, Y. Int.J.Parasitol. 9:251, 1979.
18.  Nawa, Y., and Miller, H.R.P.   Cell.Immunol. 42:225, 1979.
19.  Ogilvie, B.M., and Jones, V.E.   Prog.Allergy 17:93, 1973.
20.  Rivera-Ortiz, C-I, and Nussenzweig, R.   Expl.Parasitol. 39:7, 1976.
21.  Preston, J.M., and Allonby, E.W.   Vet.Rec. 103:509, 1978.
22.  Rothwell, T.L.W., Le Jambre L.F., Adams, D.B., and Love, R.J.   Parasitology 76:201, 1978.
23.  Sher, A., MacKenzie, P., and Smithers, S.R.   J.Inf.Dis. 130:626, 1974.
24.  Stewart. M.A., Miller, R.F., and Douglas, J.R. J.Agric.Res. 55:923, 1937.
25.  Tanner, C.E.   J. Parasit. 64:956, 1978.
26.  Wakelin, D.   Parasitology 71:51, 1975.

27. Wakelin, D. Parasitology 71:377, 1975.
28. Wakelin, D. Nature (Lond.) 273:617, 1978.
29. Wakelin, D. Adv.Parasitol. 16:219, 1978.
30. Wakelin, D. Parasite. Immunol. 1980 (in press).
31. Wakelin, D., and Wilson, M.M. Immunology 37:103, 1979.
32. Wakelin, D., and Wilson, M.M. Exp.Parasitol. 48:305, 1979.
33. Wakelin, D., and Wilson, M.M. Int.J.Parasitol. 1980 (in press).
34. Wakelin, D., and Donachie, A.M. Parasite Immunol. 1980 (in press).
35. Wassom, D.L., DeWitt, C.W., and Grundmann, A.W. J.Parasit. 60:47, 1974.
36. Wassom, D.L., David, .S., and Gleich, G.J. Immunogenet. 9:491, 1979.
37. Whitlock, J.H. Cornell Vet. 45:422, 1955.

## DISCUSSION

Eisenstein: Can Wakelin describe the response to infection with regard to mast cells? Where does he see them; in the mucosa? Is it a Jones-Mote type of reaction? Is it immunologically mediated?

Wakelin: Mast cells appear initially in the lamina propria, at the level of the crypts and, as the infection progresses, the mast cell numbers reach a peak and migrate towards the intra-epithelial position. There is a lot of dispute at the moment as to whether intra-epithelial, eosin-blue staining cells are mast cells or some other type of cells. As far as the nature of the response is concerned, it is assumed to be reagin-mediated, but there is really no experimental evidence. Assessment of the role of mast cells should be based on a dynamic footing rather than a static situation which typifies past studies. We need to know something of the rate of mast cell turnover, as absolute numbers can obscure many changes*.

---

*Editor's Comment (E.S.): The exact functional role of mucosal mast cells in the immunopathological response to intestinal nematode parasites is controversial. Genetic studies cast a doubt on decisive effector role of mast cells in this situation and consign it, probably, to the long list of immunological epiphenomena: $W/W^V$ mice have a point mutation resulting in the lack of mast cells. They, however, have nematode parasite rejection comparable to +/+ controls, in the absence of any mucosal mast cell response.

Skamene: I would comment on some conceptual similarities between the models of genetic resistance to Trichenella as presented by Wakelin and to Listeria as studied by our group (Kongshavn et al. this volume). There are similarities in the strain distribution of Trichinella-resistant and Listeria-resistant animals among inbred mice and the genetic control of resistance is exerted, in both instances, by genes that map outside H-2 and that do not express themselves in the T-cell response. The results on resistance to Trichinella and Listeria of radiation bone marrow chimeras created between the sensitive donor → resistant host and vice versa show, in both models, that the gene product expresses itself as a radio-resistant factor in the host's environment. In the Listeria model, we see it as a regulator of the bone marrow-derived macrophage response to this infection. However, we always notice the contribution of a variety of other leukocyte types (neutrophils, basophils, eosinophils) accumulating together, with macrophages, at the sites of infection or inflammation. Although the effector mechanisms in resistance to Trichinella and Listeria are ultimately different, the gene product which is responsible for their activation may be similar or even identical. This hypothesis is yet to be verified experimentally by formal linkage analysis on segregating populations.

Bradley: One of the complicating factors of working with these parasites is that some of the intestinal nematodes can alter the ability of the host to mount an immune response to parasite antigens and also to other antigens. I wonder if you have examined the immunosuppressive ability of this parasite in the Trichinella-resistant and -sensitive strains?

Wakelin: The answer is no. Trichinella is known to exert powerful immunosuppressive effects. It struck me very recently that it would be rewarding to look at the genetic control of the ability to suppress as well as the ability to mount resistance, but up to now I have not done that.

# VARIATION IN ANTI-TRICHINELLA RESPONSIVENESS IN INBRED MOUSE STRAINS

R.G. Bell and D.D. McGregor

James A. Baker Institute for Animal Health
New york State College of Veterinary Medicine
Cornell University
Ithaca, New York 14853

Infections with the nematode, Trichinella spiralis are terminated by the expulsion of the parasite from the intestine. In rats, three separate immune responses lead to worm expulsion. They have been defined as follows: Anti-adult immunity; terminates the primary infection (2). Anti-preadult immunity; has a minor role in eliminating secondary infections (2). Rapid expulsion (RE) eliminates from 90-99% of a secondary infection within 24 hours (2,13,15). In addition, the reproductive capacity of T. spiralis is controlled by two more immune responses. Anti-fecundity restricts newborn larvae production (7,8) and systemic anti larval responses inhibit the implantation of larvae in muscle. Elimination of primary infections in rats begins on days 9-10 and is usually complete by days 12-14. Secondary infections persist for 6-7 days although >90% of the challenge is expelled within 24 hours. This pattern of response is observed in both inbred and randomly-bred rats (2,10,13).

The enteral history of T. spiralis infections in mice varies from one that is essentially identical with that described for rats (1,7,9,17) to a pattern characterized by the slow elimination of a primary infection and a weak or absent secondary response (5,6,11,12,14). Technical differences may account for some strain variation, but the degree of genetic influence cannot be estimated until systematic interstrain comparative studies are undertaken.

This report examines strain variation is protective ability by submitting mice to standardized immunization regimes with T. spiralis. The response to challenge infection is compared to quantitatively demonstrate strain differences and to examine the immunological basis for these differences.

## Effect of Enteral Immunization on Worm Expulsion

Enteral immunization consists of exposing the host to T. spiralis worms derived from orally administered muscle larvae. Infections of seven or ten days duration are term-

inated by injecting methyridine (300 mg/kg) subcutaneously.
Worm reproduction is inhibited by feeding mice diets containing 0.05% thiabenadzole from day 3 until termination.
This procedure sterilizes the female but does not impair
worm longevity in the intestine (2). In rats, this is a
powerful immunization regime that primes for RE, anti-preadult immunity, anti-adult immunity and anti-fecundity responses (2).

Table 1.  Response of Inbred Mice to a Challenge Infection
After Exposure to Enteral T. spiralis for 7 days

| Mouse Strain | Intestinal T. spiralis 9 days after the challenge infection (200 muscle larvae) | | Probability |
|---|---|---|---|
| | Immune | Non Immune | |
| CBA | 9 + 11 | 74 + 18 | <.0005 |
| C$_3$H | 1 + 2 | 94 + 28 | <.0005 |
| SJL | 10 + 10 | 121 + 29 | <.0005 |
| DBA/2 | 34 + 31 | 139 + 45 | <.01 |
| A/He | 97 + 38 | 140 + 9 | <.05 |
| C$_{57}$Bl | 117 + 18 | 139 + 18 | N.S. |

Mice immunized by exposure to T. spiralis for 7 days
then challenged with 200 muscle larvae (Table 1) show wide
interstrain variation in their ability to eliminate the
challenge infection. The CBA, C3H and SJL strains respond
strongly and eliminate most of their intestinal worms by 9
days after challenge. In contrast C57BL mice fail to eliminate worms during this period. Two strains (A/He, DBA/2)
show intermediate responses. The observed differences in
worm burdens in the various strains, and between normal and
immune mice cannot be ascribed to the variation in infectivity, because such animals harbored approximately the same
number of worms 24 hours after challennge (data not shown).

Table 2.    Response of B10 Congenic Mice of Stage-specific
                        Immunization

| Strain | Immunization type | Intestinal worms 14 days after challenge with 600 M.L. | Muscle Larvae |
|--------|-------------------|--------------------------------------------------------|---------------|
| B10·D$_2$ | preadult (1 d) | | 23,440 $\pm$ 6,094[+] |
| | adult (7 d) | N.D. | 43,866 $\pm$ 11,207 |
| | combined enteral (14 d) | | 5,310 $\pm$ 4,942[+] |
| | — | | 33,920 $\pm$ 4,959 |
| B10·BR | preadult (1 d) | 24 $\pm$ 24 | 22,560 $\pm$ 14,402 |
| | adult (7 d) | 40 $\pm$ 17 | 40,750 $\pm$ 15,740 |
| | combined enteral (14 d) | 3 $\pm$ 4[+] | 1,970 $\pm$ 2,505[+] |
| | — | 36 $\pm$ 21 | 28,680 $\pm$ 5,880 |

+Significantly different from control value.

To analyze the response of the C57BL mouse in more
detail the foregoing experiment was repeated using a 14 day
enteral exposure to both preadults and adults; a 7 day exposure to adult worms alone, or exposure (24 hours) restricted to preadults. The latter two regimes induce anti-
adult and anti-preadult responses respectively. Experimental animals were members of the congenic B10.BR and B10.D2
strains. Protection was analyzed by quantitation of muscle
larvae burdens as this assesses overall protection. The results (Table 2) showed that B10.BR and B10.D2 mice did not
respond to 7 day adult immunization and only weakly to preadult immunization, although the B10.D2 group were significantly protected. Combined enteral immunization (comprising
the natural infection of preadult and adult worms) produced
a much stronger immunity than exposure to either preadults
or adults alone. It is evident from the intestinal adult
worm counts that protection in this group was primarily mediated through adult worm expulsion, although other factors,
(anti-fecundity) cannot be excluded. Since exposure to preadults is quantitatively similar during both the preadult
and complete enteral regimes, the difference in effectiveness may be due to enhanced anti-adult responses. This in-
terpreation is consistent with the reduction in adult worm
burdens.

Variations in the ability of mice to expel a challenge
infection within 24 hours

Table 3.  Worm persistence 24 hours after a Challenge
infection in ♂♂ NFR/N, NFS/N and CFW mice

| Strain | Worms 24 hours after challenge with 500 T. spiralis | | Probability |
|:------:|:-----------:|:----------:|:----------:|
| | Immune | Non Immune | |
| NFR/N | 73 + 57 | 423 + 76 | <.0005 |
| NFS/N | 16 + 15 | 396 + 131 | <.0005 |
| CFW | 27 + 34 | 414 + 54 | <.0005 |

Priming infection 400 muscle larvae, mice were placed on
thiabendazole at day 3 and taken off at day 14 (no methyridine was given).  Challenge infection of 500 per os given 21
days after the priming infection.


The RE reaction in rats has specificity for preadult
T. spiralis (3,4).  Because of this specificity it is not
surprising that mouse strains that are weakly responsive to
preadult worms do not express RE, e.g. the B10 mice.  However, the inability of other more immunologically competent
strains (CBA, C3H, SJL, Table 1) to promptly expel challenge
infection is more unexpected.  A survey was conducted to
determine whether mice of any strain were capable of expel-
ling a significant portion of a challenge infection within
24 hours.  Only three strains of the 12 tested consistently
rejected challenge worms within 24 hours after enteral stimulation (Table 3).  Two strains were inbred (NFR/N and
NFS/N) and one randomly bred (CFW), the NFR/N and NFS/N
strains are closely related as they were derived from the
same NIH stock.
To determine whether the response of the inbred mice
was kinetically similar to that of the rat a group of NFR/N
♂ mice were infected with 40 T. spiralis, and fed thiabendazole from day 3 on.  The infection was terminated by methyridine injection at days 10 and 11.  Rats subjected to this
regime and rechallenged at 14 days expel 95-99% of the chal-

lenge infection by 24 hours, with the remainder of the worms
being expelled from days 4-7. The effect of this immunization regime on a challenge infection in NFR/N mice (Table 4)
is very similar to RE in rats.

Table 4. Fate of a challenge infection in NFR/N mice
exposed to an abbreviated infection

| Time after | Number of Worms | | |
|---|---|---|---|
| challenge | Immune | Non Immune | Probability |
| 1 day | 2 + 4 | 404 + 110 | <.0005 |
| 2 days | 5 + 3 | - | - |
| 3 days | 2 + 2 | 300 + 44 | <.0005 |
| 4 days | 0.1 + 0.4 | - | - |
| 5 days | 2 + 2 | 340 + 52 | <.0005 |
| 6 days | 0.3 + 1 | - | - |
| 7 days | 0.4 + 1 | 419 + 56 | <.0005 |

Inheritance of the capacity for 24-hour expulsion of
challenge worms in mice

The unusually restricted strain distribution of 24-hour
expulsion of challenge T. spiralis suggested a genetic component. To examine this NFR/N mice were crossed with $C_3H$
and B10.BR mice. Both the B10.BR and $C_3H$ mice fail to expel
challenge T. spiralis within 24 hours, however, the $C_3H$
mouse mounts a strong slow response (days 5-9) and the B10.-
BR strain mounts weak anti-preadult responses and is poorly
protected against challenge infections. The strong reactivity of the $F_1$ resulting from crosses between ♂ $C_3H$ x ♀ NFR/N
or B10.BR x ♀ NFR/N is shown in Table 5. From these results
it is evident that 24-hour expulsion in mice can be inherited as a dominant characteristic. Strong reactivity is conferred upon two non-reactive strains irrespective of the
capacity of either strain to mount slow or anti-preadult
protective responses.

Table 5.  Twenty-four hour Response of $F_1$ hybrids to
challenge T. spiralis

| Cross | Worm Burden | | Probability |
| | Immune | Non Immune | |
|---|---|---|---|
| C₃H x NFR/N ♂♂ offspring | 46 + 34 | 364 + 46 | <.0005 |
| B10·BR x NFR/N ♂♂ offspring | 36 + 31 | 372 + 65 | <.0005 |
| B10·BR x NFR/N ♀♀ offspring | 25 + 31 | 322 + 76 | <.0005 |

In contrast to rats, extreme heterogeneity is evident
in the ability of inbred mouse strains to respond to infections with T. spiralis, this parallels similar findings in
mice infected with Trichuris muris (16). Unresponsiveness
is evident both in the failure of 'slow' worm expulsion as
well as the inability of many inbred mouse strains to reject
challenge infections with T. spiralis within 24 hours.
Crosses made between 24-hour expulsion responder strains
(NFR/N) and non-responder strains (B10.BR and C₃H) have
shown a transfer of responsiveness in the $F_1$ thus unequivo-
cally demonstrating a dominant genetic component.

REFERENCES

1.  Bass, G.K., and Olson, L.J.  J.Parasitol. 51:640, 1965.
2.  Bell, R.G., McGregor, D.D., and Despommier, D.D.
    Exp.Parasitol. 47:140, 1979.
3.  Bell, R.G., and McGregor, D.D.  Exp.Parasit. 48:42,
    1979.
4.  Bell, R.G., and McGregor, D.D.  Exp.parasitol. 48:51,
    1979.
5.  Crandall, R.B., and Crandall, C.A.  Exp.Parasitol.
    31:378, 1972.
6.  Denham, D.A.  J.Helminthol. 42:257, 1968.
7.  Denham, D.A., and Martinez, A.R.  J.Helminth. 44:357,
    1970.
8.  Despommier, D.D., Campbell, W.C., and Blair, L.S.
    Parasitol. 74:109, 1977.
9.  Despommier, D.D., and Wostmann, B.S.  Exp.Parasit.
    23:778, 1968.

10. Gursch, O.F. J.Prasit. 25:19, 1949.
11. Kozar, M. Acta Parasit.Pol. 21:513, 1933.
12. Larsh, J.E. Adv.Parasit. 1:213, 1963.
13. Love, R.J., Ogilvie, B.M., and McLaren, D.J. Immunol. 30:7, 1976.
14. Machnicka, B. Exp.Parasit. 31:172, 1972.
15. McCoy, O.R. Am.J.Hyg. 32:105, 1940.
16. Wakelin, D. Parasitol. 71:51, 1975.
17. Wakelin, D., and Lloyd, M. Parasitol. 72:173, 1976.

# MHC-LINKED GENETIC CONTROL OF THE IMMUNE RESPONSE TO PARASITES: TRICHINELLA SPIRALIS IN THE MOUSE

Donald L. Wassom, Chella S. David and Gerald J. Gleich

From the Departments of Medicine and Immunology
Mayo Clinic and Foundation
Rochester, MN 55901

Experiments conducted in a variety of host-parasite systems have confirmed that genetically controlled factors operate to influence the host's response to parasitic infection (2). Little is known, however, of the role played by MHC-linked genes in contributing to these genetic differences. To properly evaluate the role played by MHC-linked genes in controlling the immune response to parasites it is necessary to study congenic strains of hosts which are genetically identical, or nearly so, except for genes within or closely linked to the MHC. When H-2 congenic strains of mice are used for such experiments any measurable difference in the host response between the different strains can be related directly to the H-2-linked gene(s) by which they differ (1). Likewise, if one wishes to evaluate the role played by non-H-2-linked genes, strains of mice which share common H-2 haplotypes but express different genetic backgrounds can be studied. Taking such an approach we have begun to investigate the genetic difference in the host response expressed by different inbred strains of mice when infected with the helminth parasite Trichinella spiralis. We have shown that levels of resistance to infection with this parasite are influenced by several genes mapping within the H-2 complex and by one or more genes mapping outside the major histocompatibility complex (3).

In all experiments to test for strain susceptibility, age matched male mice were infected by esophageal intubation with 150 infective muscle larvae prepared by acid pepsin digestion of infected C3HeB/FeJ mice. Strain susceptibility was assessed by determining total body larval counts 30 days post-infection. Larval counts from 8-10 mice per experiment were used to calculate a mean worm count value for each strain. In early experiments the strain B10.BR($H-2^k$) was shown to be highly susceptible to infection and the strain B10.S($H-2^s$) shown to be highly resistant. The strains B10.BR and B10.S were therefore included in most experiments as susceptible and resistant controls. Mean larval counts for the strains B10.BR and B10.S were then used along with the mean worm counts for each strain tested to calculate a

resistance index for each strain according to the formula
shown in Table 1.

Table 1.  Distribution of Resistance in Strains Expressing
Independent Haplotypes

|        |           | Resistance |
|--------|-----------|------------|
| Strain | Haplotype | Index¨ |
| B10.BR | k | 0 |
| B10.P | p | -22 |
| B10.RIII | r | 33 |
| B10 | b | 68[†] |
| B10.S | s | 100[†] |
| B10.M | f | 104[†] |
| B10.Q | q | 105[†] |

$$\text{Resist.index} = \frac{(\text{mean count } H\text{-}2^k) - (\text{mean count } H\text{-}2^?)}{(\text{mean count } H\text{-}2^k) - (\text{mean count } H\text{-}2^S)} \times 100$$

an index of 0 = highly susceptible; 100 = highly resistant
†Significantly more resistant than B10.BR

Using this formula, a strain showing a mean larval count
identical to the susceptible $H\text{-}2^k$ haplotype is assigned an
index of 0 and a strain showing resistance equal to the
$H\text{-}2^S$ haplotype will have an index of 100.  Strains of mice
harboring more muscle larvae than the B10.BR (susceptible)
control are assigned a negative index value while strains
more resistant than the B10.S control are assigned indices
higher than 100.  An infection with 150 muscle larvae generally results in approximately 30,000 larvae encysted in the
muscle of B10.BR mice whereas the more resistant B10.S
strain harbors approximately 15,000.

To determine whether or not genes within the H-2 complex influence susceptibility to infection with T. spiralis,
congenic strains of mice expressing different independent
haplotypes, but sharing the C57BL/10 genetic background,

have been tested for levels of resistance. The resistance index of each strain is given in Table 1. The strains B10.BR($\underline{H-2}^k$) and B10.P($\underline{H-2}^p$) are the most susceptible of the strains tested while the strains B10.S($\underline{H-2}^s$), B10.M-($\underline{H-2}^f$) and B10.Q($\underline{H-2}^q$) are the most resistant. The strains B10.RIII($\underline{H-2}^r$) and B10($\underline{H-2}^b$) show intermediate levels of resistance. Because these strains of mice differ only a gene loci within the H-2 complex, it can be concluded that H-2-linked genes are responsible for the differences in levels of resistance observed. In a separate experiment we tested whether or not genes outside the H-2 complex might also influence resistance to infection. Five strains of mice differing in their genetic backgrounds but sharing the $\underline{H-2}^k$ haplotype and another grouping of three different strains sharing the $\underline{H-2}^q$ haplotype were infected with $\underline{T.}$ $\underline{spiralis}$ and total body larval counts determined 30 days later.

Table 2. Role of Non-H-2 Genes in Determining
Susceptibility or Resistance

| H-2 Haplotype | Strain | Mean Larval±Count SEM | p* |
|---|---|---|---|
| k | C3HeB/FeJ | 42644±3604 | ---- |
| k | CBA/J | 33663±4035 | NS |
| k | RF/J | 25813±1065 | p<0.001[†] |
| k | AKR/J | 23370±2255 | p<0.001[†] |
| k | C58/J | 21956±2548 | p<0.001[†] |
| q | DBA/1J | 19675±2758 | ---- |
| q | SWR/J | 14500±1926 | NS |
| q | BUB/BnJ | 13344±605 | p<0.05[‡] |

*Mann Whitney rank sum test
[†]Compared to larval counts for C3HeB/FeJ
[‡]Compared to larval counts for DBA/1J.

Table 2 shows that of the H-2$^k$ mice the strain C3HeB/FeJ
was significantly more susceptible to infection than were
the strains RF/J, C58/J, C58/J and AKR/J. Furthermore, the
DBA/1J mice were more susceptible than the strains SWR/J and
BUB/BnJ. These results demonstrate that genes outside the
MHC may also act to influence resistance to infection with
T. spiralis and clearly point out the need to use congenic
strains of mice in studies directed at evaluating the role
played by H-2-linked genes in this host-parasite system.

Having established that H-2-linked genes influence resistance to T. spiralis, we have begun testing H-2 recombinant strains of mice to map the genes involved. At present
at least two and probably three H-2-linked genes controlling
resistance to this parasite have been identified.

Table 3. Mapping of Gene(s) Associated with Resistance to
T. spiralis

|          |   |   |   | Haplotype |   |   |   |   |      |
|----------|---|---|---|-----------|---|---|---|---|------|
| Strain   | K | A | B | J | E | C | S | D | RI* |
| B10.BR   | k | k | k | k | k | k | k | k | 0   |
| B10.A    | k | k | k | k | k | d | d | d | -9  |
| B10.M(17R)| k | k | k | k | k | d | d | f | 6   |
| B10.S(8R)| k | k | k | s | s | s | s | s | -44 |
| B10.TL   | s | k | k | k | k | k | k | d | 6   |
| B10.S(9R)| s | s | ? | k | k | d | d | d | 219 |
| B10.HTT  | s | s | s | s | k | k | k | d | 93  |
| B10.S    | s | s | s | s | s | s | s | s | 100 |

*Resistance index, see Table 1
0=highly susceptible, 100=highly resistant

Table 3 shows the resistance indices of several congenic
recombinant strains of mice chosen to demonstrate the involvement of a gene in I-A or I-B subregion of the H-2 complex.
Strains carrying the susceptible k alleles in the I-A or I-B
subregions are uniformly more susceptible to infection with

T. spiralis than strains expressing the resistant s alleles
in these regions.


Table 4.  Evidence for the Role of D-End Genes in Resistance
to T. spiralis


| Experiment | Strain | Haplotype | | | | | | | | Mean Larval Count+SEM | RI* | p† |
|---|---|---|---|---|---|---|---|---|---|---|---|---|
| | | K | A | B | J | E | C | S | D | | | |
| 1 | B10.BR | k | k | k | k | k | k | k | k | 30286+1291 | 0 | ---- |
| | B10.A | k | k | k | k | k | d | d | d | 28680+2485 | 11 | NS |
| | B10.TL | s | k | k | k | k | k | k | d | 29300+2564 | 6 | NS |
| | B10.S | s | s | s | s | s | s | s | s | 15050+1024 | 100 | ---- |
| | B10.S(7R) | s | s | s | s | s | s | s | d | 23489+1549 | 45 | p<0.002 |
| | B10.M | f | f | f | f | f | f | f | f | 15750+1394 | 95 | ---- |
| | B10.M(11R) | f | f | f | f | f | f | f | d | 20301+1793 | 66 | p<0.05 |
| 2 | B10.DA | q | q | q | q | q | q | q | s | 19680+2221 | --- | ---- |
| | B10.T(6R) | q | q | q | q | q | q | q | d | 33100+2382 | --- | p<0.003 |


*Resistance index, see Table 1
†Mann Whitney rank sum test




Results shown in Table 4 shows that a gene on the D end of
the H-2 complex is also important.  The presence of a d
allele in the D region of the H-2 complex results in increased susceptibility of the otherwise resistant haplotypes
s, q and f yet has no effect when combined with the susceptible k-alleles at other loci.

Table 5. Heterogeneity Among H-2 D-End Recombinant Strains
of Mice in Resistance to T. spiralis

| Experiment | Strain | Haplotype | | | | | | | | Mean Larval Count$\pm$SEM | p* |
|:---:|:---:|:---:|:---:|:---:|:---:|:---:|:---:|:---:|:---:|:---:|:---:|
| | | K | A | B | J | E | C | S | D | | |
| 1 | B10.S(7R) | s | s | s | s | s | s | s | d | 27210$\pm$3367 | ---- |
| | B10.S(24R) | s | s | s | s | s | s | s | d | 17400$\pm$2336 | p<0.003[†] |
| 2 | B10.S(7R) | s | s | s | s | s | s | s | d | 26230$\pm$2500 | ---- |
| | B10.S(23R) | s | s | s | s | s | s | s | d | 17538$\pm$2109 | p<0.02[†] |
| 3 | B10.S(7R) | s | s | s | s | s | s | s | d | 23489$\pm$1549 | ---- |
| | B10.S(24R) | s | s | s | s | s | s | s | d | 13833$\pm$1283 | p<0.002[†] |
| | B10.S(23R) | s | s | s | s | s | s | s | d | 17260$\pm$1961 | p<0.012[†] |
| | B10.S | s | s | s | s | s | s | s | s | 15050$\pm$1024 | p<0.002[†] |

*Mann Whitney rank sum test
†Compared to larval counts for B10.S(7R)

Additionally, there are indications that a third gene,
perhaps mapping between the S and D regions, may influence
the outcome of infection. Table 5 shows that the strains
B10.S(7R), B10.S(23R), and B10.S(24R), which were each derived from a recombination between the s and a haplotypes
and appear to be genetically identical by methods thus far
employed to test them, show consistent differences in resistance to T. spiralis. B10.S(7R) is always more susceptible
than the other two strains which show levels of resistance
comparable to those of the strain B10.S. The most likely
explanation for this finding is that the B10.S(7R) mice
differ from the other two strains in the point of crossover
between the S and D regions.
    Thus far we have shown that several H-2-linked genes
play important roles in controlling resistance to T. spiralis infections in the mouse. We have also demonstrated that
one or more genes mapping outside of the H-2 complex are

involved in determining the outcome of these infections. We do not know, however, whether the several genes identified interact or complement one another in any way nor do we know the mechanisms whereby these genes operate to manifest their effect. Future studies will be directed at answering these questions.

## ACKNOWLEDGEMENT

This research was supported by grants from the National Institutes of Health, AI 07047, AI 9728, CA 24473, and by the Mayo Foundation.

## REFERENCES

1. Benacerraf, B., and Germain, R.W. Immunol. Rev. 38:70, 1978.
2. Wakelin, D. In Advances in Parasitology. W.H.R. Lumsden, R. Mueller, and J.R. Baker (eds). New York, Academic press, 16:219, 1978.
3. Wassom, D.L., David, C.S., and Gleich, G.J. Immunogenetics 9:491, 1979.

## DISCUSSION

**Williams:** Have you looked at backcrosses that have been typed to verify that the phenomena are under genetic control?

**Wassom:** We have not done any backcross experiments, but have concentrated exclusively on the recombinant strains.

**Karre:** Is it known whether these larvae can incorporate H-2 material from the host on their surface?

**Wassom:** We are presently exploring this matter. Despommier has indicated that muscle larvae, even after acid-pepsin-digestion, still retain a membranous structure that very likely is of host origin. We know little about the antigenic make-up of that structure, nor do we know whether the parasite picks up H-2 components while migrating through tissues. This could, I suppose, have a very important bearing on how the host responds to the parasite initially. It might have a bearing on the development of <u>H-2</u> mediated suppression, depending on the particular antigens taken up. We ourselves have no data indicating that this is the case. I should mention that it does appear to be important where the larvae come from, in terms of how well they subsequently establish themselves in the host. If outbred animals are utilized as a source of larvae, it becomes difficult to get reproducible results, whereas inbred strains as a source of larvae yield nicely reproducible results.

<u>Karre</u>: So all the results presented here were from which host?

<u>Wassom</u>: All the larvae in these experiments were taken from C3H mice, which express the <u>H-2</u>$^k$ haplotype. It may be more than coincidental that the k haplotype strains are the susceptible ones under these circumstances.

<u>Amos</u>: Anytime you implicate the D region as exerting the control of a given trait you have to consider an involvement of Q region (QA) in such a control. There are a number of recombinants involving the genetic material to the right of the D region which would be suitable for precise mapping of the locus under consideration.

<u>Wassom</u>: We have not examined the resistance to Trichinella of any of the QA recombinants. However, the congenic strains we have studied were all derived from progenitors exhibiting recombination between the s and a haplotypes.

# IMMUNOMODULATION AND ALTERED RESISTANCE TO INFECTION IN DIFFERENT MOUSE STRAINS INFECTED WITH NIPPOSTRONGYLUS BRASILIENSIS

Ann C. Vickery, Thomas W. Klein
and Herman Friedman

University of South Florida College of Medicine
Tampa, Florida

In the laboratory, Nippostrongylus brasiliensis (Nb) is one of the most extensively studied nematodes. This parasite has proven to be an invaluable tool in the elucidation of mechanisms involved in IgE production (5) as well as in the study of host resistance to intestinal nematodes (4). In this laboratory, Nb is being utilized to examine in depth parasite-mediated modulation of the host's immune responsiveness to heterologous antigens.

Although the brown, or Norway rat (Rattus norwegicus) is the natural host of Nb, the parasite can be adapted to mice by continuous passage through this host (8). In the mouse, Nb is highly immunogenic, stimulating thymus-dependent antibody and cell-mediated immune response which led to expulsion of the host's intestinal worm burden (1). Acquired resistance to subsequent reinfection can be recognized by decreased numbers of adult worms in the small intestine of the host and by their more rapid expulsion.

Very little is known about variation in the host's resistance to Nb. Both inter- and intra-strain differences in the response of mice to Nb have been observed (4), but extensive investigation of this phenomenon has not thus far been attempted. Because failure to recognize such intra-specific variability in the host's responsiveness to a parasite can complicate the interpretation of experimental results, the resistance of four strains of mice to infection with Nb have been compared.

The intestinal worm burdens of infected outbred Swiss mice, maintained in this laboratory for parasite passage, have been compared with those seen in infected inbred $BDF_1$ mice and their two parental strains, the DBA/2 and C57BL/6. A mouse adapted strain of Nb (kindly supplied by Dr. Norman Reed, University of Montana) was used for experiments.

Comparison between the life cycle kinetics of outbred Swiss and inbred $BDF_1$ mice showed that the former strain is more susceptible to Nb infection (Fig. 1 and 2). Although the initial worm burden is not significantly larger in the Swiss mice, expulsion of the adult parasite is incomplete at

GENETIC CONTROL OF NATURAL RESISTANCE
TO INFECTION AND MALIGNANCY

83

Figure 1.

Figure 2.

Figure 3.

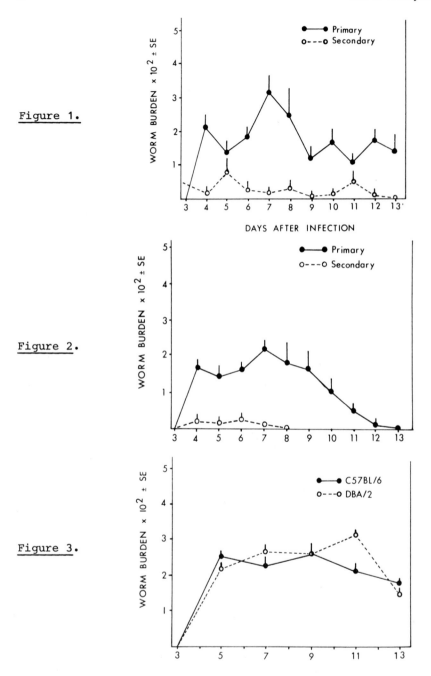

Intestinal worm burden in Swiss mice (Figure 1), $BDF_1$ mice (Figure 3) and C57BL/6 and DBA/2 mice (Figure 3).

the time when BDF$_1$ mice have completely erradicated the infection. The Swiss mice are also more susceptible to reinfection. Swiss mice show greater variations in worm numbers than do the inbred BDF$_1$ mice. An initial examination of the intestinal worm burdens of inbred DBA/2 and C57BL/6 mice showed that these strains lack the resistance to Nb apparent in the BDF$_1$ hybrid. As does the outbred Swiss mice strain, these inbred strains fail to expel a primary infection by day 13 post infection (Fig. 3).

The variations in levels of resistance to infection observed among the four strains of mice suggest that parasite-mediated modulation of the host's ability to respond immunologically to heterologous antigens could also vary with the mouse strain. An initial comparison of the splenic direct (IgM) plaque forming cell response (PFC) to the T-dependent antigen sheep red blood cells (SRBC) in Nb infected and normal Swiss and BDF$_1$ mice showed such variation (Table 1). Following an intraperitoneal injection of SRBC on various days after infection, both mouse strains showed first an enhancement and then a suppression of the PFC response. The kinetics differed however in that infected BDF$_1$ mice exhibited a prolonged enhancement of the response, while the infected Swiss mice showed a sustained suppression. Following a second infection, the PFC response of the BDF$_1$ mice remained suppressed (not shown) to less than 50% of the uninfected control.

Altered immune responsiveness was also observed in C57BL/6 and DBA/2 mice. Spleen cells from these mice, obtained at various days following Nb infection, were immunized *in vitro* against SRBC. Following a four day incubation, the cells were assayed for direct (IgM) PFC response and this was compared with the response of spleen cells from infected BDF$_1$ mice also immunized *in vitro*. The results show that alteration of the direct PFC response in these two strains following Nb infection resembles that seen in the BDF$_1$ hybrid (Table 1). An early enhancement of the response three days after infection is followed by a significant suppression comparable to that observed in BDF$_1$ mice.

Clearly, the parasite mediated modulation of an immune response to heterologous antigen is not directly related to the protective immune responses which result in worm expulsion. C57BL/6 and DBA/2 mice which fail to expel completely an initial Nb infection show similar alterations in ability to respond to SRBC as their F$_1$ hybrid which completely eliminates the primary infection.

A similar comparison can be made between outbred Swiss and inbred BDF$_1$ mice as discussed above. Swiss mice fail to expel their intestinal worm burdens show a pattern of alter-

Table 1.  DIRECT SPLENIC PLAQUE FORMING CELL RESPONSE

| Days After Infection (500 NbL3) | Direct Plaque Forming Cells per 1x10⁶ viable Spleen Cells ($\bar{X}$ ±SD of 3 mice) | | | | | | | | | |
| --- | --- | --- | --- | --- | --- | --- | --- | --- | --- | --- |
| | Swiss[a] | %C | BDF1[a] | %C | BDF1[b] | %C | C57BL/6[b] | %C | DBA/2[b] | %C |
| Day 3 | 561± 94 | 99 | ND[c] | | 1643+224 | 212 | 722+130 | 248 | 1460+ 87 | 209 |
| Control | 565± 141 | | | | 775+357 | | 291+ 96 | | 700+120 | |
| Day 5 | 1675+ 112 | 245 | 2555+509 | 180 | ND | | 351+ 60 | 143 | ND | |
| Control | 684+ 72 | | 1417+209 | | | | 245+ 76 | | | |
| Day 7 | 328+ 73 | 64 | 1494+ 96 | 200 | 852+261 | 246 | 642+ 71 | 266 | 861+200 | 123 |
| Control | 511+ 73 | | 747+ 34 | | 346+111 | | 241+ 43 | | 694+215 | |
| Day 11 | 75+ 41 | 10 | ND | | 48+ 10 | 23 | 515+ 56 | 103 | 584+ 57 | 115 |
| Control | 769+ 57 | | | | 208+ 38 | | 500+ 51 | | 507+ 56 | |
| Day 13 | ND | | 1572+108 | 309 | 106+ 7 | 45 | 445+139 | 46 | 190+ 24 | 54 |
| Control | | | 508+ 21 | | 237+100 | | 970+113 | | 350+ 98 | |
| Day 21 | 477+ 164 | 6 | 129+ 13 | 44 | 1358+338 | 94 | | | | |
| Control | 1436+ 107 | | 296+ 58 | | 1439+227 | | | | | |
| Day 28 | 605+ 80 | 6 | 287+ 92 | 43 | 1381+147 | 72 | | | | |
| Control | 1911+ 96 | | 664+147 | | 1925+196 | | | | | |
| Day 34 | 2158+ 239 | 108 | 1332+119 | 109 | 278+ 56 | 44 | | | | |
| Control | 1997+ 546 | | 1217+188 | | 636+108 | | | | | |
| Day 44 | 1279+ 86 | 147 | 817+ 92 | 58 | | | | | | |
| Control | 872+ 88 | | 1411+104 | | | | | | | |

a  Assayed 4 days after i.p. injection of 0.5 ml 4% SRBC.

b  Assayed after 4 days of in vitro culture with SRBC.

c  Not done.

ed immune responsiveness to SRBC which is similar to the
BDF$_1$ mice which do expel a primary infection. In this system, however, the kinetics differ as Swiss mice show a more
rapid onset of suppression.

The outcome of host-parasite relationships appears to
be the result of a balance between the host's immune response and parasite survival mechanisms. One of the most important factors is acquired immunity to parasite antigens.
Since the ability to respond immunologically to particular
antigens is under genetic control (2) immune mediated resistance to a parasite may be genetically determined and
account for variation between strains within a host species.
We have demonstrated such variation in resistance to Nb in
the results of the present study.

Resistance or susceptibility of a host strain to infection can be determined by the level at which such infections are initially established, or by the effectiveness of
subsequent host response. The results of this study show
that the four mouse strains examined permitted similar
levels of infection; variation was seen, however, in the
effectiveness of immune responses leading to worm expulsion.
The BDF$_1$ hybrid developed a greater degree of resistance to
the parasite than did the two parental strains or the outbred Swiss strain. Furthermore, C57BL/6 and DBA/2 animals
which differ in their H-2 histocompatibility haplotype, displayed a similar degree of resistance to Nb. This appears
to support the previous observation (3,6) that resistance or
susceptibility to infection is not determined solely by the
major histocompatibility complex, but is most probably under
polygenic control. The greater variation in worm burden and
less uniformity in worm expulsion seen with outbred Swiss
mice are consistent with results obtained using the Trichinella muris mouse model (7) and is a consequence of individual differences in immune responsiveness.

Studies of altered immune responsiveness to parasite
antigens is complicated by the extreme complexity of the
antigens themselves. While an examination of immune responses to heterologous antigens may be helpful, the significe-
ance of the altered host's response to SRBC in the outcome
of the host-parasite interrelationship is uncertain. Further study of this phenomenon is necessary in order to clar-
ify the poorly understood mechanisms involved in parasite-
mediated immunomodulation.

### REFERENCES

1.   Jones, V.E., and Ogilvie, B.M.  Im. 20:549, 1971.

2. McDevitt, H.O., and Benacerraf, B.   Adv.Im. <u>11</u>:31, 1969.

3. Mitchell, G.F., Hogarth-Scott, R.S., Edwards, R.D., Lewers, H.M., Cousins, G., and Moore, T.   Int.Arch.Al.-Appl.Im. <u>52</u>:64, 1976.

4. Ogilvie, B.M., and Jones, V.E.   Progr.Allergy <u>17</u>:93, 1973.

5. Suemura, M., and Ishizaka, K.   J.Im. <u>123</u>:918, 1979.

6. Tanner, C.E.   J.Parasit. <u>64</u>:956, 1978.

7. Wakelin, D.   Parasit. <u>71</u>:51, 1975.

8. Wescott, R.B., and Todd, A.C.   J.Parasit. <u>52</u>:233, 1966.

GENETIC CONTROL OF NATURAL RESISTANCE TO TRYPANOSOMA
RHODESIENSE IN MICE

Hellen C. Greenblatt[1], David L. Rosenstreich[2]
and Carter L. Diggs[1]

[1]Walter Reed Army Institute of Research
Washington, D.C.
[2]Albert Einstein College of Medicine
Bronx, N.Y.

Trypanosoma rhodesiense is an etiologic agent of
African sleeping sickness. This parasite, as well as other
related African trypanosomes (T. gambiense, T. brucei, T.
congolense), are extracellular protozoa predominantly confined to the blood and lymph within the mammalian host.
Natural infection occurs through the bite of the infected
tsetse fly.

The exact mechanisms by which the host resists this
class of organisms are not understood although antibodies
(3,15), perhaps in combination with components of the mononuclear phagocytic system (10 and Greenblatt et al. manuscript to be submitted), have been implicated.

Elimination of this parasite is complicated by several
evasion mechanisms possessed or initiated by the organism.
For example, African trypanosomes exhibit constant antigenic
variation (6) and can induce a profound state of host immunosuppression (1,9).

Cattle, sheep, pigs and goats exhibit considerable
variability to both natural and experimental trypanosome infections (7,14). In addition, several investigations of
murine intrastrain variation in response to African trypanosomiases have revealed genetic control of resistance to
diseases produced by T. brucei (4,5,11) and T. congolense
(12,13).

This report is an analysis of the genetic control of
resistance of mice to a causative agent of human sleeping
sickness, Trypanosoma rhodesiense.

MATERIALS AND METHODS

Animals. The inbred mouse strains listed in Table 1 were
obtained from the Jackson Laboratory, Bar Harbor, Maine.
CXB RI mice, and their progenitors BALB/cJBy and C57BL/6JBy,
were also obtained from this source. DBA/2f Mai mice were
purchased from Microbiological Associates, Bethesda, Md.
F1, F2, and backcross mice derived from BALB/cJ, DBA/2f Mai
or DBA/2J, and C57BL/6J were bred at this Institute. Mice

were infected at 3-5 months of age.

Trypanosoma rhodesiense. The EATRO No. 1886 (8) strain of
T. rhodesiense was used in these studies. (Infection of
mice with this parasite invariably results in death). The
stabilates utilized consisted of aliquots of a single clone
derived using the method of Campbell et al. (2). C57BL/6J
male mice were irradiated with 900R from a $^{137}$Cs source
immediately before an injection of a stabilate to generate
high numbers of parasites.

After 5d, mice were exsanguinated, their blood pooled
and centrifuged. Trypanosomes were gently aspirated from
the surface of the pellet to limit contamination with erythrocytes. The trypanosome suspension was diluted to the
proper concentration in RPM1 1640 (Flow Laboratories,
Rockville, MD) and held on ice until used. Mice were injected intraperitoneally, depending on the protocol with either
$10^4$ or $10^5$ live trypanosomes in a total of 0.1 ml RPM1 1640.
Nine days post-injection a daily mouse census was initiated.

## RESULTS

Thirteen inbred mouse strains were surveyed for their
susceptibility to T. rhodesiense by inoculating the mice
i.p. with $10^5$ parasites. The mean time of death ± the standard error of the mean for each strain was determined and is
listed on Table 1.

## Analysis of the genetic control of resistance to T. rhode-
siense of BALB/c x C57BL/6 progeny.

The pattern of a continuous spectrum of resistance
among inbred mouse strains suggested that resistance was under polygenic control. Mendelian analysis was performed to
further investigate the role of inheritance.

Highly susceptible BALB/c females were bred with the
more resistant C57BL/6 males and their F1 progeny tested for
their resistance to injection with $10^4$ T. rhodesiense organisms. Although greater than 99% of the F1 hybrids were "resistant" to the infection, there was a wide variation in
their survival times (Table 2). These progeny had a mean
survival time of 51.3 days (greater than that of either parent), but some of the mice succumbed to death at times in-
termediated between those obtained for the parental strains.
Others were strikingly more resistant than the C57BL/6 strains.

Although both male and female F1 progeny were resistant, there was significant (P < .001) difference in their
survival. F1 female mice survived 60.2d±2 (mean ± S.E.M.)
as compared with F1 male mice which survived 42.4d±1.5.

Table 1. Survival times of inbred mouse strains to infection with $10^5$ Trypanosoma rhodesiense[1]

| Mouse Strain | H-2 haplotype | Mean day of death ± S.E.M.[2] | Number of mice |
|---|---|---|---|
| C3H/HeJ | k | 13.8 ± 0.6 | 12 |
| CBA/J | k | 14.0 ± 1.5 | 12 |
| C3HeB/FeJ | k | 14.8 ± 0.7 | 12 |
| A/WySn | a | 15.2 ± 1.5 | 13 |
| C3H.SW/SN | b | 16.6 ± 0.4 | 12 |
| BALB/cJ | d | 17.3 ± 0.4 | 9 |
| DBA/1J | q | 17.5 ± 0.4 | 11 |
| DBA/2J | d | 19.4 ± 1.0 | 12 |
| C57L/J | b | 20.2 ± 3.0 | 16 |
| A/J | a | 20.8 ± 1.7 | 12 |
| SWR/J | q | 24.8 ± 1.5 | 12 |
| AKR/J | k | 28.3 ± 1.2 | 12 |
| C57BL/6J | b | 35.5 ± 3.8 | 12 |

[1] All mice except BALB/cJ were male and were injected on the same day. BALB/cJ females were tested at a later date.
[2] S.E.M. = standard error of the mean

Table 2. Resistance of parentals BALB/c and C57BL/6, and F1 hybrids to infections with T. rhodesiense[1].

| | Susceptible[2] | Resistant[3] | Mean Survival Time[4] | Range of Survival | No. of Mice |
|---|---|---|---|---|---|
| BALB/c (C) | 94.7 | | 19.4 ± 0.6 | 17–40d | 38 |
| C57BL/6 (B6) | | 96.8 | 45.0 ± 1.0 | 16–64d | 105 |
| F1 (C x B6) | | 99.4 | | | 156 |
| females | | | 60.2 ± 2.0 | 19–97d | 73 |
| males | | | 42.4 ± 1.5 | 25–70d | 83 |

[1] Compilation of data of several experiments of mice injected with $10^4$ T. rhodesiense.
[2] Percent of male and female mice dying on or before day 24.
[3] Percent of male and female mice surviving beyond day 24.
[4] Mean survival time (days) ± standard error of the mean.

The above data are consistent with the presence of two
resistance genes.   One that is autosomal and a second that
is X-linked.
     F1 progeny were backcrossed to each parental type, or
to each other, to produce respectively backcross and F2 progeny.   Each group was then infected with T. rhodesiense and
the survival times for individual mice were determined.   The
pooled data from several experiments are presented in Table
3.

Table 3.   Resistance of CxB6 F2 and backcross progeny to
           infection with T. rhodesiense[1]

| | Susceptible[2] | Resistant[3] | Mean Survival Time ± S.E.M.[4] | Range of Survival | No. of Mice |
|---|---|---|---|---|---|
| **Backcross** | | | | | |
| CxF1 | 64.4 | | | 15-96d | 104 |
| F1xC | 43.9 | | | 18-94d | 154 |
| B6xF1 | | 97.8 | | 22-72d | 95 |
| F1xB6 | | 98.1 | | 17-87d | 52 |
| F2 (F1 x F1) | 14.0 | 86.0 | | | 157 |
| females | | | 46.3 ± 1.9 | 20-93d | 80 |
| males | | | 38.8 ± 1.8 | 11-96d | 77 |

[1] Compilation of data of several experiments of mice injected
with $10^4$ T. rhodesiense.
[2] Percent of male and female mice dying on or before day 24.
[3] Percent of male and female mice surviving beyond day 24.
[4] Mean survival time (days) ± standard error of the mean.


     Backcross of F1 to the susceptible BALB/c parent resul-
ted in 44-64% of the progeny dying before day 24 whereas
backcrosses to the resistant C57BL/6 parent generated progeny of which greater than 97% survived beyond 24 days.
These data are consistent with a single codominant autosomal
gene that is a major determinant of survival.
     Analysis of the data obtained from the F2 generation
proved to be more complex.   Among F2 progeny derived from
matings of F1 (BALB/c x C57BL/6), only 22/157 (14%) could be
classified as susceptible.   This is substantially fewer than
the 25% predicted if only a single gene were involved.

## Analysis of the genetic control of resistance to T. rhodesiense infection of DBA/2 x C57BL/6 progeny

Further analyses were performed by crossing the resistant C57BL/6 male mice with different susceptible strain, DBA/2. When inoculated with $10^4$ parasites, DBA/2 mice had a mean survival time of 25.1d±0.9 (mean ± S.E.M.) as compared with 45.0d±1.0 of the more resistant C57BL/6 mice (Table 4).

Table 4. Resistance of hybrid progeny of DBA/2 and C57BL/6J mice to infection with **T. rhodesiense**[1]

| | Susceptible[2] | Resistant[3] | Mean Survival Time ± S.E.M.[4] | Range of Survival | No. of Mice |
|---|---|---|---|---|---|
| DBA/2 (D2) | 86.4 | | 25.1 ± 0.9 | 12–42d | 46 |
| C57BL/6J (B6) | | 96.8 | 45.0 ± 1.0 | 16–62d | 105 |
| F1 (D2 x B6) | | 96.1 | | 27–81d | 102 |
| females | | | 49.5 ± 1.2 | | 50 |
| males | | | 44.3 ± 1.4 | | 52 |
| F2 (F1 x F1) | 30.4 | 69.6 | | 20–73d | 79 |
| females | | | 48.1 ± 2.3 | | 35 |
| males | | | 39.0 ± 2.1 | | 44 |

[1] Compilation of several experiments of mice injected with $10^4$ **T. rhodesiense**.
[2] Percent of male and female mice dying on or before day 20.
[3] Percent of male and female mice surviving beyond day 30.
[4] Mean survival time (days) ± standard error of the mean.

The F1 progeny of crosses between DBA/2 and C57BL/6 mice were uniformly more resistant than the DBA/2 parent (Table 4), and as we found with the BALB/c x C57BL/6 F1 hybrids (Table 3), there was a widespread variation (27–81d) in survival times (Table 4). F1 (DBA/2 x C57BL/6) mice were bred to one another to obtain F2 mice which were infected with trypanosomes. Of this group, 30.4% were susceptible (Table 4), more than twice the percentage found when F1 (BALB/c x C57BL/6) were crossed with one another (Table 3).

DISCUSSION

As has been demonstrated in this study, the inheritance of resistance to Trypanosoma rhodesiense is complex. Inbred mouse strains exhibit a continuum of resistance ranging from high susceptibility to high resistance. Initial analysis of the data presented in this report suggests control of resistance by several genetic loci. Highly susceptible BALB/c mice appear to differ from highly resistant C57BL/6 mice in one dominant X-linked resistance gene and in at least two autosomal dominant or codominant resistance genes.

The DBA/2 strain appears to differ from the C57BL/6 strain at fewer resistance loci than do the BALB/c. F1 (DBA/2 x C57BL/6) progeny exhibited a continuous range of resistance, but the sex differences were not as striking as with the BALB/c x C57BL/6 F1 hybrids. Also, the percent of susceptible individuals in the F2 generation [F1 (DBA/2 x C57BL/6) x F1 (DBA/2xC57BL/6)], 30.4% was close to the expected 25% that would be obtained with a single autosomal gene. It is possible that the increased susceptibility of BALB/c mice is due to the presence of additional susceptibility alleles.

More precise genetic analyses will undoubtedly require resistance markers more sophisticated than survival. Recently, Morrison and Murray (12) found a similar complex pattern of inheritance of resistance in mice to another trypanosome, T. congolense. Their preliminary findings on the daily fluctuations in levels of parasitemia in parental strains and hybrid progeny suggest that this approach may prove useful.

The findings of this study are consistent with the hypothesis that resistance to T. rhodesiense in mice is controlled by several distinct gene loci. Further support for this conclusion is strengthened by observations (not detailed here), suggesting that in a group of recombinant inbred mouse strains derived from BALB/cByJ and C57BL/6By, CXB, several strains exhibited an intermediate pattern of resistance rather than being completely susceptible or resistant. Also, some strains are highly resistant (CXBH), and some highly susceptible (CXBD).

Examination of data derived from these RI lines as well as analyses of other existing groups of congenic mice should prove useful in delineating the inheritance of resistance to Trypanosoma rhodesiense.

REFERENCES

1. Albright, J.F., Albright, J.W., and Dusanic, D.G. J.Reticul.Soc. 21:31, 1977.
2. Campbell, G.H., Esser, K.M., Wellde, B.T., and Diggs, C.L. Am.J.Trop.Med.Hyg. 28:974, 1979.
3. Campbell, G.H., and Phillips, M. Infect.Immun. 14:-1144, 1976.
4. Clarkson, M.J. Parasitology 73:(prt 2)viii, 1976.
5. Clayton, C.E. Exp.Parasitol. 44:202, 1978.
6. Cross, G.A.M. Proc.R.Soc.Lond.B. 202:55, 1978.
7. Dargie, J.D., Murray, P.K., Murray, M., and McIntyre, W.I.M. Res.Vet.Sci. 26:245, 1979.
8. Duxbury, R.E., Sadun, E.H., and Anderson, J.S. Am.J.-Trop.Med.Hyg. 21:885, 1972.
9. Eardley, D.D., and Jayawardena, A.N. J.Immunol. 119:-1029, 1977.
10. Ferrante, A., and Jenkin, C.R. Cell.Immunol. 42:327, 1979.
11. Herbert, W.J., and Lumsden, W.H.R. Trans.Roy.Soc.Med.-Hyg. 61:140, 1967.
12. Morrison, W.I., and Murray, M. Exp.Parasitol. 48:364, 1979.
13. Morrison, W.I., Roelants, G.E., Mayor-Withey, K.S., and Murray, M. Clin.Exp.Immunol. 32:25, 1978.
14. Ormerod, W.E. Pharm.Ther. 6:1, 1979.
15. Takayanagi, T., and Enriquez, G.L. J.Parasitol. 59:-644, 1973.

# GENETIC CONTROL OF RESISTANCE TO PARASITIC INFECTIONS

Chairman's Summary

David L. Rosenstreich

Departments of Medicine, Microbiology
and Immunology
Albert Einstein College of Medicine
Bronx, New York, N.Y. 10461.

The organisms that fall under the general heading of mammalian parasites are complex and require multiple host defense mechanisms for their eradication. This complexity is due in part to their relatively large size and possession of multiple surface antigens. It also reflects their complex life cycles and the presence of morphologically and antigenically distinct stages within a single infected host. In addition, many of these organisms have evolved sophisticated mechanisms for evading host defenses, such as the antigenic variation of the African trypanosomes, or the profound state of immunosuppression induced by these and other protozoans.

This complexity virtually ensures that host resitance will be controlled by multiple genes. Nevertheless, a careful analysis of genetic control mechanisms is more important with this class of infection than with any other because it is the powerful tool of genetic analysis that will enable us to distinguish between primary and ancillary defense mechanisms. The current state of knowledge in this area has been concisely summarized in the excellent overviews by Bradley and Wakelin; accordingly it is intended to devote most of this report emphasizing the important points that emerged from the workshop discussions.

A major problem in this area is to develop strategies for analyzing systems that are under polygenic control. Most of the parasitic infections of mice fall into this category and this is especially true when one uses as an experimental parameter a late effect of infection, such as death. One approach to this problem lies in carefully analyzing the life history of the parasite in the host and the host defense mechanisms that are called into play. By dividing the infection into stages, it is possible to analyze the genetic control of individual segments that are more likely to be under the control of a single gene.

Such an approach is illustrated by the fine work of Bradley and his co-workers on L. donovani (this volume). By analyzing the distinctive parameter of early growth of the organism in the liver and spleen, they were able to define a single murine gene locus, Lsh, with a resistant and susceptible allele. By controlling variation in resistance induced by the Lsh locus, they then analyzed the genetic control of the late phase of the infection and could demonstrate that resistance in this phase was controlled by an H-2 linked gene. A similar analytic technique is illustrated by the studies on resistance of mice to T. spiralis (this volume) which identified several distinct types of resistance to this helminth; although these studies are only now emerging, this approach looks extremely promising. In contrast, analysis of genetic control of resistance to T. rhodesiense-induced lethality revealed a polygenic pattern of inheritance (this volume). Clearly, attaining an understanding of this type of infection will require a step-wise approach. In fact, recent studies by Morrison and Murray (Exp.Parasitl. 48:364, 1979) on a related organism, T. congolense, suggest that the initial number of parasites in the blood, and the ability to eliminate parasites for one or more cycles, might be controlled by distinct genes.

One of the major goals of genetic analysis is to identify the mechanism of gene action. Although we are far from identifying the biochemical effects of even a single resistance gene, work from several laboratories on resistance to L. tropica, suggests that progress in this area is taking place. Unlike most inbred mouse strains, Balb/c mice develop a progressive, non-healing cutaneous lesion after inoculation with L. tropica, that eventually visceralizes and produces death. Convincing evidence was presented by Howard that this suceptibility of Balb/c mice was due to the effect of a single, co-dominant, non-H-2 linked autosomal gene. Mice that carry the susceptibility allele of this gene develop high levels of leishmania-specific T suppressor cells. This suppression interfers with the host's ability to mount an effective cell-mediated immune response; consequently the organism grows unchecked. It is not clear whether the development of these T-suppressors is the primary defect, or whether they merely constitute a manifestation of the excessive growth of the organism due to some earlier defect. In fact the feeling was that the primary defect lies in the inability of the macrophage to control the early growth of the organism.

These findings are interesting for a number of reasons. One is that the suggestion of an initial failure of macrophage function is analogous to the defect postulated by Bradley for the Lsh locus, even though these genes are clearly distinct. Interestingly, a number of other resistance genes (i.e. Ity, Ric) are also thought to be expressed in macrophages. The development of suppressor cells in infected, susceptible hosts also appears to be a common mechanism, being reported at this workshop for Mycobacteria bovis BCG, Mycobacteria lepremurium as well as for a number of viruses. These findings suggest that many distinct resistance genes may well be expressed in a similar fasion.

The last point that bears emphasis concerns the relationship of genes that control natural resistance and responsiveness to therapeutic agents. Balb/c mice develop a progressive, and ultimately fatal infection after inoculation with L. mexicana, while C57BL/6 mice are much more resistant. Treatment with the antimonial, Glucantime, cures infected C57BL/6 mice whereas Balb/c mice carrying this infection do not respond to this chemotherapy. This observation is qualitatively similar to earlier work by Robson and Vas (J.Infect.Dis. 126:378, 1972) which indicated that susceptible mice could not be protected against S. typhimurium lethal infection by means of the usual types of vaccines that were protective for resistant strains. These findings suggest that therapeutic or preventive manouevers that prove to be only partially effective, as is the case with many parasitic infections, really need to be tailored to the genetic background of the host if their effectiveness is to be improved. In the long run, the contribution of genetic variation to responsiveness to therapy, not given a great deal of attention thus far, may prove to be much more relevant to these health problems than the attribute of innate resistance.

Given the complex nature of this class of organisms, it is encouraging that so much progress has been made. It is clear, however, that further progress in the near future will depend on the close cooperation of scientists from the relevant disciplines. Should these proceedings give rise to a workable interaction between parasitologists, immunologists and geneticists, this workshop will then have amply fulfilled its function.

DIFFERENTIAL SENSITIVITY OF INBRED MICE TO SALMONELLA
TYPHIMURIUM: A MODEL FOR GENETIC REGULATION OF INNATE
RESISTANCE TO BACTERIAL INFECTION

Alison D. O'Brien[1], David L. Rosenstreich[2],
Eleanor S. Metcalf[3], and Irwin Scher[4]
From the Departments of Microbiology[1,3] and Medicine[4]
Uniformed Services University of the Health Sciences
Bethesda, Maryland 20014
The Department of Medicine[2]
Albert Einstein College of Medicine
New York, New York 10046
and The Department of Immunology[4]
Naval Medical Research Institute
Bethesda, Maryland 20014.

Inbred strains of mice exhibit a dose-dependent susceptibility to the agent of murine typhoid, Salmonella typhimurium (12,13,27,30). For example, mice of certain strains
such as A/J (12,30) survive parenteral challenge with >$10^4$
bacteria, whereas other strains such as C57BL/6J (12,25,27,-
30) die after infection with fewer than 20 organisms. In
the 1930's, Webster demonstrated, by the selective breeding
of salmonella-susceptible and salmonella-resistant strains
from outbred strains, that this differential sensitivity was
genetically controlled (44). Recent studies have verified
these original observations and have extended the findings
by the indentification of three distinct genetic loci which
affect the course and outcome of murine typhoid. The first
salmonella-response gene described was Ity for immunity to
typhimurium (27,28). Two allelic forms of Ity are known.
Mice which are homozygous or heterozygous (F$_1$ mice) for the
dominant allele Ity$^r$ are resistant to S. typhimurium
whereas mice homozygous for the recessive allele Ity$^s$ are
susceptible to the bacterium (27). While the alleles of Ity
are broadly distributed among inbred strains of mice, the
two other salmonella response genes, Lps$^d$ and xid, are
mutant alleles and are expressed (susceptible) by only a few
strains of mice (24,25).

In this communication, two areas of investigation on
the genetic control of murine resistance to S. typhimurium
will be discussed. The genetic analysis which led to the
delineation of these three loci will be described. In addition, the available information on the mechanisms controlled by salmonella-response genes will be summarized. Finally, a comprehensive model that describes the mechanisms responsible for S. typhimurium reistance based on these genetic studies will be proposed.

GENETIC CONTROL OF NATURAL RESISTANCE
TO INFECTION AND MALIGNANCY

THE ITY LOCUS:    A CHROMOSOME 1 GENE WHICH INFLUENCES THE
INITIAL REPLICATION OF S. TYPHIMURIUM IN THE SPLEEN AND
LIVER.

Previous studies by Robson and Vas (30) and Plant and
Glynn (27) suggested that inbred strains of mice could be
classified as either innately resistant or susceptible to
S. typhimurium by a calculation of the 50 percent lethal
dose ($LD_{50}$) of the bacterium for various strains. Similar
studies were reported by Hormaeche (12). A summary of the
findings of these investigators and some observations from
this laboratory is shown in Table 1. It should be noted
that the salmonella-susceptible and salmonella-resistant
phenotypes of mice listed in Table 1 were determined from
the $LD_{50}$ of S. typhimurium following parenteral (i.v., s.c.,
i.p.) infection. Since the natural route of acquisition of
the organism is by ingestion, the assessment of salmonella-
sensitivity by parenteral challenge has been criticized (8).
However, our findings and those of other researchers (30)
indicate that the relative susceptibility of murine strains
to salmonellae is similar, regardless of the inoculation
route.

Plant and Glynn identified a non-H-2 linked gene, which
they subsequently designated Ity (28), that governs the resistance of CBA mice and $F_1$ and backcross mice derived from
matings of CBA and S. typhimurium-susceptible BALB/c animals
(27). Recently, these investigators mapped the Ity locus to
Chromosome 1 by an analysis of the linkage between specific
phenotypic markers and salmonella resistance in hybrid murine populations (29). Results from this laboratory on the
salmonella-susceptibility of over 30 recombinant inbred strains of mice derived from $Ity^r$ and $Ity^s$ progenitor strains have confirmed the Chromosome 1 location of Ity
(O'Brien, A.D., D.L. Rosenstreich, and B.A. Taylor; manuscript submitted for publication).

It is not as yet clear how Ity regulates the murine response to S. typhimurium infection. Although Plant and
Glynn suggested a correlation between the extent of the delayed hypersensitivity footpad response to an extract of
salmonellae and the degree of resistance to the bacterium
(27), Hormaeche found no relationship between innate resistance and footpad reactivity (12). However, we have observed, as have Plant and Glynn (27), Robson and Vas (30), and
Hormaeche (12), that $Ity^s$ mice are unable to contain the
early net multiplication of salmonellae in either their spleens or livers, and, as a consequence, these animals usually
die early (< 10 days) after infection. This suggests that
Ity may affect the initial uptake or subsequent killing of

Table 1.    Response to various inbred strains of mice to S. typhimurium infection.

| STRAIN | REFERENCE |
|---|---|
| Salmonella-resistant[a] | |
| C3H/He | 30 |
| C3H/HeN | 24 |
| C3H/St | 24 |
| C3H/Bi | 24 |
| CBA | 12, 27 |
| CBA/Ca | 25 |
| BRVR | 44, Personal Obs. |
| A/J | 12, 30 |
| A/HeN | Personal Obs. |
| SWR/J | Personal Obs. |
| DBA/2[c] | 12, 25, 27, 30 |
| C57/L[c] | 29, Personal Obs. |
| Salmonella-susceptible[b] | |
| BSVS | 44, Personal Obs. |
| DBA/1 | 30 |
| BALB/c | 12, 25, 27, 30 |
| C57BL/6 | 12, 25, 27, 30 |
| B10.D2 | 12, 30 |
| C3H/HeJ | 24, 30 |
| CBA/N | 25 |

a   Resistant = $LD_{50} > 1 \times 10^3$ s.c., i.v., or i.p.
b   Susceptible = $LD_{50} < 2 \times 10^1$ s.c., i.v., or i.p.
c   These mice are resistant when infected s.c. but respond intermediately when challenged i.p.

this facultative intracellular bacterium by splenic and hepatic macrophages.  Presently, there is no direct proof that a macrophage deficit is responsible for the salmonella sus-

ceptibility of Ity$^S$ mice.  Nonetheless, two lines of indirect evidence support the hypothesis.  First, Maier and
Oels demonstrated that macrophages from S. typhimurium resistant inbred BRVR mice kill salmonellae better than do
macrophages from S. typhimurium sensitive inbred BSVS animals (18).  Since the replication of salmonellae in either
the spleens or livers of these mice has not, to our knowledge, been examined, one can only presume that BRVR and
BSVS are Ity$^r$ and Ity$^S$ mice, respectively.  In support
of such an assumption is the observation from this laboratory that F$_1$ hybrids from BSVS and C57BL/6J [Ity$^S$ (28)]
parents are salmonella-susceptible (unpublished result).
Furthermore, unrestriced initial net multiplication of S.
typhimurium is observed in the spleens of salmonella-resistant mice that have been pretreated with the macrophage-toxic
agent, silica (26).  Since such treatment also converts these mice to a salmonella-susceptible phenotype, it appears
that macrophages must control bacterial growth early in the
infectious process if the animals are to survive.

## THE Lps$^d$ LOCUS:  A CHROMOSOME 4 ALLELE WHICH RENDERS MICE ENDOTOXIN-UNRESPONSIVE AND SALMONELLA-SUSCEPTIBLE

The murine response to lipopolysaccharide (LPS) is controlled by the Chromosome 4 locus, Lps (43).  Two alleles at
this locus have been described.  The Lps$^n$ allele which is
expressed by most inbred strains of mice renders them sensitive to the biological effects of endotoxin.  In contrast,
some inbred strains such as C3H/HeJ and C57BL/10/ScCr carry
the mutant allele Lps$^d$ which results in a poor response to
LPS (19,43).  For example, C3H/HeJ mice are abnormally refractory to such LPS-induced effects as lethality (41), mit-
ogenicity (42), polyclonal antibody formation (40), and non-
specific resistance to infection (6).  In vitro studies have
demonstrated that the Lps$^d$ phenotype is expressed by a
variety of cell types which include T cells (16,20), B cells
(10), fibroblasts (35), and macrophages (31,34).

Two apparently contradictory reports in the literature
prompted us to examine the possibility that the Lps$^d$ allele might affect the murine response to salmonellosis.
Plant and Glynn observed that C3H/He mice were salmonella-
resistant (27) while Robson and Vas had found that C3H/HeJ
mice were sensitive to murine typhoid (30).  Since all C3H/
He mice examined to date except C3H/HeJ mice are LPS responsive (9), we speculated that the discrepancy between the observations of these two groups of investigators might reflect differences in the LPS phenotypes of the animals.
Therefore, we performed a series of genetic analyses to de-

termine whether Lps[d] influences murine resistance to S. typhimurium (24). First, we determined the $LD_{50}$ of the bacterium for various C3H substrains. We found that of the genetically related animals tested (C3H/HeN, C3H/Bi, C3H/St, C3H/HeDub, and C3H/HeJ), only C3H/HeJ were S. typhimurium-susceptible ($LD_{50} < 2$); All the other strains were resistant ($LD_{50} > 2 \times 10^3$). Furthermore, C3H/HeJ mice were unable to contain the initial net multiplication of salmonellae in their spleens, whereas C3H/St mice did control splenic replication of the bacteria.

To determine whether the C3H/HeJ response to S. typhimurium could reflect the expresion of Ity[s], we tested the sensitivity of hybrid mice to the organism. We reasoned that if C3H/HeJ mice are of the Ity[s] genotype, $F_1$ progeny from crosses of C3H/HeJ with the Ity[s], S. typhimurium-susceptible C57BL/6J strain should also be sensitive to the bacterium. Since (C3H/HeJ X C57BL/6J)$F_1$ mice were S. typhimurium resistant ($LD_{50} > 8 \times 10^3$) it appeared that gene complementation had occurred. Thus, the C3H/HeJ and C57BL/6J susceptibility genes must be distinct. Moreover, C3H/HeJ susceptibility is not X-linked, since both (C3H/HeJ X C3H/HeN) $F_1$ male and female mice were resistant to murine typhoid ($LD_{50} > 8 \times 10^3$).

The elimination of the influence of either Ity[s] or X-linked genes (notably xid) on the salmonella-susceptibility of C3H/HeJ mice indicated that another gene(s) was responsible for bacterial sensitivity. To determine if the Lps[d] gene was in fact influencing the response of C3H/HeJ mice to murine typhoid, a backcross linkage analysis was performed with the progeny obtained from crosses of C3H/HeJ and (C3H/HeJ X C57BL/6J)$F_1$ mice. These studies revealed a close correlation between the phenotypic expression of Lps[d], as measured by the low proliferative response of peritoneal B cells to LPS, and salmonella sensitivity since 13/14 LPS-unresponsive mice died whereas only 2/13 LPS-responsive animals succumbed to the infection. These observations suggested that Lps[d] and a salmonella-sensitivity gene were either linked or identical. The chromosomal location of this salmonella-sensitivity gene was confirmed by its association with another Chromosome 4 locus, Mup-1[a] (43). Based on these findings, our working hypothesis is that the C3H/HeJ susceptibility gene and Lps[d] are identical. Further studies may, however, reveal that the two loci are distinct.

The mechanism by which Lps[d] confers S. typhimurium susceptibility on C3H/HeJ mice is not known, but the rapid initial net splenic multiplication of the bacterium (24) after low dose challenge (50 organisms) resembles the phenotype of $Ity^S$ mice. Moreover, other aspects of the response of $Ity^S$ and $Lps^d$ are also similar. For example, we found that C3H/HeJ mice cannot be protected from otherwise lethal infection by standard vaccines, but protection is possible if they are lethally irradiated and reconstituted with syngeneic C3H/HeN ($Lps^n$) bone marrow (O'Brien, A.D., and D.L. Rosenstreich; manuscript in preparation). Similarly, C57BL/6J mice cannot be protected by vaccination (22,30), and Hormaeche showed that the phenotype of $Ity^S$ mice (early net splenic replication of $S$. typhimurium) can be altered by adoptive transfer of $Ity^r$ bone marrow cells (14). Nevertheless, differences between the expression of $Ity^S$ and $Lps^d$ must exist, since gene complementation occurs when C57BL/6J and C3H/HeJ mice are crossed (24). If one assumes that the inability of mice to contain bacterial growth in RES organs reflects a macrophage dysfunction, then one must also presume that the macrophage defects of $Ity^S$ and $Lps^d$ mice differ. This corollary is supported indirectly by the observation that $Lps^d$ macrophages, unlike $Ity^S$ macrophages, are poorly tumoricidal in vitro and cannot be stimulated by the lymphokine MIF (34). A comparison of the capacity of $Lps^d$ and $Ity^S$ macrophages to phagocytize and kill salmonellae is in progress.

## THE XID LOCUS: AN X-LINKED GENE WHICH ALTERS B-CELL FUNCTIONS AND RENDERS CBA/N MICE SALMONELLA-SUSCEPTIBLE

The X-linked recessive allele xid (for X-linked immunodeficiency) confers a B lymphocyte functional defect on CBA-/N mice and $F_1$ male mice obtained from crosses of CBA/N females with immunologically normal male mice of another inbred strain (1,2,38). Thus, (CBA/N X DBA/2N) $F_1$ male mice are immune-defective but (CBA/N X DBA/2N) $F_1$ female mice and (DBA/2N X CBA/N) $F_1$ male and female animals appear to be immunologically normal. Some of the B-lymphocyte dysfunctions of xid mice include poor or absent antibody responses to certain T-independent and T-dependent antigens (1,15,36-38), defective splenic proliferative responses to some B-cell mitogens(36), increased susceptibility to in vitro tolerance induction (21,23), and low levels of serum IgM (1). In contrast to many of the B-cell functions of these animals, most of their T-cell activities are not impaired. Thus, xid mice reject grafts and their splenic lymphocytes respond to concanavalin A and mediate T-cell cellular cytotoxicity reactions as well as control mice (36). In general, the T-cell helper functions of these mice also appear to be normal (15), although two recent reports suggest that T-cell help is suboptimal for certain responses [LPS-induced polyclonal antibody formation (11) and phosphorylcholine T-15 antibody response (4)]. In addition, CBA/N macrophages respond normally to endotoxin (32).

We have examined the effect of the xid-conferred B-cell defect on the susceptibility of CBA/N mice to murine typhoid (25). The $LD_{50}$ of S. typhimurium was 10 for CBA/N mice but $1 \times 10^4$ for the immunologically normal, genetically related, CBA/CaHN strain, which suggested that expression of xid might render mice salmonella-sensitive. Further genetic analyses confirmed this supposition. First, in lethal dose studies with crosses of CBA/N mice and DBA/2N or BALB/c mice, only immune-defective $F_1$ male mice were highly susceptible to murine typhoid ($LD_{50} < 10$); immunologically normal $F_1$ female littermates and reciprocal $F_1$ male mice were salmonella-resistant ($LD_{50} > 5 \times 10^3$). Secondly, linkage analyses revealed a close association between expression of xid (low serum IgM levels) and susceptibility to salmonellosis among backcross and $F_2$ mice derived from CBA/N parents; 93% (52/53) of xid mice died compared to a 44% incidence of death (22/50) among backcross and $F_2$ mice with normal serum IgM levels.

Recently, we investigated the mechanism of xid-conferred salmonella sensitivity (O'Brien, A.D., I. Scher, and E.S. Metcalf; manuscript in preparation). We first compared the mean time to death (MTD) of xid mice of $Ity^s$ mice and of $Lps^{d}$ mice after intraperitoneal inoculation with 10 $LD_{50}$ s of S. typhimurium. While the MTD for xid mice was 16 days, the MTD for $Ity^s$ and $Lps^d$ mice was 7 and 6 days, respectively. Thus, in contrast to $Ity^s$ and $Lps^d$ mice, xid mice die late in the course of the infection. The survival of xid animals early in salmonellosis reflects the ability of their spleens to contain initial bacterial replication. By day 7 after i.p. infection with 50 bacteria, the geometric mean number of S. typhimurium per spleen of (CBA/N X DBA/2N) $F_1$ male mice was $2 \times 10^4$. In contrast, the geometric mean number of organisms per spleen of BALB/c ($Ity^s$) mice was $2 \times 10^6$. Taken together, these results indicate that at least two mechanisms of resistance to murine typhoid are operative, an early phase which is presumably macrophage-dependent, and a late phase for which xid mice are defective.

We next examined the nature of the xid-conferred defect in the late phase of innate resistance to S. typhimurium. We considered the possibility that expression of xid might affect T-cell dependent cell-mediated immunity to S. typhimurium, since such a mechanism has been proposed as the means by which outbred mice acquire immunologically specific resistance to murine typhoid (3,7). A T-cell dependent immune mechanism is also essential in murine resistance to another facultative intracellular bacterium, Listeria mono-cytogenes (17). The possibility of an xid-controlled gener-alized defect in cell-mediated immunity was eliminated by our previous observation that B-cell-defective (CBA/N X BALB/c) $F_1$ male mice were as resistant as immunologically normal $F_1$ female littermates to L. monocytogenes (25). How-ever, it is still conceivable that an S. typhimurium-specific defect in cell mediated immunity could be respon-sible for the salmonella sensitivity of xid mice. Current-ly, we are testing this hypothesis by a determination of the delayed hypersensitivity-footpad responsiveness of salmo-nella-sensitized xid mice and control mice to an extract of the organism.

Another explanation for the late deaths of salmonella-infected xid mice could be a deficient antibody response to the bacterium. Indeed, xid mice have well documented abnor-malities in their antibody responses to certain antigens (1,15,36-38), and some investigators have proposed a role for antibody in resistance to murine typhoid (33). There-fore, we measured the anti-S. typhimurium IgG titers of sera from (CBA/N X DBA/2N) $F_1$ male and female mice immunized with a killed preparation of the bacterium. Killed rather than live bacteria were used to elicit antibody because most xid mice fail to survive even low doses of the live organism for more than 3 weeks. Antibody titers were quantitated by a solid-phase radioimmunoassay (Metcalf, E.S., and A.D. O'Brien; manuscript in preparation). We found that the anti-Salmonella mean IgG titers of $F_1$ female sera were 64-fold and 40-fold higher than titers of $F_1$ male sera by 3 and 4 weeks after immunization, respectively. That such reduced antibody titers might affect salmonella sensitivity was sug-gested by the marked increase in salmonella resistance of $F_1$ male mice when given $F_1$ female serum or a gamma globulin portion of the serum before challenge. Moreover, the pro-tective substance in $F_1$ female serum was removed by adsorp-tion with the bacterium. The resistance of $F_1$ male mice to murine typhoid was also significantly increased by adoptive transfer of immunologically normal $F_1$ male bone marrow cells. These data support the hypothesis that the salmo-nella susceptibility of xid mice is a consequence of a delayed and diminished antibody response to the bacterium.

A MODEL FOR GENETIC CONTROL OF INNATE RESISTANCE OF MURINE TYPHOID: EFFECT OF SIMULTANEOUS EXPRESSION OF SALMONELLA-RESPONSE GENES ON SURVIVAL OF THE HOST

From the studies reviewed in this report, it is clear

that the final outcome of infection with <u>S. typhimurium</u>, i.e. death or survival, depends not only on the dose, route of challenge, and virulence of the salmonella strain, but also on the genotype of the murine host. Although each of the distinct salmonella response genes was discussed individually, it is important to emphasize that resistance or susceptibility to murine typhoid is a reflection of the simultaneous expression of alleles at these loci.

## A MODEL FOR THE GENETIC REGULATION OF THE
## MURINE RESPONSE TO <u>S. typhimurium</u>

**<u>Salmonella</u> phagocytized by
hepatic and splenic macrophages**

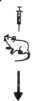

**Control of early replication (<u>Ity, Lps</u>)**

**Control of antibody formation and
late replication (<u>xid</u>)**

<u>Fig. 1.</u> A model for genetic control of innate resistance to murine typhoid.

The model depicted in Fig. 1 is our view of how each of these genes affects natural immunity to murine typhoid. In this model, the infectious process is divided into two phases, early (< 10 days) and late (> 10 days). The first requirement for expression of resistance is the capacity of the murine RES organs to restrict bacterial multiplication; $Ity^s$ and $Lps^d$ mice, which cannot contain the net multiplication of salmonellae, die at an early stage. Interestingly, this requisite for murine survival applies not only to S. typhimurium but also to the parasite Leishmania donovani. Indeed, we have found that the Lsh gene which controls the replication of L. donovani in the RES (5) is closely linked to the Ity locus (O'Brien, A.D., D.L. Rosenstreich, and B.A. Taylor; manuscript submitted for publication).

Mice which survive the first, apparently immunologically non-specific phase of salmonellosis ($Ity^r/Lps^n$ phenotype) must then combat the infection by immunologically specific means. We believe, as shown in Fig. 1, that at least one of the immunologically specific, late stage resistance mechanisms is antibody dependent. In support of this theory is the failure of salmonella-antibody-defective xid mice to survive this phase of murine typhoid. It seems probable that a T-cell dependent cell-mediated immune mechanism is also operative at this stage in innately salmonella-resistant mice.

The model which we have proposed was formulated from our current knowledge of the salmonella response genes and their mechanisms of action. However, there may be other, as yet undefined genes, which also influence salmonella susceptibility . The identification of additional loci may necessitate revision of this simple model. Nevertheless, this model is a logical framework on which to base further studies.

ACKNOWLEDGEMENTS

     This work was supported by the Uniformed Services University of the Health Sciences Research Protocols No. RO7313 and CO7305 and by the Naval Medical Research Development Command, Work Unit. No. M0095-PN.001-1030. The opinions and assertions contained herein are the private ones of the authors and are not to be construed as official or reflecting the views of the Navy Department or the naval service at large. The experiments reported herein were conducted according to the principles set forth in the "Guide for the Care and Use of Laboratory Animals", Institute of Laboratory Resources, National Research Council, Department of Health, Education, and Welfare, Pub. No (NIH) 78-23.

## REFERENCES

1. Ambaugh, D.F., Hansen, C.T., Prescott, B., Stashak, P.W., Bartold, D.R., and Baker, P. J.Exp.Med. 136:931, 1972.
2. Berning, A., Eicher, E., Paul, W.E., and Scher, I. Fed.Proc. 37:1396, 1978.
3. Blanden, R.V., Mackaness, G.B., and Collins, F.M. J.Exp.Med. 124:585, 1966.
4. Bottomly, K., and Mosier, D.E. J.Exp.Med. 150:1399, 1979.
5. Bradley, D., Taylor, B.A., Blackwell, J., Evans, E.P., and Freeman, J. Clin.Exp.Immunol. 37:7, 1979.
6. Chedid, L., Parant, M., Damais, C., Parant, F., Suy, D. and Galelli, A. Infect.Immun. 13:722, 1976.
7. Collins, F.M. Bact.Rev. 38:371, 1974.
8. Collins, F.M., and Carter, P.B. Infect.Immun. 6:451, 1972.
9. Glode, L.M., and Rosenstreich, D.L. J.Immunol. 117:2061, 1976.
10. Glode, M.S., Scher, I., Osborne, B., and Rosenstreich, D.L. J.Immunol. 116:454, 1976.
11. Goodman, M.G., and Weigle, W.O. J.Immunol. 123:2484, 1979.
12. Hormaeche, C.E. Immunology 37:311, 1979.
13. Hormaeche, C.E. Immunology 37:319, 1979.
14. Hormaeche, C.E. Immunology 37:329, 1979.
15. Janeway, C.A., and Barthold, D.R. J.Immunol. 115:898, 1975.
16. Koenig, S., Hoffman, M.K., and Thomas, L. J.Immunol. 118:1910, 1977.
17. Lane, F.C., and Unanue, E.R. J.Exp.Med. 135:1104, 1972.
18. Maier, I., and Oels, H.C. Infect.Immun. 6:438, 1972.
19. McAdam, J.P.W.J., and Ryan, J.L. J.Immunol. 120:249, 1978.
20. McGhee, J.R., Farrar, J.J., Michalek, S.M., Mergenhagen, S.E., and Rosenstreich, D.L. J.Exp.Med. 149:793, 1979.
21. McKearn, J.P., and Quintans, J. J.Immunol. 124:77, 1980.
22. Medina, S., Vas, S.J., and Robson, H.G. J. Immunol. 114:1720, 1975.
23. Metcalf, E.S., Scher, I., and Klinman, N.R. J.Exp.Med. 151:486, 1980.
24. O'Brien, A.D., Rosenstreich, D.L., Scher, I., Campbell, G.H., MacDermott, R.P., and Formal, S.B. J.Immunol. 124:20, 1980.

25. O'Brien, A.D., Scher, I., Campbell, G.H., MacDermott, R.P., and Formal, S.B. J.Immunol. <u>123</u>:720, 1979.
26. O'Brien, A.D., Scher, I., and Formal, S.B. Infect.Immun. <u>25</u>:513, 1979.
27. Plant, J., and Glynn, A.A. J.Infect.Dis. <u>133</u>:72, 1976.
28. Plant, J., and Glynn, A.A. In Mouse New Letter, Jackson Laboratory, Bar Harbor, Maine <u>57</u>:38, 1977.
29. Plant, J., and Glynn, A.A. Clin.Exp.Immunol. <u>37</u>:1, 1979.
30. Robson, G.G., and Vas, S.J. J.Infect.Dis. <u>126</u>:378, 1972.
31. Rosenstreich, D.L., Vogel, S.N., Jacques, A.R., Wahl, L.M., and Oppenheim, J.J. J.Immunol. <u>121</u>:1664, 1978.
32. Rosenstreich, D.L., Vogel, S.N., Jacques, A., Wahl, L.M., Sher, I., and Mergenhagen, S.E. J.Immunol. <u>1212</u>:685, 1978.
33. Rowley, D., Turner, K.J., and Jenkin, C.R. Aust.J.Exp. Biol.Med.Sci. <u>42</u>:237, 1964.
34. Ruco, J.L., and Meltzer, M.S. J.Immunol. <u>120</u>:329, 1978.
35. Ryan, J.L., and McAdam, K.P.W.J. Nature <u>269</u>:153, 1977.
36. Scher, I., Ahmed, A., Strong, D.M., Steinburg, A.D., and Paul, W.E. J.Exp.Med. <u>141</u>:788, 1975.
37. Scher, I., Berning, A.K., and Asofsky, R. J.Immunol. <u>123</u>: 477, 1979.
38. Scher, I., Franz, M.M., and Steinburg, A.D. J.Immunol. <u>110</u>:1396, 1973.
39. Scher, I., Steinburg, A.D., Berning, A.K., and Paul, W.E. J.Exp.Med. <u>142</u>:637, 1975.
40. Skidmore, B.J., Chiller, J.M., Morrison, D.C., and Weigle, W.O. J.Immunol. <u>114</u>:770, 1975.
41. Sultzer, B.M. Nature (Lond) <u>219</u>:1253, 1968.
42. Sultzer, B.M., and Nilsson, B.S. Nature (Lond) New Biol. <u>240</u>:198, 1972.
43. Watson, J., Kelly, K., Largen, M., and Taylor, B.A. J.Immunol. <u>120</u>:422, 1978.
44. Webster, L.T. J.Exp.Med. <u>57</u>:793, 1933.

## DISCUSSION

<u>Hormaeche</u>: What happens in these experiments when O'Brien administers the Salmonella intravenously? Or are all these data derived from experiments based on i.p. route of infection?

<u>O'Brien</u>: The LPS response gene data have been affirmed by

oral challenge, i.v. challenge, and subcutaneous challenge. The C3H/HeJ mice were susceptible in all instances. The xid gene data was also examined and confirmed by intravenous challenge.

Plant:  We have also confirmed our Ity findings by giving Salmonella orally, and the results correlate very well with the intravenous route.  Intraperitoneally, we get some discrepancy and I think this is peculiar to DBA/2 and C3H strains, possibly because in these mice, other genes also play a part in the resistance to infection.

Ruco:  I was wondering if O'Brien noticed any changes in inflammatory reaction following Salmonella infection in C3H/HeN and C3H/HeJ mice involving cells other than macrophages.

O'Brien:  This was not done.  My suspicion, based on some unpublished observations, is that the C3H/HeJ mice make a poor inflammatory response to Salmonella compared to C3H/HeN controls.

Collins:  With regard to the LPS-sensitive and resistant mouse strains:  Do they show a difference as regards the $LD_{50}$ dose for purified LPS?  Is there a difference in their susceptibility to heat-killed Salmonella typhimurium, which of course might be attributable to complexed LPS?  Does this correlate with the $LD_{50}$ data that O'Brien has for the viable organisms?

O'Brien:  It does, somewhat, in a reciprocal manner.  The C3H/HeJ strain is highly resistant to the lethal effects of endotoxin. The other strains are pretty much equal in their LPS sensitivity, although i have not done the experiment.  I have not taken other C3H substrains and challenged them with phenol-water LPS extracts to ascertain mortality data.  But my understanding is, at least in terms of toxicity of LPS for macrophages (not exactly the same thing), that they are rather similar in their response.

Collins:  I would just expect, since one has a 1000-to-10,000-fold difference in the lethal effects of the challenge, that there would be a very substantial difference in the $LD_{50}$ for the LPS itself, or for the heat-killed organisms.

O'Brien:  There is a substantial difference, but it is the reverse of what one would expect.  In other words, the mice apparently are not dying of LPS toxicity, as they are instead refractory to the effect of LPS.

Collins:   How can you explain that?

O'Brien:   I can only offer a theory, based on absolutely no
facts at all.  It goes this way - during the interaction of
a Gram-negative organism with a macrophage, for example,
something on the cell surface of that macrophage, not necessarily a receptor really, is required for uptake of that
organism by the macrophage.  Certainly, there is evidence
with C3H/HeJ mice and purified endotoxin, that the macrophages are not triggered by endotoxin;  they do not really
perceive it as a normal animal would.  So, if one could
envision that the LPS gene is coding for some kind of a receptor and that the C3H/HeJ animals are missing that recept-
or on a lot of cell types, that they fail to perceive the
bacterium in the usual fashion, i.e., do not take it up
properly;  but they also do not see LPS and consequently are
not triggered to release their pharmacologically active substances which may well be responsible for endotoxin action.
As you see - all theory, no facts.

Bennett:   Has O'Brien tested her hypothesis about C3H/HeJ
macrophages by doing cell transfer experiments between
genetically-resistant and susceptible animals?

O'Brien:   Yes we surely have.  We have not done it with the
Ity-s/Ity-r combination.  Hormaeche has, and has been able
to transfer a change in the early net multiplication, by BM
cell reconstitution of lethally irradiated animals.   We
have done BM transfer, spleen cell transfer, peritoneal cell
transfer, between C3H/HeJ and C3H/HeN mice, and between
(CBA/N x DBA/2N) $F_1$ males and $F_1$ females.  To sum it up, one
can make a C3H/HeJ mouse Salmonella-resistant if one transplants BM from a C3H/HeN mouse;  but this will not go with
spleen cells or peritoneal cells.  You can make a xid male
mouse Salmonella-resistant, i.e., you can increase the resistance, by giving it $F_1$ female BM.  This involves complete
reconstitution if one is to change the resistance to Salmonella.  Though one can give the C3H/HeJ mouse spleen cells
and make it respond to the mitogenic stimulus of LPS, that
does not make it Salmonella-resistant.  This also holds for
CBA/N mice.

THE C3HeB/FeJ MOUSE, A STRAIN IN THE C3H LINEAGE WHICH
SEPARATES SALMONELLA SUSCEPTIBILITY AND IMMUNIZABILITY FROM
MITOGENIC RESPONSIVENESS TO LIPOPOLYSACCHARIDE

Toby K. Eisenstein,[1] Lynn W. Deakins,[1]
and Barnet M. Sultzer[2]

[1] Department of Microbiology and Immunology
Temple University School of Medicine
Philadelphia, Pennsylvania 19140
and
[2] Department of Microbiology and Immunology
State University of New York
Downstate Medical Center
Brooklyn, New York 11203

It has been recognized since the 1930's that susceptibility to Salmonella infection in mice is under genetic control (4,12). Recent studies show that three separate loci
control Salmonella resistance (5) although none is H-2 linked (9). Studies on mice in the C3H lineage have identified
a locus on chromosome 4 which determines Salmonella susceptibility in the C3H/HeJ mouse (5). It has been mapped to a
locus closely linked or identical to the Lps gene (7,10)
which controls responsiveness to a variety of bioloical
effects of lipopolysaccharides (LPS) of gram-negative
bacteria (5). Although C3H/HeJ mice are Salmonella susceptible, they are resistant to the toxic effects of lipopolysaccharide and carry the Lps$^d$ allele. Other mice in the
C3H lineage, such as the C3H/HeN, C3H/St, and the C3H.Bi,
have been found to be Salmonella resistant, but LPS sensitive (5). Breeding experiments by these investigators suggested a genetically controlled relationship in which Salmonella susceptibility segregated with the Lps$^d$ allele in
mice of the C3H lineage. As part of our studies on susceptibility and immunity to murine salmonellosis in C3H/HeJ
mice, we used C3HeB/FeJ mice as positive controls, since
these animals have been reported to give normal mitogenic
and immune responses to lipopolysaccharide (11). In the
course of these studies we found that the C3HeB/FeJ mouse is
Salmonella susceptible, but endotoxin sensitive, thus providing at least one example of a strain in the C3H lineage
where the Salmonella-susceptible phenotype is not associated
with LPS-nonresponsiveness (Lps$^d$). Vaccination studies
also showed that these mice are poorly protected by lipopolysaccharide vaccines.

For these studies C3H/HeJ and C3HeB/FeJ mice were purchased from Jackson Laboratories, Bar Harbor, Maine. C3H

Copyright © 1980 by Academic Press, Inc.
All rights of reproduction in any form reserved.
ISBN 0-12-647680-2

and CD-1 mice were purchased from Charles River Breeding
Laboratories, Wilmington, Mass. (C3H mice were derived by
the breeder from C3H/HeN mice which are maintained at NIH).
All animals, unless specified, were females weighing 19-21
g. For any given experiment, all animals were received in
the same shipment. Salmonella typhimurium, strain W118-2,
was used for experimental infection. This organism has been
used extensively by our laboratory in previous studies in
CD-1 and C3H/HeJ mice (1,2). To determine $LD_{50}$ values, log-
-phase cultures were used. Bacterial numbers were estimated
by Petroff-Hauser counts and the actual number of organisms
injected calculated from duplicate spread plates on blood
agar. As shown in Table 1, the C3HeB/FeJ mouse, like the
C3H/HeJ mouse, is hypersusceptible to Salmonella infection,
with a theoretical lethal dose approaching a single cell.
In contrast, mice of the C3H strain are approximately a
thousand times more resistant to an intraperitoneal Salmonella infection, with an $LD_{50}$ of $1.2 \times 10^3$ cells.

**Table 1.**   Intraperitoneal $LD_{50}$ of S. Typhimurium, W118-2, in
Various Mouse Strains

| Mouse Strain | Breeder | $LD_{50}$ Number of Cells |
|---|---|---|
| C3H/HeJ | Jackson Laboratory | <7 |
| C3HeB/FeJ | Jackson Laboratory | <2 |
| C3H | Charles River | $1.2 \times 10^3$ |
| CD-1 | Charles River | $1 \times 10^4$ |

Spleen cells of the three different mouse strains in
the C3H lineage were all tested on the same day for ability
to incorporate $H^3$-thymidine in response to three different
mitogens. All three substances were extracts from a single
batch of S. typhimurium W118-2. Trichloracetic acid extracted lipopolysaccharide (TCA-LPS) was prepared by the method
of Boivin as described by Sultzer (6). A portion of this
TCA-LPS was further extracted with hot phenol (8). Phenol-
water extracted lipopolysaccharide (PW-LPS) was recovered
from the aqueous phase. Endotoxin protein (EP) was recovered from the phenol phase.

As expected from previous reports (8), C3H/HeJ mice did
not give a mitogenic response to PW-LPS, but did respond to
TCA-LPS and to EP (Table 2). C3HeB/FeJ and C3H mice responded to all of the mitogens tested. The C3HeB/FeJ mouse was
than compared with the others strains for its sensitivity to
endotoxemia. Table 3 shows the mortality data for groups of

Table 2.  H[3]-Thymidine Uptake by Spleen Cells In Vitro of
Three Different Mouse Strains in the C3H Lineage

| Mitogen[a] | Dose (µg/well) | C3H/HeJ Mean CPM ± S.D.[b] | S.i.[c] | C3HeB/FeJ Mean CPM ± S.D. | S.I. | C3H Mean CPM ± S.D. | S.I. |
|---|---|---|---|---|---|---|---|
| None | – | 780 ± 51 | – | 541 ± 27 | – | 1,141 ± 88 | – |
| PW–LPS | 5 | 2,953 ± 506 | 3.8 | 36,024 ± 471 | 67 | 47,149 ± 4,360 | 41 |
|  | 25 | 5,683 ± 957 | 7.5 | 43,921 ± 5,336 | 81 | 55,281 ± 665 | 48 |
| EP | 1 | 36,643 ± 1,990 | 47 | 35,617 ± 8,900 | 66 | 39,350 ± 3,470 | 35 |
|  | 5 | 38,091 ± 3,067 | 49 | 55,069 ± 893 | 102 | 58,373 ± 1,208 | 51 |
|  | 25 | 36,916 ± 5,549 | 47 | 61,779 ± 1,475 | 114 | 63,968 ± 724 | 56 |
|  | 100 | 34,603 ± 2,367 | 44 | 37,709 ± 3,289 | 70 | 43,674 ± 1,590 | 38 |
| TCA–LPS | 1 | 27,730 ± 2,028 | 36 | 39,470 ± 3,390 | 73 | 40,429 ± 2,858 | 35 |
|  | 5 | 33,649 ± 6,508 | 43 | 44,446 ± 5,662 | 82 | 50,197 ± 470 | 44 |

[a]All mitogens derived from S. typhimurium, strain W118-2.-
PW-LPS = phenol-water extracted lipopolysaccharide;EP = endotoxin protein; TCA-LPS = trichloroacetic acid extracted lipopolysaccharide.
[b]Uptake of 0.25 µCi of H[3] - thymidine by triplicate cultures of $4 \times 10^5$ spleen cells.
[c]S.I.= $\dfrac{\text{Mean cpm of mitogen}}{\text{Mean cpm without mitogen}}$

Table 3.  Toxicity of Phenol-Water Extracted Lipopolysaccharide for Various Mouse Strains in the C3H Lineage

| Dose LPS (µg)[a] | Survival (alive/total)[b] Mouse Strain C3H/HeJ | C3H | C3HeB/FeJ |
|---|---|---|---|
| 2000 | 4/6 | N.D. | N.D. |
| 1000 | 6/6 | 0/6 | 0/6 |
| 500 | 6/6 | 3/6[c] | 1/6[c] |
| 250 | N.D. | 6/6 | 0/6 |
| 100 | N.D. | 6/6 | 6/6 |
| TD$_{50}$[d] | >2000 | 500 | 250<100 |
| Classification | R | S | VS |

[a]Phenol-water extracted lipopolysaccharide from Salmonella typhimurium (Difco lot #1604064)0.5 ml suspended in sterile, nonpyrogenic saline (Cutter Medical) and injected ip.
[b]Mortality scored 48 hours post injection.
[c] An additional mouse succumbed 3 days post injection.
[d] TD$_{50}$=Toxic dose for 50% of the animals
[e]R = Resistant, S = Sensitive, VS = Very Sensitive

6 mice receiving graded doses of commercially prepared PW-
LPS. C3HeB/FeJ mice were the most sensitive of the three
strains tested, with 100% of the animals succumbing to the
250-μg dose. It is evident that they respond very differently from C3H/HeJ mice, which are exceptionally resistant
to the lethal effects of LPS, the $LD_{50}$ being greater than
2000 μg. Thus, the C3HeB/FeJ mouse is hypersusceptible to
Salmonella infection, but sensitive to the toxic effects of
PW-LPS, and mitogenically responsive to this substance
(Table 4).

Table 4. Summary

| Mouse Strain | Salmonella Susceptibility[a] | Endotoxin Sensitivity[b] | Mitogenic Responsiveness |
|---|---|---|---|
| C3H/HeJ | Sus | R | — |
| C3HeB/FeJ | Sus | VS | + |
| C3H | Res | S | + |

[a]Based on $LD_{50}$ determinations
[b]Based on $TD_{50}$ determinations

We had previously shown that C3H/HeJ mice are poorly
protected by PW-LPS (2) and by endotoxin protein (EP) (3).
However, their mean time to death is prolonged by vaccination with TCA-LPS (3). In contrast, CD-1 mice are well protected by PW-LPS, with 1 μg affording protection against a
challenge of 500 $LD_{50}$ doses (1). The results presented in
Table 5 show that C3HeB/FeJ mice respond like C3H/HeJ mice,
in that they are poorly protected by EP or PW-LPS, but show
a prolonged mean time to death when vaccinated with TCA-LPS
and challenged 21 days later. The poor immunizability of
C3HeB/FeJ mice was not expected, as these mice have been reported to give normal in vitro and in vivo immune responses
to PW-LPS (11). In contrast, Salmonella-resistant C3H mice
are protected by PW-LPS and EP vaccines (unpublished observations).

Table 5. Survival and Antibody Titers of C3HeB/FeJ Mice Vaccinated and Challenged ip

| Vaccine[a] | Dose (μg) | Survival[b] 30 Day | 30 Day MTD[c] | 61 Day | 61 Day MTD | | Whole Cell Agglutination Titers |
|---|---|---|---|---|---|---|---|
| EP | 10 | 10% (1/10) | 15 | 10% (1/10) | 15 | pre[d] | <2 |
| | | | | | | 12 | <2 |
| | | | | | | 21 | <2 |
| | 25 | 10% (1/10) | 12 | 0% (0/10) | 17 | pre | <2 |
| | | | | | | 12 | <2 |
| | | | | | | 21 | <2 |
| | 100 | 20% (2/10) | 15 | 0% (0/10) | 21 | pre | <2 |
| | | | | | | 12 | 4 |
| | | | | | | 21 | 2 |
| PW–LPS | 10 | 0% (0/10) | 11 | 0% (0/10) | 11 | pre | <2 |
| | | | | | | 12 | <2 |
| | | | | | | 21 | <2 |
| | 25 | 0% (0/10) | 13 | 0% (0/10) | 13 | pre | <2 |
| | | | | | | 12 | <2 |
| | | | | | | 21 | 4 |
| | 100 | 40% (4/10) | 16 | 10% (1/10) | 27 | pre | <2 |
| | | | | | | 12 | 4 |
| | | | | | | 21 | 2 |
| TCA–LPS | 10 | 10% (1/10) | 20 | 10% (1/10) | 22 | pre | <2 |
| | | | | | | 12 | 16 |
| | | | | | | 21 | 16 |
| | 25 | 0% (0/10) | 25 | 0% (0/10) | 25 | pre | <2 |
| | | | | | | 12 | 4 |
| | | | | | | 21 | 16 |
| | 100 | 89% (8/9) | – | 22% (2/9) | 38 | pre | <2 |
| | | | | | | 12 | 16 |
| | | | | | | 21 | 32 |
| PBS | | 0% (0/10) | 11 | 0% (0/10) | 11 | | <2 |
| | | | | | | | T.S. = 16[e] |

[a]Mice immunized ip
[b]Mice challenged 21 days post vaccination with 24 cells of W118-2 given ip
[c] MTD = Mean time of death
[d]Pre = preimmunization titer; 12 and 21 = titers on designated days post vaccination. Pooled sera of 4 mice.
[e]T.S. = typing serum titer.

These studies establish that C3HeB/FeJ is a mouse strain in the C3H lineage which is Salmonella susceptible, but sensitive to the toxic and mitogenic effects of lipopolysaccharide. Thus, in this mouse strain, Salmonella susceptibility is not associated with the defective LPS responsiveness controlled by the $\underline{Lps}^d$ allele. Whether susceptibility is controlled by a very closely linked locus, or by one of the other two loci known to determine Salmonella susceptibility, is currently being investigated using appropriate genetic crosses. The studies presented here also show that the C3HeB/FeJ strain does not behave like the resistant CD-1 or C3H mouse strain in ability to be protected against Salmonella infection by vaccination with PW-LPS, TCA-LPS or EP.

ACKNOWLEDGEMENT

This work was supported by NIH grant A1-15613 from the National Institute of Allergy and Infectious Diseases. The assistance of Ms. Loran Killar in carrying out the toxicity studies is appreciated.

REFERENCES

1.  Angerman, C.R., and Eisenstein, T.K.   Infect. Immun. 19:575, 1978.
2.  Eisenstein, T.K., and Angerman, C.R.   J.Immunol. 121:-1010, 1978.
3.  Eisenstein, T.K., Angerman, C.R., and Deakins, L.W.   In Immunomodulation by bacteria and Their Products.   H. Friedman, (ed).   Baltimore, Md: University Park Press, 1980 (in press).
4.  Hill, A.B., Hatswell, J.M., and Topley, W.W.C.   J.Hyg. 40:538, 1940.
5.  O'Brien, A.D., Rosenstreich, D.L., Scher, I., Campbell, G.H., MacDermott, R.P., and Formal, S.B.   J.Immunol. 124:20, 1980.
6.  Sultzer, B.M.   J.Immunol. 103:32, 1969.
7.  Sultzer, B.M.   Infect.Immun. 13:1579, 1976.
8.  Sultzer, B.M., and Goodman, G.W.   J.Exp.Med. 144:821, 1976.
9.  Vas, S.I.   In Infection, Immunity, and Genetics.   H. Friedman, et al (eds).   Baltimore,Med: University Park Press, p39, 1978.
10. Watson, J., Kelly, K., Largen, M., and Taylor, B.A. J.Immunol. 120:422, 1978.
11. Watson, J., and Riblet, R.   J.Immunol. 114:1462, 1975.
12. Webster, L.T.   J.Exp.Med. 65:261, 1937.

# NATURAL RESISTANCE TO MOUSE TYPHOID: POSSIBLE ROLE OF THE MACROPHAGE

Carlos E. Hormaeche, James Brock and Richard Pettifor
Microbiology Division, Department of Pathology,
University of Cambridge
Cambridge, England

## INTRODUCTION

There is increasing evidence that natural resistance to certain parasites may depend on genetically determined host factors, as yet poorly understood. Marked differences in resistance can be found among inbred strains of mice.

Genetic differences in natural resistance to mouse typhoid have been known for many years (1,6,23). The matter is being reinvestigated and several groups have found important differences among currently used strains of laboratory mice (15,16,20,22). Plant and Glynn (17,18) studied natural resistance to subcutaneous challenge with S. typhimurium C5 and were able to group 7 different mouse strains as resistant or susceptible (LD 50); resistance was controlled by a single autosomal gene or gene cluster located on chromosome 1 (19) which follows exactly the same mouse strain distribution as the Lsh leishmania resistance gene (2). There was an apparent correlation between high natural resistance and the development of delayed hypersensitivity (footpad test) to a salmonella extract.

Studies in this laboratory (8,9,10) using S. typhimurium C5 given i/v have shown that natural resistance is under polygenic control; that the host defence mechanisms operating during the early and late phases of the infection are under separate genetic control; and that susceptibility to infection can be due to different genetic defects occurring at different stages of the infection.

One host defence gene is of prime importance. This is almost certainly the same gene described by Plant and Glynn, and may also be the one responsible for Webster's original results. This gene operates very early in the course of the infection and determines the in vivo net growth rate of the salmonellae in the liver and spleen. Mouse strains can be grouped as "fast" or "slow" net growth rate, the latter trait following simple autosomal dominant inheritance. The gene is not H-2 linked and is not related to the development of a positive footpad test in mice immunized either i/v or s/c.

"Slow" net growth rate is essential for resistance, but insufficient. Not all strains of the "slow" category are

121

equally resistant, due to the existence of additional genetic defects. These modifier genes can alter the later
course of the infection and make some strains unable to suppress the bacterial load and lead to increased susceptibility (8,9).

## THE NET GROWTH RATE PHENOTYPE OF RADIATION CHIMERAS

The net growth rate phenotype was shown to be transferable to lethally irradiated recipients by bone marrow grafts
from the appropriate donor; the recipient then expresses
the net growth rate phenotype of the donor (10). This paper
reports the results obtained with a similar system, using
(Balb/c X C3H)F1 ("fast" X "slow")F1 which are of "slow"
phenotype. Lethally irradiated F1 mice were reconstituted
with T-depleted (anti-Thy 1,2 and complement) bone marrow
from Balb/c, C3H or F1 bone marrow and challenged with S.
typhimurium C5 i/v 3 months later. Fig. 1 shows that the
resulting in vivo net growth rate in the different groups is
essentially similar to that reported earlier with the B10-
-A/J model: the donor net growth rate phenotype determines
the phenotype of the recipient.

In addition, recipient F1 mice were given a mixture of
equal amounts of bone marrow from Balb/c and C3H. The result, also shown in Fig. 1, was essentially similar to that
seen with Balb/c cells alone: the actual counts were
slightly lower than in mice getting only Balb/c but the net
growth rate was very similar and clearly different from that
in mice getting C3H or F1 bone marrow.

The degree of chimerism was checked using a dye exclusion microcytotoxicity test on peripheral blood samples.
The single chimeras were found to have no detectable cells
of the host type. However, the double chimeras which had
been given equal amount of Balb/c and C3H bone marrow were
found to be approximately 90% Balb/c ("fast"). The experiments were therefore repeated, but giving the irradiated F1
recipients 10% Balb/c and 90% C3H T-depleted bone marrow.
This resulted in approximately 50% chimeras and preliminary
experiments showed that they did not significantly differ
from the 90% Balb/c chimeras when challenged with salmonellae. Fig. 2 shows the results of several experiments in
which individually typed mice were challenged with $10^4$ salmonellae and assayed 5 days later. Similar high counts were
obtained with mice carrying either 50% or 90% Balb/c cells.

Summarizing, radiation chimeras express the "fast"
phenotype whether they are carrying predominant "fast" type
cells or equal amounts of "fast and "slow". We have obtain-

ed comparable results in the B10-A/J model, alhough in the latter case the transfer of equal amounts of both parental bone marrows resulted in approximately 50% chimeras.

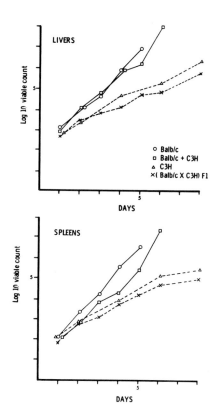

Fig. 1. Growth of S. typhimurium C5 ($10^4$ i/v) in livers and spleens of (Balb/c x C3H)$F_1$ radiation chimeras. $F_1$ recipients received 850 R and approximately $5.10^6$ T-depleted bone marrow from Balb/c (circles), C3H (triangles), $F_1$ (crosses) or equal amounts of Balb/c and C3H (squares).

IN VIVO FATE OF TEMPERATURE SENSITIVE (TS) SALMONELLA
MUTANTS

The mechanisms by which in vivo net growth rate is controlled is unknown. More specifically, there is no evidence

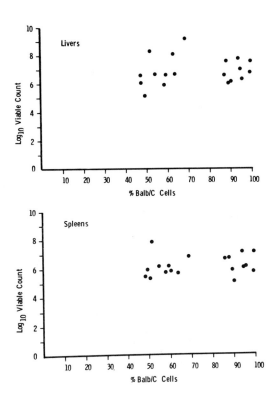

**Fig. 2.** Growth of salmonellae in (Balb/c x C3H) $F_1$ double chimeras carrying different amounts of donor cell types. Viable counts in liver and spleen 5 days after $10^4$ $\underline{S}$. $\underline{typhimurium}$ C5 i/v.

to indicate whether the difference between the "fast" and "slow" phenotypes is or is not due to a bactericidal mechanism. While a greater macrophage bactericidal activity has been found in some resistant mice (13), this has not been confirmed in other strains (21). Similar experiments in this laboratory (unpublished) have also failed to show a consistently higher killing of salmonellae $\underline{in}$ $\underline{vitro}$ by macrophages of resistant mice. An attempt was made to estimate the RES bactericidal efficiency $\underline{in}$ $\underline{vivo}$, using non-replica-

ting TS mutants.    Five salmonella strains were used, the
highly virulent S. enteritidis 5694, the virulent S. typhimurium C5, the intermediate S. typhimurium M525 (8,9) and
M526 (14) and the non-virulent S. typhimurium M206 (11).
The in vivo net growth rate of the parent strains in Balb/c
mice is greatest in the highly virulent 5694 and negative in
the non-virulent M206, the other strains being arranged in
between in order of virulence (Fig. 3).

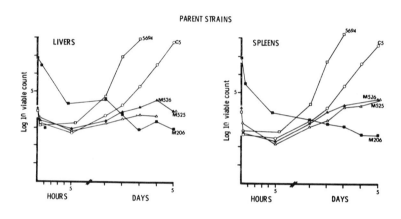

Fig. 3.    Growth  of  parent  salmonellae  in  Balb/c  mice.
Viable  counts  in  liver  and  spleen  following  intravenous
challenge with $10^3$ S. enteritides 5694, S. typhimurium C5,
M525 or M526, or $10^7$ M206.

TS mutants were prepared from all these strains by a method
similar to that described by Hooke et al. (7).   These mutants grew normally at 26°C, but ceased to divide at 37°C;
they were non-virulent.    Fig. 4 shows the fate of these TS
mutants in the livers and spleens of Balb/c mice injected
i/v.   A challenge of $10^7$ organisms is initially inactivated
but then reaches a plateau;   the plateau level is highest
for the more virulent mutants, and arranges them according
to the virulence of the parent strains.

A clear  pattern  therefore  exists  in  the  fate  of  the
different TS mutants in vivo, with Balb/c mice clearing TS

mutants from less virulent parents more efficiently than those derived from virulent parent strains.

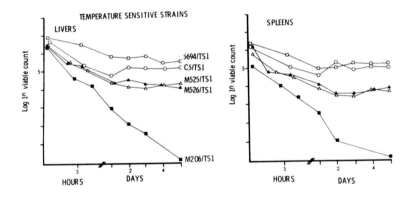

**Fig. 4.** Fate of TS mutants in Balb/c mice. Viable counts following intravenous challenge with TS mutants of strains 5694, C5, M525, M526 and M206.

The TS mutant of S. typhimurium C5 was injected into groups of mice of 7 different inbred and F1 strains, three of the "fast" and four of the "slow" phenotype. Fig. 5 shows the result: there was no consistent difference in the pattern of clearance according to the "fast" or "slow" phenotype. Counts reached a plateau between approximately $10^4$ and $10^5.^5$, but the different strains did not consistently separate into two groups, as might have been expected if the "slow" phenotype were due to a more efficient bactericidal mechanism.

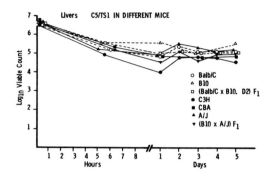

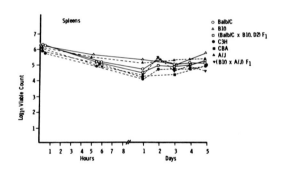

**Fig. 5.** Fate of a TS mutant from S. typhimurium C5 in different mouse strains injected with $10^7$ organisms i/v. Mice of "fast" phenotype (Balb/c, B10, (Balb/c x B10.D2)$F_1$) in open symbols, "slow" phenotype (C3H, CBA, A/J, (B10 x A/J)$F_1$) in solid symbols.

## DISCUSSION

The present results show that chimeric mice carrying both resistant and susceptible cells behave like susceptible mice, and that resistant mice do not consistently clear non-replicating salmonellae better than susceptible mice.

The results on chimeric mice suggest that the gene regulating in vivo net growth rate may not be acting by inducing
an earlier immune response (Ir gene?) in slow net growth
rate mice.    There is comparatively little data on cellular
interactions operating in salmonella infections.    However,
it is generally believed that a major mechanism in resistance to mouse typhoid is the development of a T-cell mediated immune response, possibly assisted by antibody (4,24).
If  the  same  conditions  of  cellular  interactions  seen  in
other systems also apply to the salmonella immune response,
then T cells from the putative high responder parent ("slow"
net growth rate) maturing in an F1 thymus could be expected
to cooperate with cells (including macrophages) of either
parent and slow net growth rate should result.    The observed
high bacterial counts in these double chimeras appears to
negate this hypothesis and is more in keeping with the view
that net growth rate is not mediated by an immune response
but is the direct result of macrophage function, and that
the observed fast net growth rate in double chimeras is in
fact taking place largely in the macrophages of the "fast"
parental type.    Clearly additional data on cellular interactions in salmonella infections could be desirable to shed
more light on this question.
The results with temperature sensitive mutants appear to
suggest that the differences in net growth rate seen in mice
of different strains may not be due to marked differences in
in vivo bactericidal activity, but that perhaps other differences in microenvironment may be important.    It is known
that TS salmonellae are non-virulent (5) and that E. Coli TS
mutants are killed by macrophages in vitro (7).    The present
studies show that TS mutants of salmonellae of different
virulence do not survive equally well in vivo, as mutants
from virulent parents survived better than those from less
virulent ones.    It is known that only salmonellae that can
survive in macrophages are pathogenic.    The present studies
showed that the degree of survival in vivo arranges them in
the order of virulence of the parents suggesting that the
degree of virulence, which appears to be due in great part
to the overall growth rate of the parent strain in the RES,
may be associated with susceptibility to in vivo bactericidal systems.

    On the other hand, the degree of survival of one TS
mutant derived from S. typhimurium C5 did not arrange the
different mouse strains in two groups according to the net
growth rate phenotype.    Some "slow" strains inactivated the
TS mutant better than some "fast" strains, but this was not
the general case.    This contrasts with the clear arrangement
seen when different TS mutants were injected in one mouse

strain, and suggests that - at least under these experimental conditions - the degree of natural resistance may not be due to a clear higher bactericidal efficiency in resistant mice.

Additional information from other non-replicating mutants would be desirable to shed more light on this question. It was observed that mice injected with TS mutants can develop septic arthritis from which live TS mutants can be cultured; that is, however, a late-developing complication (2-3 weeks) and is unlikely to influence the short term experiments described in this report. It is known that salmonellae divide _in vivo_ much more slowly than they do _in vitro_, and are very resistant to the bactericidal effect of macrophages (3,12,14). More detailed knowledge of the conditions governing replicating and inactivation in the macrophage microenvironment will be required before a definite conclusion on the mode of action of the net growth rate controlling gene can be established.

## REFERENCES

1. Bohme, D.H. Bull N.Y.Acad.Med. 46:499, 1970.
2. Bradley, D.J., Taylor, B.A., Blackwell, J., and Evans, E.P. Clin.Exp.Immunol. 37:7, 1979.
3. Carrol, M.E.W., Jackett, P.A., Aber, V.R., amd Lowrie, D.B. J.Gen.Microbiol. 110:421, 1979.
4. Collins, F.M. Bacteriol.Revs. 38:371, 1974.
5. Fahey, K.J., and Cooper, G.N. Infect.Immun. 1:263, 1970.
6. Gowen, J.W. Bact.Revs. 24:192, 1960.
7. Hooke, A.M., Oeschger, M.P., Zeligs, B.J., and Bellanti, J. Infect. Immun. 20:406, 1978.
8. Hormaeche, C.E. Immunology 37:311, 1979.
9. Hormaeche, C.E. Immunology 37:319, 1979.
10. Hormaeche, C.E. Immunology 37:329, 1979.
11. Jenkin, C.R., Rowley, D., and Auzins, I. Aust.J.Exp.-Biol.Med.Sci. 42:215, 1960.
12. Lowrie, D.B., Aber, V.R., and Carrol, M.E.W. J.Gen.-Microbiol. 110:409,, 1979.
13. Maier, T., and Oels, H.C. Infect.Immun. 6:438, 1972.
14. Maw, J., and Meynell, G.G. Brit.J.Exp.Pathol. 49:597, 1969.
15. Medina, S., Vas, S.J., and Robson, H.C. J. Immunol. 114:1720, 1975.
16. Miseldt, M.L., and Johnson, W. Infect.Immun. 14:652, 1976.
17. Plant, J, and Glynn, A.A. Nature (Lond). 248:345, 1974.

18. Plant, J., and Glynn, A.A.  J.Infect.Dis. 135:72, 1976.
19. Plant, J., and Glynn, A.A. Clin.Exp.Immunol. 37:1, 1979.
20. Robson, H.C., and Vas S.J. J. Infect.Dis. 126:378, 1972.
21. Vas, S.J. "Infection, immunity and genetics" H.
    Friedman, J.E. Prier, Eds. University Park Press,
    Baltimore, p39, 1978.
22. Von Jeney, N., Gunther, B., and Jann, K. Infect.Immun.
    15:26, 1977.
23. Webster, L.T. J.Exp.Med. 57:793, 1933.
24. Zinkernagel, R.M. Infect.Immun. 13:1069. 1976.

## DISCUSSION

Bennett: It seems to me that there is one control experiment Hormaeche would have to do before he can say that the
mixture of Balb/c and C3H cells allows the growth of the
permissive cell. What would happen if he were to put in two
H-2 incompatible BM cell types, both of which were genetically resistant, so as to rule out any H-2 allogenetic effect? In other words, the effect he is getting, the increased bacterial growth, could theoretically be due to H-2 nonidentical cells interacting with each other in the same
host.

Hormaeche: I have not checked for that. I simply depleted
the BM of T cells. All I can say is that these experiments
were done three months after transfer; the mice appeared
healthy; the spleens were small. They did not appear to be
undergoing a GVH reaction. I have no further data.

Eisenstein: In connection with an earlier comment by
Collins, I would like to know a but more about the relationship between Salmonella susceptibility and endotoxin resistance. This is an issue that has been around for a long time
and, while some have very strong opinions on it, I rather
think it remains unresolved. Personally, I feel that in the
C3H/HeJ mouse we see an animal that is Salmonella-susceptible and LPS-resistant while, in most of the other C3H strains, the animals are Salmonella-resistant but endotoxin
sensitive. What we have discovered is that there is another
mouse strain C3HeB/FeJ, which is Salmonella-susceptible, but
endotoxin sensitive, thus apparently dissociating these two
parameters. So I think that perhaps endotoxin sensitivity
and Salmonella-resistance are not necessarily linked. If
that is the case, we do not have much of a handle, at the
moment, on what causes a mouse to die of Salmonella.

Hormaeche: I would agree. I think one little clue may derive from the findings on the effects of endotoxin in human typhoid fever. I think it is now fairly clear that the symptoms of typhoid are not due to endotoxemia. In the same way, I believe the cause of death of the mouse infected with Salmonella is not circulating endotoxin. If I could just turn to your results on the C3H/HeJ mice, I find that another, similar, approach confirms O'Brien's results with silica increasing the microbial growth rate by knocking out the macrophages. One can get pretty much the same results by giving LPS. A large dose of LPS, or dead organisms, given together with the Salmonella challenge pushes up the growth rate and the mice die. That does not happen in C3H/HeJ mice if one uses phenol-water-prepared LPS; but it does occur if one uses Boivin type LPS or killed organisms.

Amos: In the experiments in which Hormaeche transplanted mixtures of bone marrow cells, did he evoke a chronic GVH reaction in the recipients?

Hormaeche: I did not check for GVH. The mice appeared healthy and there was no visible spleen enlargement when the mice were sacrificed one day after infection with Salmonella. They appeared completely normal.

Amos: I do not see why you would not have had a GVH going on, especially as you are putting in mixtures of H-2 incompatible cells.

Cudkowicz: Was Hormaeche using BM-cells pretreated with anti-theta serum?

Hormaeche: Monoclonal anti-Thy-1 plus complement, yes.

Cudkowicz: That would explain why Hormaeche did not get detectable GVH. But that still does not mean that the two cells types had not interacted somehow. His finding is unusual in that he got only 10% of one population persisting. Could he say again how he determined chimerism? What cell was he typing for?

Hormaeche: First I want to say that I got exactly the same results with the B10.A-A/J system. But in these, giving equal amounts of B10.A and A/J BM, we got 50:50 chimeras. It is only with the Balb/c and C3H that I got this imbalance. The typing was done on peripheral blood leucocytes obtained from buffy coat and separated by carbonyl iron and Ficoll-Hypaque; results of microcytotoxicity tests were judged by eosin exclusion.

Cudkowicz:   Although it is unusual, there are precedents for
Hormaeche's findings.   I mentioned that Lengerova has been
working with mixtures, and she has been looking at cells
much earlier than 90 days, and found evidence for interaction between certain genotypes leading to the prevalence
of one population over the other.   Also, some 10-15 years
ago, there was a report that (this was not a cell mixture
experiment) cells transplanted into irradiated animals, for
no well-identified reason, at some point ceased to persist
and, given enough time (in your case it is a long time), the
host cells returned.   So that the mixture is established between the donor and the host cells.

    I would like also to make a short comment about the
silica experiment.   Everyone seems to imply that silica administered in vivo results in the elimination of macrophages, essentially.   I think that was the guiding principle
for everyone doing experiments until a few years ago, but
there are quite strong opinions now that this is not necessarily the case.   Silica particles are certainly injurious
to macrophages but they do not destroy them.   And I would
say perhaps that the more interesting data now emerging is
that injured macrophages, or macrophages that have been exposed to silica, turn into suppressor macrophages; suppressors for a number of immune responses, and also suppressors
for NK cells or cytotoxic macrophages such as are likely to
be involved in these phenomena.   So most of those experiments may have to be reconsidered.

O'Brien:   The silica studies we did were in vivo.   And
Cudkowicz is right, we did not see a decrease in macrophage
numbers;   in fact, we saw an increase in macrophage numbers
but it appeared that they were not functioning as they had
been before.

    Coming back to the subject of murine typhoid and the
old question of why Salmonella typhi is not virulent for
mice:   I want to point out that C3H/HeJ mice are resistant
to Salmonella typhi and that silica treatment does not render a mouse susceptible to Salmonella typhi.   So at present
there is no evidence that the macrophage sets the groundwork
for natural resistance to Salmonella typhi.

# CONTROL OF RESISTANCE TO SALMONELLA TYPHIMURIUM IN HYBRID GENERATIONS OF INBRED MICE AND BIOZZI MICE

Janet E. Plant and Alan A. Glynn

Bacteriology Department
Wright-Fleming Institute
St. Mary's Hospital Medical School
London W2 1PG, England.

We have found that resistance to Salmonella typhimurium injected subcutaneously into mice is largely controlled by a single gene locus on chromosome 1 - Ity. Resistance gene $Ity^r$ is dominant and sensitive inbred mouse strains are homozygous $Ity^s$ (7). This paper investigates the completeness of this dominance in various hybrid generations of mice.

The parental mice were either the commonly used inbred mouse strains (5) or the Biozzi mice from Selection I, i.e. selected for high or low antibody responses to sheep red blood cells (2).

The mice were evaluated for resistance to S. typhimurium s.c.i. by three methods. Firstly the $LD_{50}$ was estimated in groups of mice challenged subcutaneously. Secondly individual mice were distinguished as sensitive or resitant by the viable bacterial count per liver or spleen on day 10 (VC10) after infection with $10^3$ organisms s.c.i. (6). Thirdly, groups of mice given $10^3$ S. typhimurium s.c. on day 0 were killed at intervals up to 4 weeks to determine the kinetics of their infection in the organs.

The $LD_{50}$ values for inbred mice and their $F_1$ hybrids are shown in Table 1.

All hybrids with at least one resistant parent were resistant with $LD_{50}$ of $10^6$-$10^7$. All sensitive-sensitive hybrids were susceptible to <10 organisms. The viable counts of bacteria in the organs after a dose of $10^3$ S. typhimurium confirmed these results (Table 1). Although bacteria in the spleen are shown, these correspond to those found in the liver, hybrids with at least one resistant parent having $10^3$-$10^4$ and sensitive-sensitive hybrids having $10^6$-$10^7$ bacteria per organ, as demonstrated previously for inbred parental strains (6).

The kinetics of infection in the resistant-sensitive hybrids closely paralleled infection in resistant mice over 3-4 weeks and was further evidence that no major complementation had occurred between resistant, $Ity^r$ $Ity^r$, and sensitive, $Ity^s$ $Ity^s$, parental mice.

GENETIC CONTROL OF NATURAL RESISTANCE
TO INFECTION AND MALIGNANCY

## Table 1

| | $LD_{50}$ S.typhimurium (C5) s.c.i. | Spleen VC10* |
|---|---|---|
| BALB/c | <10 | $1 \times 10^6$ |
| C57BL | $2 \times 10$ | $7 \times 10^7$ |
| DBA/1 | <10 | |
| | | |
| DBA/2 | $2 \times 10^5$ | $8 \times 10^3$ |
| A/J | $2 \times 10^6$ | $5 \times 10^2$ |
| CBA/Ca | $1 \times 10^7$ | $2 \times 10^3$ |
| C57L | $5 \times 10^6$ | $2 \times 10^4$ |
| SENSITIVE x SENSITIVE | | |
| BALB/c x DBA/1 | <5 | $2 \times 10^7$ |
| C57BL x DBA/1 | <5 | $2 \times 10^7$ |
| BALB/c x C57BL | <20 | $2 \times 10^6$ |
| SENSITIVE x RESISTANT | | |
| BALB/c x C57L | $1 \times 10^7$ | $9 \times 10^3$ |
| C57BL x DBA/2 | $5 \times 10^6$ | $2 \times 10^4$ |
| BALB/c x CBA | $3 \times 10^6$ | $3 \times 10^3$ |
| CBA x C57BL | $1 \times 10^7$ | $2 \times 10^4$ |
| RESISTANT x RESISTANT | | |
| CBA x A/J | $2 \times 10^7$ | $1 \times 10^3$ |

*Viable bacteria/spleen on day 10 of infection with $10^3$ S. typhimurium s.c.i.

 

The Biozzi mice are denoted as High line or Low line according to their antibody responses to sheep erythrocytes 92). We have compared these mice and hybrid generations for responses to S. typhimurium using BALB/c and CBA as our sensitive and resistant inbred mouse strains respectively. The High and Low lines showed clear differences in their responses to subcutaneous S. typhimurium (Table 2). The High line were as susceptible as BALB/c mice and the Low line resistant, confirmed by the $LD_{50}$ and VC10 values shown. Although no significant difference was apparent from these data in the resistance of Low line and CBA mice (Table 2), when the kinetics of infection were studies over 3-4 weeks in the two pairs of strains, their responses differed.

Table 2.

| | $LD_{50}$ S. typhimurium s.c.i. | Spleen VC10 | Liver VC10 |
|---|---|---|---|
| BALB/c | <10 | $1 \times 10^6$ | $1 \times 10^5$ |
| CBA | $1 \times 10^7$ | $2 \times 10^3$ | $4 \times 10^3$ |
| BALB/c x CBA | $3 \times 10^6$ | $3 \times 10^3$ | $3 \times 10^3$ |
| HIGH line | <20 | $3 \times 10^7$ | $9 \times 10^7$ |
| LOW line | $3 \times 10^6$ | $1 \times 10^3$ | $1 \times 10^3$ |
| HIGH x LOW | $5 \times 10^6$ | $2 \times 10^4$ | $2 \times 10^4$ |
| BALB/c x LOW | $6 \times 10^6$ | $3 \times 10^3$ | $4 \times 10^3$ |
| CBA x LOW | $5 \times 10^6$ | $2 \times 10^3$ | $3 \times 10^3$ |
| BALB/c x HIGH | <20 | $2 \times 10^7$ | $5 \times 10^7$ |
| CBA x HIGH | $4 \times 10^5$ | $3 \times 10^5$ | $2 \times 10^6$ |

CBA mice had levels of $10^3-10^4$ bacteria in the organs at 3 weeks (6) and remained carriers until at least 8 weeks after infection. In contrast, Low line mice were able to clear the organs of detectable bacteria within 3 weeks (Fig. 1). This must either be a modification of expression of Ity in the Low line mice or alternative genetic control of resistance. The resistance of the (High x Low)$F_1$ mice as demonstrated by the $LD_{50}$ and VC10 results (Table 2) indicated that this control was inherited and able to overcome the sensitivity of High line mice.

We have crossed the Biozzi mice with BALB/c or CBA: $LD_{50}$ and VC10 results are in Table 2. The results for the BALB/c or CBA hybrids with Low line showed both were as resistant as Low line, so the resistance factor in Low line had been inherited, and moreover could modify both Ity$^r$ and Ity$^s$ to an equal degree.

The High line hybrid results showed that their susceptibility factor was also inherited. The BALB/c-High line hybrid had VC10 values equivalent to High line indicating a modification even of Ity$^s$ expression. The CBA-High line hybrid demonstrated clearly that the suceptibility factor in High line was also able to modify Ity$^r$. The mice were apparently intermediate in resistance compared with parental $LD_{50}$ and VC10 data. The genetic inheritance from High line is unable to modify Ity$^r$ completely, as was demonstrated more obviously in the kinetics of infection in the CBA, High line and hybrid mice (Fig. 2).

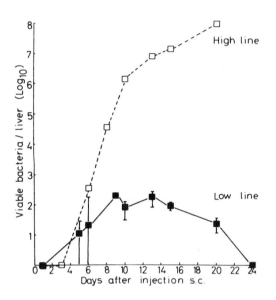

**Figure 1.** Viable bacteria in livers of High line and Low line mice infected with $10^3$ S. typhimurium s.c.i. on day 0. Counts in groups of at least 4 mice expressed as G.M.±SD.

 The resistance of the High-Low hybrid suggests a fairly simple genetic control of resistance or modification of Ity with no evidence of polygenic inheritance.

 The inheritance of the Low resistance factor in BALB/c and CBA hybrids and therefore its equal modification of $Ity^r$ or $Ity^s$ was confirmed by the kinetics of infection in these hybrids (Fig. 3) which showed them to be more resistant even than the CBA parent and comparable to the High-Low hybrid (Fig. 2).

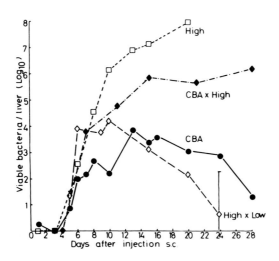

Figure 2. Viable bacteria in livers of CBA x High and High x Low mice.

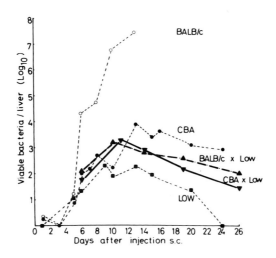

Figure 3. Viable bacteria in Low line hybrid mice.

We therefore postulate that

1)  In inbred mouse strains $Ity^r$ is the dominant gene
    largely controlling resistance to S. typhimurium s.c.i.
    (unpublished data demonstrates similar results for in-
    travenous and oral routes of infection).
    There was no evidence of complementation between the
    strains.
2)  Low line mice possess an additional or alternative re-
    sistance factor which is able to modify the effect of
    $Ity^r$ and $Ity^S$ in the hybrid mice.
3)  High line mice possess a susceptibility factor which is
    able to modify the effect of $Ity^r$, but incompletely.
    It also modifies $Ity^S$ to some extent. However, the
    resistance factor of Low line is dominant. The two
    factors may or may not be genetically correlated.

In view of the fact that infections in which Low line
mice are resistant, the immunity is postulated to be macrophage mediated, the mechanisms of the susceptibility/resis-
tance factor for S. typhimurium may be dependent on the
macrophages in the two lines (1). This may or may not be in
addition to whatever is controlled by Ity in the mice. We
received the mice after 20-24 generations and they have subsequently been inbred for 5 years, so should theoretically
be genetically stable. They are thought to differ at 6-10
loci, which may inc. 1de the H-2 locus (4).
The close parallel between Leishmania resistance and
Salmonella resitance (3) indicates the possibility of a controlling locus for certain infections or Chromosome 1. The
involvement of macrophages in the mechanism of control of
either Lsh or Ity has not been eliminated. The modifica-
tions of Ity by High and Low line mice, which can be
genetically compared, may lead to clarification of these
mechanisms.

## REFERENCES

1.  Biozzi, G.   In Genetic Control of Immune Responsive-
    ness. H.O. McDevitt and M. Landy (eds). New York:
    Academic Press, p317, 1972.
2.  Biozzi, G., Stiffel, C., Mouton, D., Bouthillier, Y.,
    and Decreusefond, C.  In Protides of the Biological
    Fluids Proc. Colloq Bruges. H. Peeters (ed.). Oxford:
    Pergamon Press, p161, 1970.
3.  Bradley, D.J., Taylor, B.A., Blackwell, J., Evans,
    E.P., and Freeman, J.  Clin.exp.Immunol. 37:7, 1979.

4.   Mouton, D., Bouthillier, Y., Mevel, J.C., Prouvost-
     Danon, A., and Biozzi, G.   Ann.Immunol. (Inst.Pasteur)
     128C:20, 1977.
5.   Plant, J., and Glynn, A.A.   Nature (Lond) 248:345,
     1974.
6.   Plant, J., and Glynn, A.A.   J.Infect.Dis. 133:72, 1976.
7.   Plant, J., and Glynn, A.A.   Clin.exp.Immunol. 37:1,
     1979.

## DISCUSSION

**Wake:**   Low line mice produce low levels of antibody against
SRBC.   What about the antibodies against Salmonella antigens?

**Plant:**   Well, they are supposed to produce low levels of
antibody to Salmonella antigens.   Right now we have not got
very good testing mechanisms for Salmonella antibodies,
assessing only hemagglutination, in both high-and-low line
mice, and in the hybrids.   There did not seem to be any
correlation between the antibody levels in these mice and
their resistance or susceptibility.

**Rosenstreich:**   Concerning gene linkage studies with respect
to the high and low line genes, are there alleles of Ity?
Are they on chromosone 1?

**Plant:**   We do not know yet.   We have got as far as the $F_1$'s
and were hoping to do some backcross experiments to see the
extent of this correlation.

**Skamene:**   The curves of bacterial growth in the high and the
low line do not really differ very much during the first
week, a time at which one would expect to see a difference
were it linked to Ity.

**Plant:**   Well, in fact, mice differing in the Ity gene do not
show much difference in the actual counts in the first week,
although something must be happening.   If you take Balb/c
and CBA as an example, it is just after day 6 that the Balb-
/c really shoots up, while the CBA stays at a lower level.

**Collins:**   Do CBA mice mount a DTH response to Salmonella infection and does this correlate at all with the antibody?
Also, I noticed with both Balb/c and Plant's high-responder
mice, that the infection went up to a microbial count of $10^8$
or more.   It is feasible to assess the infection-immunity in

the half of the mice that survive your $LD_{50}$ dose; can the animal eventually eliminate the infection or is the situation such that but one organism constitutes the $LD_{50}$ and you kill the animal?

Plant: CBA mice do produce good DTH but the problem is comparing the sensitive and resistant mice. How would one get good DTH in the sensitive mice without killing them? As to the second point, if one gives a dose of less than 10, some mice do survive. Whether this is because some have received no Salmonella at all is hard to say. But if they are given a slightly larger dose, they all die.

# A SINGLE GENE (Lr) CONTROLLING NATURAL RESISTANCE TO MURINE LISTERIOSIS

Christina Cheers[a], I.F.C. McKenzie[b]
T.E. Mandel[c] and Yu Yu Chan[a]

[a]Department of Microbiology
University of Melbourne
Parkville, Victoria, 3052, Australia
[b]Department of Medicine
University of Melbourne
Austin Hospital, Heidelberg
Victoria, Australia
[c]The Walter and Eliza Hall Institute
University of Melbourne
Parkville, Victoria, 3052, Australia

Recently there has been a renewal of interest in the genetics of resistance to infection, spurred by the current interest in the genetics of immune responses in general, and fed at the experimental level by the availability of a variety of inbred strains of mice. These include congenic, recombinant, recombinant inbred and mutant strains. Much emphasis has been placed on the fundamental role in the immune response of the major histocompatibility complex (MHC) linked genes, and on their function in resistance to viruses (5) and parasites (6). However, it is now becoming apparent that there are more genes to consider in resistance to infection.

The genetics of resistance to some infections is complex, but others have shown more readily definable patterns. Experimental or natural murine infections in which a single gene or small number of non-MHC linked genes have been implicated include murine hepatitis (4), salmonellosis (9), Corynebacterium kutcheri infection (3) and listeriosis (2).

We chose to study the genetics and mechanisms of resistance to Listeria monocytogenes because it represents an acute, potentially lethal infection, the immune response to which is already well defined. It is an intracellular bacterium, readily phagocytosed by macrophages but not by polymorphs (10). The early stages of resistance apparently require a bone marrow derived cell (7), while later acquired immunity rests on T cell activation and recruitment of macrophages and monocytes (8). Antibody plays no role in immunity. Resistant or susceptible mice could differ in any of these stages.

Mice fell into two distinct categories when challenged

141

intravenously with Listeria (Table 1).

Table 1.  Mouse strains resistant or susceptible to Listeria
          monocytogenes

| Resistant | Susceptible | |
|---|---|---|
| C57BL/6J | Balb/cJ | LP.RIII |
| C57BL/10 ScSn | CBA | WB.Re |
| NZB/WEHI | DBA/1J | 129J |
| SJL/WEHI | A/J | C3H |

Resistant mice had an $LD_{50}$ of about $5 \times 10^5$, while susceptible strains showed an $LD_{50}$ of about $5 \times 10^3$.  C57B1/10 and
BALB/c were chosen for detailed study of genetics and mechanisms of resistance.  Methods have been described elsewhere
(1,2).
        BALB/c x C57BL)$F_1$ were relatively resistant.  (BALB/c x
C57BL)$F_1$  x  C57BL)$N_1$  backcrosses  were  96%  resistant  and
[(BALB/c x C57B1)$F_1$ x BALB/c]$N_1$ backcross was 52% resistant,
showing a single gene or closely linked group of genes (2).
(BALB/c x C57BL)$F_2$ were 79% resistant, confirming this estimate (1).  Furthermore (CBA x BALB/c)$F_1$ were fully susceptible, showing that there was no complementation between
these two susceptible strains and that they had the same
genetics with respect to listeria resistance.  We have named
this gene Lr for listeria resistance, since it differs from
host  resistance  genes  for  other  intracellular  bacteria,
Salmonella and Brucella (9 and below), thus having some
functional specificity, although probably not immunolo-gical
specificity.
        No linkage has yet been established for Lr.  Linkage to
H-2, Ig and to 9 other genes listed in Table 2 have been excluded (2).  There was no difference in the response of male
and female mice.
        When listeria organisms are injected I/V they are rap-
idly phagocytosed by the reticuloendothelial system, mainly
in the liver and spleen.  Ninety percent are trapped in the
liver and could be seen in the Kupffer cells by light or
electron microscopy within 3 hours of injection (2).  Resistant and susceptible strains showed no difference in numbers
of viable Listeria in livers and spleens at this time.  Subsequently the growth of Listeria in the resistant strain was
slower, especially in the liver, leading to a ten fold

Table 2.  Known mouse genes excluded for linkage to listeria
          resistance (Lr) gene (2).

| Gene | Chromosome | System Studied |
|------|-----------|----------------|
| H-2 | 17 | Backcross, congenics on resistant and susceptible backgrounds |
| Ig | ? | Backcross |
| H-1 | 7 | Congenics on resistant |
| H-3 | 2 | backgrounds |
| H-4 | 7 | |
| H-7 | ? | |
| H-8 | ? | |
| Hc | 2 | Congenics on resistant background |
| Thy-1 | 9 | Congenics on resistant and susceptible background |
| Coat Colour | | |
| B | 4 | Backcrosses |
| C | 7 | |

difference in bacterial numbers between resistant and susceptible mice by 24 hours.  (Compare intact BALB/c and B10-
D2, which behave like C57B1, in Figure 1).  Acquired immunity can be measured by the down turn in bacterial numbers
during infection, by the ability to adoptively transfer
immunity, and by the appearance of delayed type hypersensitivity (DTH).  All these occurred at 2-3 days in resistant
and 3-5 days in susceptible mice (1).  However, once immunity was established there was no deficiency in the BALB/c
mice, either in resistance to subsequent challenge ($LD_{50}$ in
BALB/c and C57BL/10 mice surviving infection 1 month earlier
was $2 \times 10^6$ and $5 \times 10^6$ respectively) or in their ability to
adoptively transfer immunity (1).

It appears then that the critical events determining
survival or death of the mouse may occur in the first 24-48
hours.  To test whether these were independent of acquired
immunity, i.e. of T lymphocytes, chimeric mice were prepared.  Mice of the BALB/c or H-2 congenic but resistant strain
B10D2 were neonatally thymectomized ($NNT_x$) and received

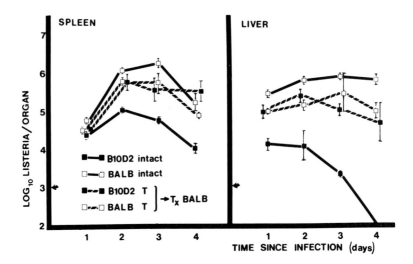

Figure 1. Growth of Listeria monocytogenes in the spleen
(left) and liver (right) of intact BALB/c or B10D2 mice or
in neonatally thymectomized BALB/c mice reconstituted with
thymocytes from BALB/c or B10D2. $10^3$ listeria organisms
were injected I/V. Each point represents the geometric mean
and standard deviation of 4 mice.

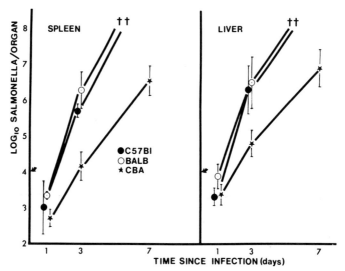

Figure 2. Growth of Salmonella typhimurium in spleens
(left) and livers (right) of C57BL/10, BALB/c and CBA mice
after $10^5$ organisms were injected I/V. Each point represents the geometric mean and standard deviation of 5 mice.
C57B1/10 and BALB/c mice were rapidly killed.

weekly intraperitoneal injections of 100 x $10^6$ thymocytes
for 6 weeks, while receiving tetracycline in their drinking
water. Antibiotics were then withdrawn and the mice challenged with 1 x $10^3$ <u>Listeria</u>. In Figure 1, which shows
chimeras based on $NNT_x$ BALB/c, it may be seen that the
growth of <u>Listeria</u> in the chimeras followed that of intact
BALB/c rather than B10D2, regardless of the source of T
lymphocytes. Subsequently it was checked by adoptive
transfer of immunity using the chimeric mice as donors of
spleen lymphocytes, that T lymphocytes in the chimeric mice
had indeed become immune during infection.

Although the difference between the resistant and susceptible strains thus does not involve the specific immune
response, it is apparently functionally specific. Figure 2
shows that while CBA mice were relatively resistant to
<u>Salmonella typhimurium</u>, both BALB/c and C57BL/10 were sus-
ceptible. Another experiment showed no difference in growth
of <u>Brucella abortus</u> in spleen and liver of BALB/c or C57BL/
10 mice for the first 14 days of infection. Both these
bacteria grow predominantly within the macrophages.

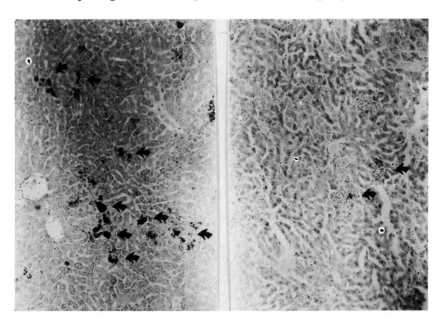

<u>Figure 3</u>. Foci of infection in livers of BALB/c (left) and
C57BL/10 (right) mice 16 hours after injection of $10^8$
listeria organisms. Foci (arrowed) comprise polymorphs surrounding Kupffer cells packed with organisms and are more
numerous in BALB/c. Magnification 100 X. Gram strain.

To try to localize the early events of the response to
Listeria, the cellular response was monitored by blood
smears and histology of the spleen and liver. C57BL/10 mice
showed a marked rise in monocytes in the blood within 24
hours of infection, while the BALB/c mice showed a predominantly polymorph response. In the liver and spleen, however, both strains mounted a strong polymorph response 24
hours post infection. In the liver these could be seen
clustered around the foci of infecting bacteria which, at
the high dose necessary in order to see them in sections,
packed the cytoplasm of Kupffer cells. Figure 3 shows that
there were many more of these foci in BALB/c than in C57BL/
10 mice. Whether or not non-resident macrophages and monocytes play a role in determining the numbers of these foci,
we are not able to tell from these studies. Certainly
incoming monocytes did not form a significant portion of the
population in the inflammatory foci until 3 or 4 days post
infection.

ACKNOWLEDGEMENT

This work is supported by the National Health and
Medical Research Council of Australia.

REFERENCES

1.    Cheers, C., Mandel, T.E., and McKenzie, I.F.C.    In
      Function and Structure of the Immune System.    W.
      Muller-Rucholtz and H.K. Muller-Hernelink (eds).    New
      York: Plenum Press, p. 703, 1978.
2.    Cheers, C., and McKenzie, I.F.C.    Infect. Immun. 19:
      755, 1978.
3.    Hirst, R.G., and Wallace, M.E.    Infect. Immun. 14:475,
      1976.
4.    Levy-Leblond, E., Oth, D., and Dupuy, J.M.    J.Immunol.
      122:1359, 1979.
5.    McDevitt, H.O., Oldstone, M.B.A., and Pinkus, T.
      Transplant Rev. 19:209, 1974.
6.    Mitchell, G.F.    Adv. Immunol. 28, 1980 (in press).
7.    Mitsuyama, M., Takeya, K., Nomoto, K., and Shimatori,
      S. J. gen. Microbiol. 10:165, 1978.
8.    North, R.J.   In Mechanisms of Cell Mediated Immunity.
      R.T. McClusky and S. Cohen (eds).   New York, John Wiley
      and Soons, p. 185, 1974.
9.    Plant, J., and Glynn, A.A.    Clin.exp.Immunol. 37:1,
      1979.
10.   Tatsukawa, K., Mitsuyama, M., Takeya, K., and Nomoto,
      K. J.gen.Microbiol. 115:161, 1979.

## DISCUSSION

O'Brien: Does Cheers have any idea where the Lr is located; has she looked at recombinant inbred strains?

Cheers: We expect later on to have a look at the recombinant inbreds.

O'Brien: I want to verify Cheer's remark that antibody has never been shown to be important in terms of Listeria immunity by making the comment that the xid mice I mentioned earlier, both males and females, are equally resistant to Listeria infection.

Wake: Would Cheers tell us whether there are any strain differences in specific immune resistance to Listeria?

Cheers: Not that we can detect. The specific immune response appears to be the same in the C57BL/6 and in the Balb/c. We have measured this in terms of $LD_{50}$, of mice surviving a sublethal infection, and we have also measured it by adoptive transfer, where we have looked at the extent of protection over a period of time after transfer of the cells. We have also titrated the numbers of cells required to adoptively transfer immunity; by these criteria, there is no strain difference.

Mogensen: Cheers said that there were no sex differences in her system. Has she tested the $F_1$ generation males and females in resistant male x female crosses?

Cheers: Yes. We have also tested the backcrosses, and they all behave the same way.

Mogensen: I say this because her intermediate resistance in her $F_1$ generation might be this random-X inactivation, if it were X-linked.

Cheers: No, resistance is the same in the $F_1$'s; it is also the same in the backcrosses.

CELLULAR MECHANISMS OF GENETICALLY DETERMINED RESISTANCE TO
LISTERIA MONOCYTOGENES

Patricia A.L. Kongshavn, Chitra Sadarangani
and Emil Skamene

Montreal General Hospital Research Institute
and
Department of Physiology,
McGill University
Montreal, Quebec, Canada

## INTRODUCTION

The murine model of host resistance to infection with the intracellular bacterial pathogen, Listeria monocytogenes (L. monocytogenes), has been established as a model of an acute bacterial infection in which host resistance is brought about by a cellular form of immunity (1,2). Resistance to infection is provided initially by fixed macrophages (3), such as the Kupffer cells, but it is the bactericidally activated macrophage, generated from an immature precursor during the course of an infection, that provides the crucial antibacterial protection (4). From studies in athymic mice, it is apparent that the production of this cell can be stimulated by T cell independent mechanisms (5-8), although the most efficient mechanism of activation is undoubtedly that mediated by T cells once they have become sensitized (9-12). T cells emerge in detectable numbers some time after the second day of infection (12) so that the early (0-48 hour) response of the host is T cell independent. This is normally followed by a T cell dependent phase of macrophage activation which is responsible for the rapid elimination of bacteria seen over the next 3-4 days during the normal course of events. Thus, during the early phase of the anti-listerial response, any protection generated in the host is due to T cell independent mechanisms of macrophage activation, that is, to "natural immunity" using this term in a broad sense.

Recent studies from our laboratory (13,14) and elsewhere (15,16,17) have shown that genetically-determined differences in resistance to infection with L. monocytogenes exist amongst various inbred strains of mice. This trait is apparently controlled by a single, autosomal, dominant non H-2-linked gene (or a closely-linked gene cluster) termed Lr (13,16,17). The work to be described here was done to analyse the cellular basis for the observed genetically-deter-

149

mined differences in host resistance to listeriosis. The
C57BL mouse was selected as representative of a Listeria-
resistant strain and the A/J mouse as a Listeria-sensitive
strain.

Our studies were commenced with an analysis of the various facets of host defense against infection with L. monocytogenes elicited in the sensitive A/J (A) and resistant
C57BL/6 (B6) mouse strains using the methods and materials
already described (14).

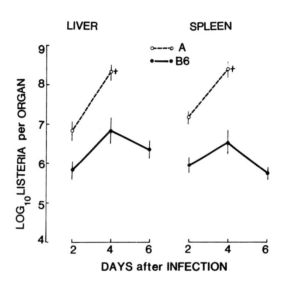

Figure 1. Growth curves of L. monocytogenes following primary challenge with 4 x 10$^4$ CFU organisms in A (o---o) and B6
(●——●) strain mice. Each point represents mean of 6-8 mice
± s.e.m. † denotes 4 of 6 mice died by day 4.

First, the bacterial growth kinetics in the spleen and
liver were compared in both strains over a wide range of infective doses. Differences in bacterial growth kinetics
develop progressively between the strains as the inoculating
dose is increased (14). This point is well illustrated in
Figure 1, which shows the bacterial proliferation in the
livers and spleens of A and B6 strain hosts infected with 4
x 10$^4$ colony forming units (CFU) Listeria. As can be observed, with this dose of Listeria (lethal for the A strain),
bacterial growth is at least two logs higher in the A than
in the B6 strain host. This marked difference in bacterial

growth kinetics is already seen by day 2, during the T cell independent phase of the response. Listeria-resistant B6 strain mice, furthermore, exhibit a greatly enhanced ability to clear Listeria challenge in a secondary response, and their genetic advantage is also obvious in the adoptive transfer of resistance to naive recipients using Listeria-immune splenocytes (14).

From these experiments it could safely be concluded that the anti-listerial response of the resistant B6 strain mouse was clearly superior but formal proof was still lacking as to which of the two cell types, the T cell or the macrophage, involved in anti-listerial resistance, was being influenced by the Lr gene. Accordingly, experiments were designed to test this point, using the adoptive transfer technique in which Listeria-immune T cells from sensitive or resistant type donors were tested for their ability to adoptively protect naive sensitive or resistant recipients against listerial infection, by activating the macrophages of the recipients. Since T cell-macrophage cooperation requires H-2 compatibility (18), A and B10.A strains were used for this study. B10.A, like B6, strain mice carry the allele expressing high resistance to Listeria. In these experiments, mice of both strains were inoculated with splenocytes from 7-day immune A or B10.A strain donors, following challenge 2 hours previously with 1 x $10^4$ CFU Listeria. The number of bacteria in the spleens of the recipients was determined 48 hours later. The results of these experiments (19) are summarized in Table 1.


Table 1. Ability of Listeria-immune T cells from B10.A or A strain donors to adoptively protect B10.A or A strain naive recipients. Donors were primed 7 days previously with 1 x $10^3$ CFU Listeria. Each recipient received half an organ equivalent of splenocytes (non-adherent fraction).


| Donor Strain (Immune T Cells) | Recipient Strain (Macrophage Response) | Protection |
|---|---|---|
| A | A | + |
| A | B10.A | +++ |
| B10.A | A | + |
| B10.A | B10.A | +++ |

As can be observed (Table 1), both A (sensitive) and
B10.A (resistant) strain Listeria-immune T cells are able to
activate macrophages in the naive recipient and provide some
protection against listerial infection.   However, much better protection is obtained when the B10.A rather than the A
strain recipient is used.   For example, transfer of A type T
cells into an A strain recipient gives some protection, but
the same A strain T cells transferred into a B10.A recipient
gives much greater protection.   Thus, it is the macrophages
in the B10.A strain host that are the cell component responsible for providing the enhanced anti-listerial resistance.
This finding is further supported by the earlier observation
that differences in anti-listerial resistance are already
detectable by the second day of infection, during the T cell
independent phase of the response (Fig. 1).   Thus, the gene
controlling anti-listerial resistance is expressed phenotypically in the response of the mononuclear phagocyte system
(MPS) to infection with L. monocytogenes.

In order to discover more about how the Lr gene was
actually being expressed in the macrophage response to this
infection, we compared the characteristics of the MPS in the
two strains.   In these studies, we used the early, T cell
independent phase of the response, in order to simplify interpretation of the results.   Figure 2 depicts the normal
sequence of events leading to macrophage activation and the
next section details some of the steps in this activation
sequence that have been compared in Listeria-sensitive and
resistant strains.

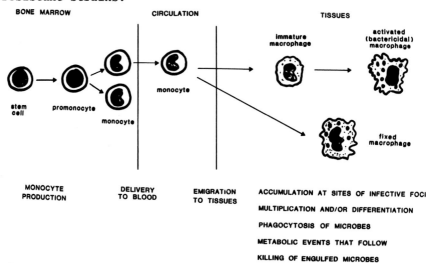

Figure 2.   Response to Mononuclear Phagocyte System (MPS) to
Infection.

   The total bone marrow cellularity is about double in
the Listeria-resistant strain. Furthermore, autoradiograph-
ic studies done in collaboration with Galsworthy indicate
that in the B10.A strain there is a marked decrease in the
generation time of monocyte precursors (20) following stimulation with a saline extract of Listeria monocytogenes (21),
suggesting that there may be an accelerated production of
monocytes and delivery to the blood following listerial
infection in the Listeria-resistant strain. This is further
corroborated by the observation that injection of such saline extract elicits a dramatic monocytosis 48 hours later in
the blood of the Listeria-resistant mouse, whereas the Listeria-sensitive mouse responded not at all (20). Similar
results are seen following infection with live Listeria
(Fig. 3).

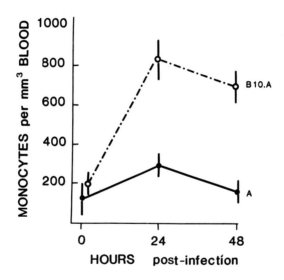

Figure 3. Monocyte kinetics in A and B10.A strain mice following primary intravenous infection with 1 x 10$^4$ CFU Listeria. Mean of 6-8 mice ± s.e.m.


   The chemotactic ability of thioglycollate-induced peritoneal macrophages to respond to endotoxin activated mouse
serum (EAMS) has also been compared in both mouse strains by
Stevenson (see this volume). Whilst the macrophages of the
Listeria-resistant B10.A strain exhibited very good migration, the Listeria-sensitive A strain macrophages exhibited

only low baseline levels of chemotaxis (22). Thus, the
ability of mononuclear phagocytes to emigrate to the tissues
appears to be better in the resistant mouse strain.

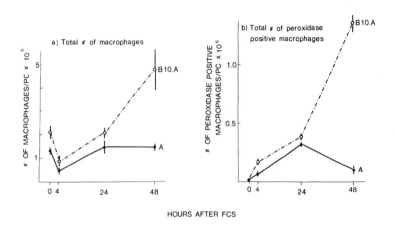

HOURS AFTER FCS

**Figure 4.** Kinetics of macrophage accumulation in peritoneal
cavity of A and B10.A strain hosts following intraperitoneal
injection of 1 ml fetal calf serum (FCS). Total and differential counts were performed according to standard techniques and the percentage of peroxidase positive cells enumerated using the method of Kaplow (23).

The ability of mononuclear phagocytes to accumulate at
the site of an inflammatory stimulus, fetal calf serum
(FCS), introduced into the peritoneal cavity for convenience, was also examined (Pietrangeli, unpublished observation). As shown in Figure 4, the accumulation of macrophages in the peritoneal cavity is much greater in the B10.A
than in the A strain mice, 48 hours after introducing the
FCS. Very recently, essentially the same experiment was repeated but using live Listeria as the inflammatory stimulus
and similar results obtained.

All of these results, thus provide strong circumstant-
ial evidence that the enhanced anti-listerial resistance of
the C57BL mouse could be due to the ability of these mice to
produce and mobilize adequate numbers of young mononuclear
phagocytes very promptly at the site of the infection during
the early phase of the response.

If this were the case, one would predict that the early anti-listerial response of the resistant, but not the sensitive, strain would be highly radiosensitive.  Accordingly, the sensitivity of the anti-listerial response of both strains to ionizing radiation (900 rads) was examined (24).

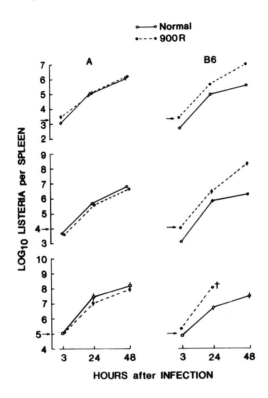

Figure 5.  Growth of Listeria in the spleens of normal (solid line) and 900R-irradiated (dotted line) A and B6  strain mice infected with $3 \times 10^3$, $10^4$ and $10^5$ CFU Listeria respectively.  Mean of 6-8 mice per group ± s.e.m. † denotes death of mice before 48 hours.

As can be observed, iradiation has no effect on the early phase of the anti-listerial response of the Listeria-sensitive A strain mice, even when very high doses of Listeria are administered.  In contrast, irradiation markedly enhances the bacterial growth in the Listeria-resistant B6 strain mice, the difference between irradiated and non-irradiated mice becoming more pronounced with increasing numbers of organisms injected. In fact, the irradiated B6 strain mouse has now become more susceptible to the growth of Listeria than the A strain mouse! The effect of irradiation is present even by 3 hours post-infection, indicating that a radiosensitive cell plays a role very early in the anti-listerial response in the resistant host. This effector cell mediating anti-listerial resistance is highly radio-sensitive (less than 200R) and appears to be of bone marrow origin (24). Presumably, therefore, it is a monocytic precursor, such as a promonocyte or monoblast.

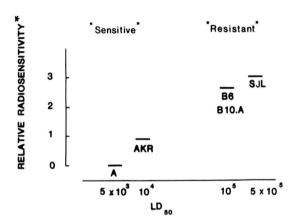

*Difference in $\log_{10}$ Listeria per spleen between normal and irradiated (900R) hosts infected with $5 \times 10^4$ CFU.

Figure 6. Relationship between radiosensitivity of early anti-listerial response and resistance of mouse strain to listerial infection.

We have recently extended this study and examined the radiosensitivity of the anti-listerial response in other mouse strains, namely, the AKR strain which is relatively sensitive to listerial infection, and the SJL strain which is a resistant type of host. When one compares the relationship between the radiosensitivity of the early anti-listerial response (as measured by the difference in the 48-hour CFU Listeria per spleen between normal and 900R irradiated hosts) and the relative sensitivity or resistance of the mouse strain to infection as determined by the median lethal dose ($LD_{50}$) shown on the abscissa, one can see that there is a very clear relationship between the two (Figure 6). The response of the Listeria-sensitive mouse is radio-resistant; that of Listeria-resistant mouse is radiosensitive and, the more resistant the mouse, the greater the radiosensitivity of its early anti-listerial response.

Table 2. Characteristics of mononuclear phagocyte system in Listeria-sensitive and -resistant strains.

| | B10.A | A |
|---|---|---|
| 1. Bone Marrow Cellularity | | |
| High | + | - |
| 2. Inflammatory Response of MPS to Sterile Irritants (48 Hr.) | | |
| Increase in Peritoneal Macrophages | + | - |
| Increase in Immature (Peroxidase Positive) Macrophages | + | - |
| Chemotactic Response to EAMS | + | - |
| 3. Early Response (0-48 Hr.) of MPS to Listeria | | |
| Sensitivity to Ionizing Radiation | + | - |
| Blood Monocyte Response to Infection | + | - |

Table 2 summarizes the essential differences we have observed between the Listeria-sensitive and -resistant mouse strains, particularly those seen during the early anti-listerial response. From the data, it is suggested that the enhanced anti-listerial resistance of mice bearing the high resistance allele is due to a vigorous early response of the mononuclear phagocyte system to infection with Listeria; in other words the Lr gene seems to be expressing itself in some fashion by regulating the production, maturation and/or

activation of mononuclear phagocytes in response to L. monocytogenes.

This leads to the last point to be discussed, namely,
whether the Lr gene is being expressed (i) as an autonomous
property of the mononuclear phagocyte per se, or (ii) by
some factor in the micro-environment of the hematopoietic
tissues, imposing the property of high or low anti-listerial
resistance on the mononuclear phagocyte as it develops and
carries out its function. This question was answered by
preparing radiation bone marrow chimeras between A and B10.A
strain mice and testing their anti-listerial resistance
(25).
Chimeras were prepared by lethal irradiation and repopulation with syngeneic or allogeneic bone marrow. After
waiting 9 weeks, by which time the entire lymphoreticular
system should have been replaced by cells of donor origin,
radiation chimeras from each group were tested for chimerism. Thus, cytotoxicity tests were performed on spleen
cells (SC) and peritoneal exudate cells (PEC) from the chimeras and normal control hosts using appropriate allo-anti-
sera against the LyM-1.1 and -1.2 alloantigens which differ
between the A and B10.A strains (26). The great majority,
if not all, of the PEC and SC were donor derived (25).
Anti-listerial resistance was then measured in the
radiation bone marrow chimeras on day 3. As can be observed
in Figure 7, the degree of anti-listerial resistance obtained in the chimeras corresponds to that exhibited by the
mouse strain of the host not to that of the mouse strain
which provided the macrophage precursors (bone marrow cells)
used to reconstitute the chimeras. This is demonstrated by
the fact that anti-listerial resistance remains superior in
the B10.A strain host repopulated with A strain bone marrow
(A → B) and inferior in the A strain host repopulated with
B10.A strain marrow (B → A). Thus, the superior anti-listerial response of the resistant strain macrophages is apparently not due to an inherent property of these cells per se,
but rather it is the environment of the host in which the
stem cell re-develops into the mononuclear phagocyte that
confers a high level of anti-listerial resistance onto these
cells.
To conclude, it appears that the gene determining relative resistance or susceptibility of different mouse strains to infection with Listeria is expressed phenotypically
in the environment of the host, exerting its influence during maturation, from bone marrow progenitors, of the macrophages that provide the anti-bacterial activity in this infection. In the Listeria-resistant host, the Lr gene pro-

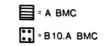

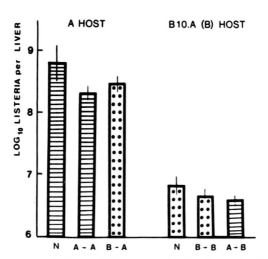

Figure 7. Bacterial proliferation of Listeria in the livers of A and B10.A strain radiation bone marrow chimeric hosts repopulated with A (hatched bars) and B10.A (stipled bars) bone marrow respectively, and normal control hosts (N). Mice were infected intravenously with $5 \times 10^4$ CFU Listeria and the bacterial organ counts performed 3 days later. Each value represents mean of 8 mice ± s.e.m.

duct appears to promote the early arrival of immature macrophages that develop potent anti-bacterial activity, thus producing the high level of anti-listerial resistance seen in these mice.

ACKNOWLEDGEMENT

This work was supported by NIH Contract NO1-CB-84269 and MRC Grants 5448 and 6431.

REFERENCES

1.  Mackaness, G.B.  J.Exp.Med. 116:381, 1962.
2.  Mackaness, G.B.  J.Exp.Med. 129:973, 1969.
3.  Mitsuyama, M., Takeya, K., Nomoto, K., and Shimotori, S.  J.Gen.Microbiol. 106:165, 1978.
4.  North, R.J.  J.Exp.Med. 132:521, 1970.
5.  Emmerling, P., Finger, H., and Bockemuhl, J.  Infect.-Immun. 12:437, 1975.
6.  Cheers, C., and Waller, R.  J.Immunol. 115:844, 1975.
7.  Chan, C., Kongshavn, P.A.L., and Skamene, E.  Immunol. 32:529, 1977.
8.  Takaya, K., Shimotori, T., Taniguchi, T., and Nomoto, K.  J.Gen.Microbiol. 100:373, 1977.
9.  North, R.J.  J.Exp.Med. 138:342, 1973.
10. Takaya, K., Shimotori, T., Taniguchi, T., and Nomoto, K.  J.Gen.Microbiol. 100:373, 1977.
11. Lane, F.C., and Unanue, E.R.  J.Exp.Med. 135:1104, 1972.
12. Zinkernagel, R.M., Blanden, R.B., and Langman, R.E. J.Immunol. 112:496, 1974.
13. Skamene, E., Kongshavn, P.A.L., and Sachs, D. J.Infect.Dis. 139:228, 1979.
14. Skamene, E., and Kongshavn, P.A.L.  Infect.Immun. 25:345, 1979.
15. Robson, H.G., and Vas, S.I.  J.Infect.Dis. 126:378, 1972,
16. Cheers, C., and McKenzie, I.F.C.  Infect.Immun. 19:755, 1978.
17. Cheers, C. this volume.
18. Farr, A.G., Dorf, M.E., and Unanue, E.R.  Proc.Natl.-Acad.Sci.USA. 74:3542, 1977.
19. Kongshavn, P.A.L., and Skamene, E.  J.Res. 24:51a, 1978.
20. Galsworthy, S.B., Sadarangani, C., and Kongshavn, P.A.L. Unpublished observation.
21. Galsworthy, S.B., Gurofsky, S.M., and Murray, R.G.E. Infect.Immun. 15:500, 1977.
22. Stevenson, M., Kongshavn, P.A.L., and Skamene, E. this volume.
23. Kaplow, L.S. Blood 26:215, 1965.
24. Sadarangani, C., Skamene, E., and Kongshavn, P.A.L. Infect.Immun. 28:381, 1980.
25. Kongshavn, P.A.L., Sadarangani, C., and Skamene, E. Cell. Immunol. (in press).
26. Tonkonogy, S.L., and Winn, H.J.  Immunogenetics 5:57, 1977.

## DISCUSSION

Cudkowicz:    I am certain that most of us want you to define this "environment" a little further.

Kongshavn:    You understand, of course, we do not actually know what the environment really is.  It is very intriguing and we do have some data which may, or may not, be relevant. This could be an epiphenomenon.  An observation made by us a few years ago was that splenectomized mice were very resistant to Listeria infection.  We splenectomized our resistant and sensitive mouse strains, and then followed the growth of Listeria over 48 hours in the two sets of splenectomized hosts.  We found that the curves of bacterial proliferation were almost superimposable.  In other words, removal of the spleen seems to have turned resistant mice into sensitive mice.  Also, splenectomized A strain (sensitive) mice have now become resistant and these mice have also become radiosensitive in their response to Listeria (like the normal B6 host).  One can reverse this radiation effect by reconstituting them with syngeneic bone marrow.  My own view is that there is something in the spleen which inhibits the monocytes or stem cell → promonocyte → activated macrophage differentiation.  In the resistant strain, normally there is less of this inhibitory effect of the spleen, and more of it in the sensitive strain.  So, it appears that the spleen or some splenic factor is the "environment" that I was talking about.  But this might well be an entirely different phenomenon.

Rosenstreich:    Did Kongshavn ascertain sensitivity and resistance in re-irradiated bone marrow chimeras?

Kongshavn:    No, but we think it should be done.

Shearer:    It was not clear to me how Kongshavn typed her chimeras in the last experiments.  Was it by Ly typing?

Kongshavn:    LyM, yes.

Shearer:    Is that typing for a T cell or a monocyte?

Kongshavn:    It is present in hematopoietic tissues, but we actually looked at spleen cells and peritoneal exudate cells.  The LyM-1.1 allotype is present in the A strain and the LyM-1.2 in the B10.A.  And it is on about 75% of spleen cells and peritoneal exudate cells.  When we did the cytotoxicity assay with the anti-LyM-1.1, for example, about 75%

of the cells were killed in the A and in the A repopulated with A, and in the B10.A repopulated with A.   With both antisera, we got the results that we would expect.

Shearer:   You are concluding that there was monocyte replacement by the donor-derived stem cells?   Is that so?

Kongshavn:   That is correct.   In the mouse the Kupffer cells are usually replaced within 3 weeks.   We waited 9 weeks to do our experiments, so I think that it would be fair to say that, by that time, the mononuclear phagocyte system had been replaced entirely.   We also examined NK activity, which we know goes with the donor, and not with the host, in these chimeras.   I was able to show that the NK activity had gone with the donor marrow (just the opposite of what we found with Listeria).   So those are the two items of evidence for our having, in fact, the chimera we claim.

Cudkowicz:   I would be cautious about that conclusion, because Kongshavn has used A/J mice.   I think the data of Haller (I checked this earlier) were obtained with A/Sn mice.   The two sublines do differ with respect to NK activity.   So, maybe that part needs a bit of caution.

Kongshavn:   Perhaps, but then both antisera gave the appropriate results.

Participant:   I want to get one point straight as I do not know if it was brought out.   Is the gene Kongshavn has been looking at in the A mice, and the gene in the Balb/c that Cheers was discussing, the same gene?   Has anyone looked at the $F_1$ to see if these two genes might complement each other?   Balb/c x A?

Kongshavn:   No.   I am not at all sure it is the same gene.

Bennett:   When (B6 x DBA/2)$F_1$ (BDF$_1$) hybrid mice are lethally irradiated, they do not manifest greater susceptibility to the growth of bacteria during the first 2 days.   Has Kongshavn tested any other $F_1$ hybrids to ascertain whether there is more than a mere quantitative increase in production of monocytes after the first 2 or 3 days?

Kongshavn:   No, we have not tested the radiosensitivity of other $F_1$ hybrids.

Lopez:   Some of the inbred strains of mice that Kongshavn finds susceptible are known to have complement deficiences or deficiences in chemotactic factor. The A mouse, I think, is one of those. Some of the other sensitive mice are not. Has she examined the monocytosis and recruitment of monocytes in some of the other susceptible mice to show whether similar patterns are involved?

Kongshavn: No, we have not looked at it, but we are aware of this work. What I have reported here could, in fact, be an epiphenomenon. One might also explain the results on the basis of, say, lack of chemotactic ability; a C5 deficiency. That is possible; we cannot rule it out, yet.

Cheers: We compared the B10.D2 (old and new) which differ in respect to a C5 deficiency but we did not find gross differences in susceptibility and resistance to Listeria. There are subtle differences that other people have reported, but perhaps these have quite a different mechanism.

Kumar: This query is devoted to Skamene and Kongshavn. I want to find out if any formal genetic studies have been done to ascertain whether the Lr gene and the monocyte-stimulating response that they see, are linked as related phenomena.

Skamene: The monocyte-stimulating response is under unigenic control thus resembling the genetic resistance to Listeria (Stevenson et al., this volume). The strain distribution of Listeria-resistant strains corresponds to that of strains with effective monocyte-stimulating response. The formal linkage of these two traits in segregating populations is under investigation.

# GENETIC CONTROL OF NATURAL RESISTANCE TO RICKETTSIA TSUTSUGAMUSHI INFECTION IN MICE

Michael G. Groves, David L. Rosenstreich
and Joseph V. Osterman

From the Department of Rickettsial Diseases,
Walter Reed Army Institute of Research,
Washington, D.C. 20012
and the
Laboratory of Microbiology and Immunology
National Institute of Dental Research
National Institutes of Health
Bethesda, Maryland 20014.

## INTRODUCTION

We became interested in natural resistance while performing intraperitoneal (IP) 50% mouse lethal dose ($MLD_{50}$) determinations with the Gilliam strain of Rickettsia tsutsugamushi, the causative agent of scrub typhus. Death patterns with this strain were very erratic and could not be related to the dosage given (Table 1). Because the Gilliam titrations were done in outbred Wrc: (ICR) mice, we felt that one possible explanation for their unpredictability was the existence of natural resistance in some of the mice.

Table 1. Intraperitoneal titration of the Gilliam strain in Wrc: (ICR) mice.

| Dilution of 20% infected yolk sac | Deaths/Total |
|---|---|
| $10^{-3}$ | 1/5 |
| $10^{-4}$ | 4/5 |
| $10^{-5}$ | 5/5 |
| $10^{-6}$ | 0/5 |
| $10^{-7}$ | 2/5 |
| $10^{-8}$ | 2/5 |
| $10^{-9}$ | 1/5 |

<u>Surveys of inbred mice</u>:  In our initial studies on natural resistance, we surveyed 16 strains of inbred mice for susceptibility to IP Gilliam infection and found resistance to be widespread (5).  Six strains were resistant, nine susceptible, and one strain could not be classified resistant or susceptible (A/J).  Subsequent studies have brought the number of resistant strains to 15 and susceptible strains to 13 (7) (Table 2).  The pattern of resistant and susceptible strains does not corespond to the distribution of susceptibility reported for other infectious agents in inbred mice. Also, Gilliam susceptibility was not associated with the <u>H-2</u> holotypes of the mouse strains studied.

Table 2..  Response of inbred mouse strains to intraperitoneal challenge with Rickettsia tsutsugamushi strain Gilliam.

| Resistant strains | | Susceptible strains | |
|---|---|---|---|
| AKR/J[1] | C57BL/10J[2] | A/HeJ[1] | CBA/J[1] |
| AU/SsJ[2] | C57L/J[1] | BRVR/N | DBA/1J[1] |
| BALB/cDub[1] | 1/LnJ[2] | BSVS/N | DBA/2J[1] |
| BALB/cJ[1] | P/J[2] | C3H/HeDub[1] | RIII/AnN |
| BDP/J[2] | PL/J[2] | C3H/HeJ[1] | SJL/J[1] |
| CBA/HT6J[2] | RF/J | C3H/HeN[1] | WB/ReJ[2] |
| CE/J[2] | SWR/J[1] | C3H/St[1] | |
| C57BL/6J[1] | | | |

[1] Groves and Osterman, 1978
[2] Groves et al. submitted for publication

Two of the more surprising aspects of the surveys were the magnitude and specificity of resistance.  Resistant mice survived IP challenges of greater than $10^5$ $MID_{50}$ while susceptible mice succumbed to challenges of less than $10^1$ $MID_{50}$.  Also, when six strains of <u>R. tsutsugamushi</u> other than Gilliam (Kostival, Karp, Kato, TA678, TA686, and TA716) were used to challenge resistant and susceptible mouse strains,

only the Kostival strain, which is antigenically related to
the Gilliam strain, demonstrated a variable virulence that
was related to mouse strain (Table 3).

Table 3.   Response of inbred mouse strains to selected
           Rickettsia tsutsugamushi strains

| R. tsutsugamushi strain | Response observed in inbred mouse strains |
| --- | --- |
| Karp, Kato | Susceptible |
| TA678, TA686, TA716 | Resistant |
| Gilliam, Kostival | Variable depending on mouse strain |

Genetic analysis:  A genetic analysis of rickettsial resistance using BALB/c (resistant) and C3H/He (susceptible) mice
in $F_1$, $F_2$, and backcross experiments yielded simple
Mendelian ratios that indicated resistance was dominant and
controlled by a single, autosomal gene.  The study of three
additional $F_1$ crosses between resistant and susceptible mice
also supported this conclusion.  We designated the gene Ric,
with r and s representing the resistant and susceptible alleles respectively.

Mapping studies:  Armed with the knowledge that Gilliam susceptibility was controlled by a single gene, we initiated
mapping studies.  These studies were made possible through
collaboration with Dr. Benjamin A. Taylor of the Jackson
Laboratory, Bar Harbor, Maine.  Using two sets of recombinant inbred (RI) mouse strains (BXD and BXH) (1), the Ric
locus was mapped to Chromosome 5 (Table 4) (7).  The results
of the BXH RI mice studies indicated that Ric was closely
linked to the retinal degeneration (rd) locus.  This linkage
was confirmed by a backcross analysis.  The recombination
frequency between Ric and rd was estimated to be 0.015.  Because of the closeness of the two loci, attempts to place
Ric in relation to rd on the Chromosome 5 gene map were equivocal using three point crosses.  However, analysis of the
C57BL/6Ty-le congenic strain indicated that Ric was proximal
to rd and that the correct gene order was probably Pgm-1 - W
- Ric - rd - Gus.

Table 4. Recombinations between Ric and Chromosome 5
markers in the BXD and BXH recombinant inbred strains.

| RI strain | Chromosome 5 marker | Recombination with Ric (crossovers/total strains) |
|-----------|---------------------|---------------------------------------------------|
| BXD | Pgm-1 | 10/25 |
| BXH | rd | 0/13 |
|  | Pgm-1 | 2/13 |
|  | Gus | 4/13 |

**Gilliam-induced acute death:**  The intravenous (IV) inoculation of mice with large doses of certain Rickettsia spp. will
cause death in less than four hours;  this acute death syndrome (ADS) has been termed the "toxic effect".  This is considered to be a misnomer, however, since toxins capable of
causing rapid deaths in mice have never been described (3).

Toward the end of our genetic mapping studies, one of
our colleagues initiated preliminary experiments on Gilliam-
induced ADS.  To our surprise, C3H/He mice carrying the
Gilliam-susceptible ($Ric^S$) allele were completely resistant to ADS.  A subsequent study of 10 inbred strains equally
divided between $Ric^r$ and $Ric^S$ allele-bearing strains revealed that susceptibility to Gilliam-induced ADS was just
the reverse of susceptibility to IP Gilliam infection (4).
A linkage study of 50 backcross progeny produced no crossovers between ADS susceptibility and the rd locus on Chromosome 5.  Furthermore, backcross mice that survived ADS
challenge succumbed days later to infectious deaths, and
those that were resistant to infection were susceptible to
ADS.  These observations strongly suggest that Ric and the
gene controlling ADS susceptibility are the same.

**Gene mechanism studies:**  Very early in our studies, we lear-
ned that cells from $Ric^r$ and $Ric^S$ allele-bearing mice
supported similar in vitro growth of Gilliam and that there
is no apparent defect in immune recognition in susceptible
mice since they could be protected against IP infection by
prior subcutaneous vaccination with virulent Gilliam organisms (4).

We have subsequently done a number of studies contrasting Gilliam infections in BALB/c ($Ric^r$) and C3H/He ($Ric^s$) mice (6). Following Gilliam infection, C3H/He mice developed rickettsemias sooner and maintained higher rickettsemia levels until death than did BALB/c mice. Furthermore, a much higher percentage of C3H/He mice (30-70%) maintained detectable rickettsemias than did BALB/c mice (0-10%) when they were observed over a one year period. One can speculate that the rickettsemias observed in the C3H/He mice resulted from a more rapid growth of the rickettsiae, a decreased host immune response, or a combination of both. However, our studies of the sequential onset of the systemic humoral and cell mediated immune responses of BALB/c and C3H/He mice infected with Gilliam did not reveal any immunological advantage for the resistant BALB/c mice.

The findings of Natsumme-Sakai et al. (9) prompted us to investigate the role of complement in resistance to Gilliam-induced ADS. They studied the complement (C3) response of six inbred mouse strains to an acute inflammatory reaction and found it to be under genetic control. The distribution of their three high and three low complement responder mice corresponded to the known distribution in inbred strains for $Ric^r$ and $Ric^s$ respectively. Our investigations proved unrewarding, however (4). Serum C3 levels in BALB/c ($Ric^r$) and C3H/He ($Ric^s$) mice challenged IV with Gilliam were comparable. Furthermore, C5 deficient mice and mice depleted of C3 with cobra venom factor from resistant and susceptible backgrounds reacted identically to their normocomplementemic counterparts when assessed for susceptibility to Gilliam-induced ADS.

The failure to find obvious differences in the systemic immune responses of resistant and susceptible mice does not preclude a difference in the local immune response. Indeed, reports of other investigators would indicate that the localized immune reactions at the inoculation site may be one of the controlling factors differentiating lethal and non-lethal rickettsial infections. Kokorin et al. (8) have reported that BALB/c mice can suppress Gilliam proliferation in the peritoneal cavity through the evolution of rickettsiacidal macrophages whereas C3H/He mice cannot. Likewise, Catanzaro et al. (2) in contrasting lethal Karp and non-lethal Gilliam infections in BALB/c mice reported a similar immunologic mechanism was responsible for the observed virulence differences of the two rickettsial strains.

Regardless of the mechanism by which Ric controls resistance, the results of ADS studies would seem to indicate that the controlling event occurs very early in infection.

## REFERENCES

1.  Bailey, D.W.  Transplantation 11:325, 1971.
2.  Cantanzaro, P.J., Shirai, A., Hildebrandt, P.K., and Osterman, J.V. Infect. Immun. 13:861, 1976.
3.  Elisberg, B.L., and Bozeman, F.M.  In Diagnostic Procedures for Viral and Rickettsial Infections.  E.H. Lennette and N.J. Schmidt (eds).  New York: American Public Health Association, Inc. p832, 1969.
4.  Groves, M.G., Eisenberg, G.H.G.Jr., Rosenstreich, D.L., Weatherly, B.S., Weinblatt, A., and Osterman, J.V. Manuscript in preparation.
5.  Groves, M.G., and Osterman, J.V.  Infect. Immun. 19:583, 1978.
6.  Groves, M.G., and Osterman, J.V.  Manuscript in preparation.
7.  Groves, M.G., Rosenstreich, D.L., Taylor, B.A., and Osterman, J.V.  Submitted for publication.
8.  Kokorin, I.N., Kyet, C.D., Kekcheeva, N.G., and Miskarova, E.D.  Acta Virol (Engl.Ed) 20:147, 1976.
9.  Natsuume-Sakai, S., Motonishi, K., and Takahashi, M. Int.Archs Allergy Appl. Immun. 53:269, 1977.

## DISCUSSION

Wake: Does not Groves think this gene (Ric) controls the ability to kill Rickettsia intracellularly?  I say this because with low dose the mouse will survive, whereas with high dose the mouse will be killed by the toxin from Rickettsia.

Groves: I find it difficult to believe.  In my experience these animals die within 2 hours.  It is also hard for me to believe that macrophages kill Rickettsia in 2 hours.  As to the pathology of this, they give rise to a tremendous pulmonary edema;  there is a leakage into the surrounding capillaries in the lung.  The normal architecture of the lungs is distorted leaving an empty clear space.  There occurs a tremendous rise in the hamatocrit.  It all looks very much as if it might be a massive cell death and penetration.  This is not an original idea on my part, but is in the literature.

Wake: You mentioned "toxic death";  do Rickettsia produce a toxin?

**Groves:** No, they have to be viable. Our experiments establish a correlation between irradiation with penetration and the evolution of a toxic death. The penetration index into cells and the ability to cause toxic death parallel each other. As soon as the cells are killed or prevented from penetrating, all toxicity is lost.

**Gavora:** Has Groves considered the possibility of multiple alleles on the one locus he described?

**Groves:** I have not. It does not look like that would be the case.

**Gavora:** If there were more than two alleles at the locus one could possibly have more than one susceptible allele that could modify the toxin response.

# SUSCEPTIBILITY OF (CBA/N X DBA/2)F$_1$ MALE MICE TO INFECTION WITH TYPE 3 STREPTOCOCCUS PNEUMONIAE

D. Briles, M. Nahm, K. Schroer,
P. Baker and J. Davie

The Cellular Immunobiology Unit of the Tumor Institute
Department of Microbiology
and
The Comprehensive Cancer Center
University of Alabama in Birmingham
Birmingham, Alabama
and
Department of Microbiology and Immunology
Washington University School of Medicine
St. Louis, MO 63110
and
National Institute of Allergy and Infectious Diseases
National Institutes of Health
Bethesda, Maryland 20014

Recently it has been shown that mice produce the bulk of their anti-carbohydrate antibody as either IgM or IgG$_3$ (6). The mechanism and the importance of this isotype restriction is not know. It is assumed that anti-carbohydrate antibodies play an important role in the protection against many pathogens, such as Streptococcus pneumoniae (7). This assumption is based largely on studies showing that animals and man can be protected by passive transfer of antibody or immune serum. While this type of approach can readily demonstrate that anti-carbohydrate antibody can be protective, it does not prove that antibody is, in fact, necessary for immunity to the pathogen in question. An alternative way to investigate the importance of anti-carbohydrate antibodies in immunity would be to examine the susceptibility of individuals or animals lacking humoral immunity to carbohydrates. In man, individuals with the X-linked Wiskott-Aldrich Syndrome appear to be defective primarily in their ability to make anti-carbohydrate antibodies and are susceptible to a number of different bacterial and viral infections (2). Unfortunately, as these individuals age they also begin to lose cellular immunity (2). Thus, it is not clear whether the susceptibility of these individuals is the result of a lack of humoral anti-carbohydrate responsiveness or a reduction in their levels of cellular immunity. A more suitable candidate for such studies appears to be the CBA/N mouse. This strain carries an X-linked inability (xid) to produce humoral antibody response to a group of thymus-independent (TI-2) carbohydrate antigens (3). The CBA/N mouse may be unable to make high levels of anti-carbohydrate antibodies in general since, compared to other strains, it makes very low serum levels of IgM and $IgG_3$ immunoglobulin (6). CBA/N mice make nearly normal responses to proteins and hapten protein conjugates, and have relatively normal levels of $IgG_1$, $IgG_{2b}$ and IgA (6).

In order to find out if the CBA/N mouse might be useful in determining the importance of anti-carbohydrate antibodies in immunity to infection we decided to infect mice carrying the xid defect with Type 3 Streptococcal pneumoniae. Our reasons for this choice were two-fold: 1) passive immunity studies in the first half of this century had indicated that anti-SSS-III polysaccharide antibody was of paramount importance in the defense against this pathogen (7); 2) Baker and his collaborators had shown that CBA/N mice fail to respond to SSS-III capsular carbohydrate (1), and would thus be expected to be susceptible to Type 3 pneumococcal infection.

In the studies described below we have demonstrated that mice carrying the xid locus are, in fact, about 1000-fold more susceptible to infection with Type 3 pneumoniae than are normal mice. Mice carrying the xid defect could be protected with hybridoma antibodies to either the pneumococcal cell wall or capsule. Our studies also indicate that naturally occurring antibody may be a major factor in protection against pneumococcal infection.

For our experimental infections we used (CBA/N x DBA/2)$F_1$ (CxD) and (DBA/2 x CBA/N)$F_1$ (DxC) male mice. Since the xid locus of CBA/N mice is on the x chromosome, only those males with CBA/N mothers (i.e., CxD males) have defective anti-carbohydrate responses. The mice were infected i.v. with an isolate of Type III pneumoccocus obtained about 15 years ago from a patient at the Washington University Dental School. In 1978 the culture was mouse passaged three times and strain WU-1 was established from a smooth colony. After an additional mouse passage of strain WU-1 we recently isolated subline WU-2. Both of these sublines were shown to be type 3 by specific antisera. The $LD_{50}$ for each of the two pneumococcal sublines in CxD and DxC males is shown in Table 1.

Although the two sublines differ by 3 logs in their virulence, each of them kills CxD males with about a 1000-fold lower $LD_{50}$ than it kills DxC males. From the data in Table 2, it is clear that deaths caused by strain WU-1 occur as early as two days after infection. Preliminary data with the WU-2 strain indicates even more striking results; for

Table 1.   $LD_{50}$ for Mice With and Without the Defective xid Gene[a]

|  | Mice | |
|---|---|---|
|  | CxD♂ [b] | DxC♂ |
| pneumococcal[a] | | |
| strain | | |
| WU-1 | $10^4$ | $10^7$ |
| WU-2 | $10^1$ | $10^4$ |

[a]Mice were infected i.v. with sublines WU-1 and WU-2 of Streptococcus pneumoniae.
[b]CxD♂ ; male mice with CBA/N mothers and DBA/2 fathers, these mice carry the xid defective gene.   DxC♂; male mice with DBA/2 mothers and CBA/N fathers, these mice do not carry the xid defective gene.

Table 2.   Survival of Mice Infected with S. pneumoniae Sublines WU-1 and WU-2.

|  | Per cent alive | | | |
|---|---|---|---|---|
| Days | $10^5$  Strain WU-1 | | 400 WU-2 | |
| Post Infection | DxC♂ | CxD♂ | DxC♂ | CxD♂ |
| 0 | 100 | 100 | 100 | 100 |
| 2 | 97 | 65 | 100 | 0 |
| 4 | 90 | 35 | 100 | 0 |
| 9 | 90 | 18 | 100 | 0 |

[a]Mice were infected with $10^5$ WU-1 or 400 WU-2.

example, in one recent experiment 6 of 7 CxD males died within 36 hours of infection with 300 colony forming units (CFU) of subline WU-2, whereas none of the five DxC males infected at the same time died within 9 days of infection. These findings indicate that the DxC males, carrying a normal allele at the xid locus, are able to resist death from pneumococcal infection even before it would be possible for them to produce significant amounts of induced antibody. The simplest explanation for this result is that the DxC males are protected by cross-reactive ("naturally" occurring) anti-carbohydrate antibody during the first 1-3 days until a humoral anti-pneumococcal response is produced.

To investigate this possibility we attempted to protect CxD males from fatal pneumococcal infection by pre-treating the infecting dose of pneumococci at 0°C with heat-inactivated normal serum from either CxD or DxC males. The infected CxD males were then injected daily with 0.1 ml volumes of either CxD or DxC male normal mouse serum.

Table 3.  Protection of CxD Mice with Normal Mouse Serum[a]

|  | % CxD♂ Alive | |
| --- | --- | --- |
|  | Protected with NMS from | |
| Strain of | | |
| S. pneumoniae | DxC♂ | CxD♂ |
| WU-1[b] | 70 | 0 |
| WU-2[c] | 64 | 0 |

[a].1 ml normal mouse serum (NMS) per day for days 0-5.
[b]Infected with $10^5$ WU-1 in 0.1 ml NMS, % alive on day 5.
[c]Infected with 400 WU-2 in 0.1 ml NMS, % alive on day 2.

During the incubation step neither normal serum source reduced the number of viable pneumococci, as determined by plating on blood agar. From the data in Table 3 it is apparent that DxC serum, administered as described above, can indeed protect CxD mice from infection with Type III pneumococci. It seems likely that this protection is dependent on naturally occurring antibodies reactive to the pneumococcus. This conclusion is consistent with our observation that DxC males have greater than 20 times as much anti-SSS-III and anti-phosphocholine antibody as CxD males. This conclusion is also supported by our findings that CxD male mice can be protected from a fatal pneumococcal infection by pre-inject-ing them with either an IgM anti-SSS-III hybridoma, antibody CC4-8, or the anti-IgM anti-pneumococcal cell wall carbohyd-rate (anti-PC) hybridoma antibody, PAG-1.

In conclusion, three major points can be made. 1) These data suggest that naturally occurring antibodies play a major role in the protection of DxC males from experiment-al pneumococcal infection. The importance of normal immuno-globulin as a defense against pathogens has long been impli-cated by its usefulness in treating certain agammaglobulin-emias in man. However, our present data provides some of the best evidence that normal immunoglobulin is important in the protection of adult experimental animals. 2) These studies also confirm theories suggesting that anti-carbo-hydrate antibody is necessary for immunity to pneumococcal infection. 3) These studies make it clear that CBA/N mice may, in fact, be useful in determining the role of anti-carbohydrate antibody in the defense against various differ-ent pathogens. Such studies by O'Brien et al. (4) have already shown that CBA/N mice are highly susceptible to salmonella.

Correspodence should be sent to: David E. Briles, Ph.D., 224 Tumor Institute, University Station, University of Alabama in Birmingham, Birmingham, Alabama 35294.

### REFERENCES

1. Amsbaugh, D.F., Hansen, C.T., Prescott, B., Stashak, P.W., Barthold, D.R., and Baker, P.J. J.Exp.Med. 136:931, 1972.
2. Cooper, M.D., Chase, H.P., Lowman, J.T., Krivit, W., and Good, R.A. Am.J.Med. 44:499, 1968.
3. Mosier, D.E., Zitron, I.M., Mond, J.J., Ahmed, A., Scher, I., and Paul, S.E. Immunological Rev. 37:89, 1977.
4. O'Brien, A.D., Scher, I., Campbell, G.H., MacDermott, R.P., and Formal, S.B. J.Immunol. 123:720, 1979.
5. Perlmutter, R.M., Hansburg, D., Briles, D.E., Nicolotti, R.A., and Davie, J.M. J.Immunol. 121:566, 1978.
6. Perlmutter, R.M., Nahm, M., Stein, K.E., Slack, J., Zitron, I., Paul, W.E., and Davie, J.M. J.Exp.Med. 149:993, 1979.
7. White, B. In The Biology of Pneumococcus. New York: The Commonwealth Fund, p1-799, 1938.

GENETICALLY CONTROLLED NATURAL RESISTANCE OF MICE TO PLAGUE
INFECTION AND ITS RELATIONSHIP TO GENETICALLY CONTROLLED
CELL-MEDIATED IMMUNE RESISTANCE

Akira Wake

First Department of Bacteriology
National Institute of Health
Tokyo, Japan

In the plague infection of mouse and guinea pig,
Yersinia pestis organisms invades the host's body causing
septicemic death within such a short time that specific protective immunity cannot develop. Therefore, the model of
murine resistance to Y. pestis seems to be useful for the
analysis of genetically controlled natural resistance to
this infection.

Specific immunity is thought to have developed during
the process of evolution in addition to mechanisms of natural resistance. Previously we reported a method of
immunization that induces specific cell-mediated protective
immunity against plague (2).

The purpose of this study is the comparison of the
differences among vrious inbred and hybrid mouse strains
with regard to natural resistance as well as specific cell-
mediated immunity to plague infection. In addition, strain
differences among inbred guinea pigs in their natural resistance to plague infection was also investigated.

EXPERIMFNTAL RESULTS

Strain differences in natural resistance of mice against
plague.

Various mouse strains were infected subcutaneously with
different doses of a fully virulent Y. pestis strain Yreka.

When animals were infected with the dose as low as 62
CFU, BALB/C mice had the longest mean survival time (5.1
days); C57BL/6J, the shortest (4.3 days), and their hybrid
intermediate (4.4 days). Nu/nu mice (BALB/C background, 3.6
days) are regarded as exceptional, because of their deficiency in mature T-cells (Fi·. 1). Although the differences
in survival time were hardl statistically significant in
this single experiment, the ɔrder from the longest to the
shortest survivors was never changed among these strains in
subsequent four experiments (Fig. 2 and 3).

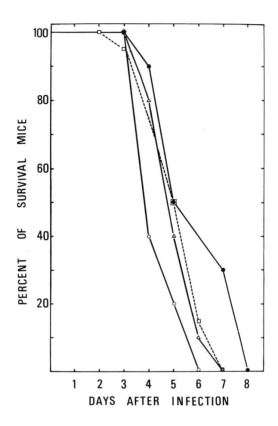

**Figure 1.** Mouse strain differences in natural resistance to
<u>Y. pestis</u> infection. Daily survival percents of 10 BALB/C
(●——●), 10 C57BL/6J (△——△), 20 (C57BL/6J x BALB/C)F1
(□----□), and 19 nu/nu-BALB/C background (○——○) mice after
s.c. infection with 62 CFU of <u>Y. pestis</u> Yreka.

The exceptional length of mean survival time in DD/S mice
could be explained by more complicated genetic control of
resistance mechanisms in outbred mouse strains.   Taken together, these results suggest that natural resistance in
mice against plague is under genetic control.

Strain differences in specific cell-mediated protective
immunity in mice

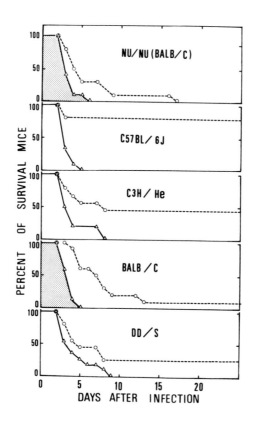

**Figure 2.** Mouse strain differences in natural and cell-mediated immune resistance to Y. pestis infection (Experiments 2 and 3). Experiments 2 (without shadowing) and 3 (with shadowing) were carried out separately. Each mouse group consisted of 10-11 animals. Daily survival percents of non-immunized (△——△) and immunized (○----○) mice after s.c. challenge with 420,000 CFU of Y. pestis are shown.

In all experiments shown in Fig. 2 and 3, parallel
groups of mice were primed subcutaneously with 2-3 hundreds
organisms of a live VW+ <u>Yersinia pseudotuberculosis</u> suspended in 0.1 ml of chondroitin sulfate colloidal $FeCl_3$, 14
days prior to the challenge with <u>Y. pestis</u>. Here, VW
designates the presence of one pair of common antigens between <u>Y. pestis</u> and <u>Y. pseudotuberculosis</u>. Immunized mice
were challenged simultaneously with the corresponding non-
immunized mice and daily deaths-survivals were recorded as
shown in Fig. 2 and 3 (dotted lines).

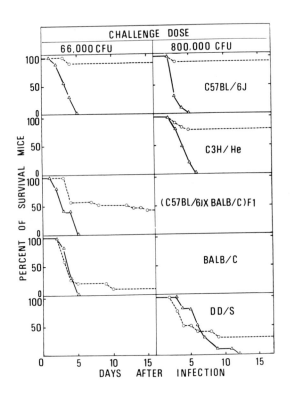

<u>Figure 3</u>. Mouse strain differences in natural and cell-
mediated immune resistance to <u>Y. pestis</u> infection (Experiments 4 and 5). Each group consisting of 10-20 non-
immunized (△——△) and immunized mice (○---○) was challenged
s.c. with 66,000 CFU of <u>Y. pestis</u> Yreka (left) or 800,000
CFU (right), respectively.

Survivors remained well until the end of observations (30th day of infection).   In detail, 80% of C57BL/6J; 50% of C3H/ He; 30th of nu/nu; 10% of BALB/C were protected from deaths by immunization (Fig. 2).   In experiment shown in Fig. 3, 91% of C57BL/6J, 10% of BALB/C and 40% of (C57BL/6J x BALB/ C)F1 were protected against the challenge with 66,000 CFU of Y. pestis.   91% of C57BL/6J, 75% of C3H/He and 30% of DD/S in the immunized groups survived until 30th day of infection with challenge dose of 800,000 CFU.

These results indicate that C57BL/6J is a high, BALB/C is a low and C3H/He is an intermediate responder to Y. pestis after priming with cross-reactive organism.

Strain differences in natural resistance of guinea pigs against plague.

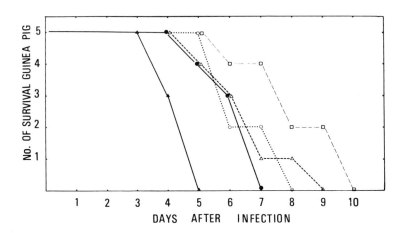

Figure 4.   Strain differences in natural resistance of in- bred guinea pig to Y. pestis infection.   Daily survivals of JY1 (△----△), JY2 (▲——▲), NIH2 (●——●) and NIH13 after in- fection with 44,000 CFU (O⋯⋯O) and 4,400 CFU (□–––□) of challenging doses of Y. pestis are shown.

Various inbred strains of guinea pigs, including 2 new- ly established ones that have originated from National Institute of Health, Tokyo, were subcutaneously infected with Y. pestis.   The daily survivals after infection with

4,400 and 44,000 CFU were recorded (Fig. 4). Significant strain differences in natural resistance were recognized between JY2(GPLA of Ia.2b,Ia.13b,P.3,P.4,P.6), and JY1(GPLA of Ia.13a,Ia.13b,P.5),NIH2(GPLA of Ia.2a,Ia.2b,P.1,P.2,P.3,P.4) and NIH13 (p<0.01). Mean survival time in these strains was 3.6, 6.8, 6.4 and 6.8 days, respectively.

## DISCUSSION

Nude mice cannot be protected from lethal infection with Y. pestis by immunization (Fig. 2) as immune T cells are necessary for such protection (3).

Our present studies would suggest that high levels of compensatory cell-mediated immune resistance might have developed in animals with low natural resistance to allow for survival in the process of evolution. This hypothesis is now being tested in the guinea pig model.

## REFERENCES

1.   Chiba, J., Otokawa, M., Nakagawa, M., and Egashira, Y. Microbiol.Immunol. 22:545, 1978.
2.   Wake, A., Morita, H., and Wake, M.   Immunology 34:1045, 1978.
3.   Wake, A.   ASM 79:E(H)11, 1979.

# GENETIC CONTROL OF DELAYED-TYPE HYPERSENSITIVITY TO MYCOBACTERIUM BOVIS BCG INFECTION IN MICE

Reiko M. Nakamura and Tohru Tokunaga

Department of Tuberculosis
National Institute of Health
Kamiosaki, Shinagawa-ku,
Tokyo, Japan

When inbred SWM/Ms mice were infected intravenously by living bacilli of Mycobacterium bovis BCG (Japanese substrain), the number of colony formers in the spleen decreased rapidly. However, the living bacilli persisted for a long time in the spleens of C3H/He mice given the same treatment (2). These two strains of mice showed quite a difference in the incidence of tumors induced by a chemical carcinogen (5,6). Furthermore, they responded differently to immunoprophylaxis and immunotherapy of autochthonous tumors with BCG (5,6). In these situations, SWM/Ms showed a low incidence of tumors, and responded well to immunoprophylaxis and immunotherapy with BCG, while C3H/He showed a high incidence of tumors and responded poorly to immunoprophylaxis and immunotherapy with BCG.

These mice were examined for their responsiveness to BCG immunization. It was found that SWM/Ms were high responders in delayed-type hypersensitivity (DTH) to BCG and C3H/He were low responders, when the immune status was measured by the footpad reaction to purified protein derivative (PPD), peritoneal macrophage disappearance test, or spleen indices after rechallenge with BCG. Since the footpad reaction is a reliable method to estimate DTH to BCG in mice, we used this method to examine the responsiveness of individual mice to BCG in F1, F2 and BC offspring (2). Table 1 shows the results. Although the values fluctuated in both high and low responders, it was clear that F1 hybrids were high responders. When the mean value minus 2 SE in F1 was set as the higher limit of the footpad reaction in low responders, F2 offspring were segregated into 3 high and 1 low responders and BC offspring were segregated into a 1 to 1 ratio (2).

Thymocytes of the hybrid mice were examined for $H-2^k$ and $H-2^d$ markers and there seemed to be no linkage between the responsiveness to BCG and H-2 (2). The results of footpad tests in various inbred and congenic strains supported this conclusion (Table 2) and was consistent with the results of Allen et al. (1).

Table 1. Number of mice showing high or low response to BCG in footpad reaction to 10 µg of PPD 2 weeks after immunization.

| Mouse strain | No. of low responders FPR* (0 - 5.0) | No. of high responders FPR (5.0 - 15.0) |
|---|---|---|
| SWM/Ms | 0 | 60 |
| C3H/He | 35 | 0 |
| (C3H x SWM)F1 | 0 | 34 |
| F2 | 11 | 36 |
| (F1 x C3H)BC | 24 | 29 |

*Footpad reaction: 0.1 mm units.

Table 2. Footpad reaction in various inbred and congenic strains of mice receiving BCG sc 2 weeks earlier.

| Mouse strain | H-2 (KISD) | FPR to PPD at 48 h (0.1 mm ± SE) |
|---|---|---|
| SWM/Ms | d??? | 10.17 ± 2.54 |
| C3H/He | kkkk | 0.71 ± 0.76 |
| B10.BR | kkkk | 6.14 ± 2.75 |
| SJL/J | ssss | 10.55 ± 3.70 |
| A.SW | ssss | 2.12 ± 0.80 |

The mechanism of the low responsiveness to BCG in C3H/He mice was found to be due to the inhibition by suppressor cells of the induction of DTH. This fact was confirmed by adoptive transfer of the spleen cells of C3H/He mice receiving BCG iv 6 days earlier into the syngeneic recipients pretreated with cyclophosphamide (3). The recipients were injected with BCG immediately after the cell transfer and tested for the footpad reaction 2 weeks later. Table 3 shows that the suppression was T-cell mediated and BCG specific.

Table 3. Suppression of footpad reaction by adoptive transfer of the suppressor cels in BCG-infected C3H/He mice.

| CY[*] | Transferred cells | FPR (0.1 mm ± SE) to | |
|---|---|---|---|
| | | PPD | SRBC[**] |
| − | − | 2.95 ± 1.04 | 2.93 ± 1.65 |
| + | − | 7.52 ± 0.36 | 7.97 ± 1.11 |
| + | Suppressor cells[***] | 3.83 ± 1.45 | 6.36 ± 1.71 |
| + | Suppressor cells + anti-θ + C | 6.40 ± 1.45 | 8.09 ± 1.57 |

*Cyclophosphamide 200 mg/kg ip 2 days before BCG injection.
**Sheep red blood cells.
***Whole spleen cells of C3H/He receiving BCG iv 6 days earlier.

The antigen-presenting ability of spleen macrophages to BCG-sensitized lymphocytes of (C3H x SWM)F1 mice was examined in C3H/He and SWM/Ms mice. The macrophages were pulsed with PPD and mixed in a culture with F1 lymphocytes to determine the antigen-induced DNA synthesis or yield of macrophage activating factor (MAF) (4). It was found that the macrophages of the low responder, C3H/He, did not present the antigen of F1 lymphocytes sensitized to BCG, while those of the high responder, SWM/Ms, did so well. Table 4 shows the results.

Table 4.   Antigen-presenting ability of macrophages (4).

| BCG-sensitized lymphocytes | Macrophages | PPD-pulse | DNA syn-thesis (cpm) | MAF[*] (% cytotox.) |
|---|---|---|---|---|
| (C3H x SWM)F1 | - | - | 2375 | -5.7 |
| " | C3H/He | - | 3088 | -11.2 |
| " | C3H/He | + | 2810 | 8.4 |
| " | SWM/Ms | - | 2900 | -9.8 |
| " | SWM/Ms | + | 6310 | 83.4 |

*MAF activity was estimated as percent cytotoxicity of tumor cells by macrophages activated with MAF.

These results suggest that the strain difference may lie in the macrophages.  The spleen cells of BCG-infected SJL/J mice produced MAF well with SJL/J macrophages pulsed with PPD, while they did not produce MAF with A.SW macrophages pulsed with PPD in spite of their matching in major histocompatibility antigens.  On the other hand, the spleen cells of BCG-infected A.SW mice did not produce MAF with SJL/J or A.SW macrophages pulsed with PPD.  These facts suggest that only SJL/J macrophages, not A.SW macrophages, are effective in antigen presentation in both primary and secondary DTH response to BCG.  It would be interesting to know whether or not the antigen-presenting ability of macrophages plays an important role in the deviation between helper-T and suppressor-T induction in DTH.

REFERENCES

1.    Allen, E.M., Moore, V.L., and Stevens, J.O.   J.Immunol. **119**:343, 1977.
2.    Nakamura, R.M., and Tokunaga, T.   Infect.Immun. **22**:657, 1978.

3.   Nakamura, R.M., and Tokunaga, T.   Infect.Immun., 1980
     (in press).
4.   Nakamura, R.M., Tokunaga, T., and Yamamoto, S.
     Infect. Immun. 27:268, 1980.
5.   Tokunaga, T., Yamamoto, S., Nakamura, R.M., and
     Kataoka, T.  J.Natl.Cancer Inst. 53:459, 1974.
6.   Tokunaga, T., Yamamoto, S., Nakamura, R.M., Kurosawa,
     A., and Murohashi, T.   Jap.J.Med.Sci.Biol.  31:143,
     1978.

## DISCUSSION

Collins:  I am not clear on how much PPD Nakamura used in
her footpad tests for delayed type hypersensitivity.  How
much swelling reaction did she elicit at 3 hours in her high
and low responders?  In the ones showing very little delayed
type hypersensitivity, did she find pronounced 3 hour footpad reactions, indicative of immediate hypersensitivity?

Nakamura:  I used 10 µg of PPD in the footpad reaction.  And
in the case of both C3H and SWM, the immediate type reaction
was in no way remarkable, but 24-48 hours later the SWM
yielded a nice reaction.

Ralph:  In the suppressor assay done by Nakamura, did this
involve only in vivo adoptive transfer?

Nakamura:  C3H mice are low responders and subsequently only
minimal footpad reaction can be detected in control BCG-
infected animals.  Cyclophophamide treatment of C3H mice 2
days before BCG infection leads to subsequent development of
nice footpad reaction.  Transfer of syngeneic BCG-immune
splenocytes to this, now high responder host leads to diminution of footpad reactivity.  We interpret this as suppress-
or cells involvement.  Such cells were characterized as T
cells.

Ralph:  They were T cells as judged by anti-theta sensitivity?

Nakamura:  Yes.  Treatment with anti-Thy 1.2 serum and complement caused the disappearance of the suppressor effect.

Ralph:  Did Nakamura explore suppression in vitro?

Nakamura:  Yes, we did.  I did the antigen-presenting experiment utilizing both blastogenesis and MAF activity. And in both, we could demonstrate an effect of suppressor cells in vitro. But is there really a subpopulation of suppressor cells? In the in vitro system we hesitate to say that we have characterized the suppressor cells.

Ralph: The cyclophosphamide treatment probably reduces the natural level of suppressor cells in the HeJ. Is that why Nakamura did that? Can you now turn the HeJ into a responsive mouse by treating with cyclophosphamide and then administering BCG? Have you tried that?

Nakamura: No, not yet, but we will.

# GENETIC CONTROL OF BCG-INDUCED CHRONIC GRANULOMATOUS INFLAMMATION AND ANERGY

Vernon L. Moore, John L. Sternick, Denis J. Schrier,
Benjamin A. Taylor* and Elizabeth M. Allen

Immunology Laboratories, Research Service
Wood VA Medical Center;
Departments of Medicine and Pathology
The Medical College of Wisconsin, Milwaukee, WI 53193
and The Jackson Laboratory*, Bar Harbor, ME 04609

Killed BCG administered by the intravenous (i.v.) route in oil or in an oil-in-saline emulsion produces chronic granulomatous inflammation (CGI) in the lungs of rabbits (13) and in the lungs and spleen of certain strains of mice (1). The pathology of this model resembles several human diseases such as sarcoidosis and hypersensitivity pneumonitis (HP). Therefore, studies on its induction, mechanisms of pathogenesis, and either resolution or progression should provide a better understanding of this type of inflammation.

Information already available on this model, primarily in the rabbit, is as follows: (i) an accelerated pulmonary inflammatory response elicited in sensitized rabbits is immunospecific (11), (ii) bronchoalveolar cells obtained from BCG-inflammed rabbits are inhibited from migrating in the presence of PPD, a test considered an in vitro correlate of T-cell mediated delayed hypersensitivity (DH) (5), and (iii) several studies have shown that lymphokines are produced by cells from the pulmonary lesions; these include migration inhibitory factor (12), macrophage fusion factor, a material which causes giant cell formation (6), and macrophage agglutinating factor, a glycosaminoglycan which agglutinates alveolar macrophages (7). Thus, most studies suggest that these pulmonary lesions are due mainly to DH.

We have been interested in the differential response in inbred mice to killed BCG in an oil-in-saline emulsion (BCG-E) because of the probable genetic predisposition of some individuals to develop certain granulomatous lung diseases (9) and because of the occurrence of HP in only certain individuals of a group with uniform exposure to environmental antigens (14). Initial studies have shown that the differential response of BCG in inbred mice is dose related and not controlled by genes within the H-2 complex (1). Similar data have been reported by another group (17). In order to obtain further information about the genetics of BCG-induced CGI in the lungs and spleen, we studied BXD recombinant inbred (RI) strains which were independently derived by in-

breeding from the $F_2$ progeny of (C57BL/6 x DBA/2)$F_1$ animals. DBA/2J and C57BL/6J (B6) mice are low and high responders respectively to BCG-E (1).

Table 1. Response of BXD Recombinant Inbred Mice to BCG-E*

| Strain (No. Tested) | Genotype H-2 | Genotype Ig | LW/BW $)10^{-3})^{\dagger}$ | SW/BW $(10^{-3})$ |
|---|---|---|---|---|
| C57BL/6 (10) | b | b | 22.4 (1.6)$^{++}$ | 33.7 (0.8) |
| DBA/2 (10) | d | c | 9.0 (0.6) | 4.0 (0.6) |
| BXD 2 (4) | b | b | 24.0 (3.1) | 23.3 (2.3) |
| 30 (6) | d | c | 22.2 (1.3) | 19.6 (1.1) |
| 29 (4) | b | b | 18.5 (2.4) | 14.9 (3.2) |
| 22 (8) | d | b | 18.4 (1.1) | 35.8 (1.4) |
| 25 (4) | d | b | 16.7 (4.0) | 13.5 (6.4) |
| 14 (6) | b | b | 15.4 (1.9) | 29.6 (5.7) |
| 12 (6) | b | c | 15.3 (2.7) | 15.7 (3.0) |
| 1 (5) | d | b | 14.7 (2.4) | 37.1 (3.1) |
| 13 (2) | b | b | 13.9 (2.9) | 18.2 (8.3) |
| 5 (5) | d | b | 13.5 (1.3) | 14.6 (2.8) |
| 19 (6) | b | b | 12.7 (1.3) | 12.1 (3.4) |
| 27 (6) | d | c | 12.3 (1.5) | 13.4 (2.8) |
| 8 (4) | b | b | 12.1 (1.5) | 15.4 (0.50) |
| 15 (3) | b | c | 11.8 (1.9) | 4.1 (0.57) |
| 11 (6) | d | c | 10.9 (2.9) | 11.2 (2.4) |
| 6 (4) | d | c | 10.7 (0.32) | 4.5 (0.13) |
| 9 (4) | d | c | 9.9 (0.55) | 7.0 (2.7) |
| 24 (4) | d | c | 9.7 (1.9) | 4.5 (0.57) |
| 28 (7) | d | c | 9.6 (1.1) | 7.6 (1.1) |
| 18 (6) | d | c | 8.9 (2.2) | 8.8 (1.7) |
| 23 (6) | b | b | 8.2 (0.6) | 7.3 (1.6) |
| 16 (6) | d | c | 8.0 (0.48) | 8.4 (1.8) |

*Animals were injected i.v. with 300 µg of killed BCG in an
oil-in-saline emulsion. They were killed 28 days later and
lung weight/body weight and spleen weight/body weight were
calculated. Ratio of organ weight to body weight are used
to quantify the intensity of inflammation (1).
†Lung weight/body weight values were used instead of organ
indices because we do not have lung and spleen weight/body
values for normal BXD mice.
++Mean and S.E.

The data in Table 1 are informative for two reasons. First,
the various BXD strains showed a wide variation in lung and
spleen indices suggesting that more than one gene is involved in responsiveness. In addition, an analysis of the data,

using Wilcoxin's Two Sample Rank Test showed that BXD strains which were $Igh^b$ had significantly greater responses in both the lungs and spleen to BCG-E (P<0.05 for both). There were no significant differences in the responses of $H-2^b$ and $H-2^d$ BXD strains (P>0.05). These data suggest that gene(s) influencing responsiveness to BCG-E are linked to the Igh allotype.

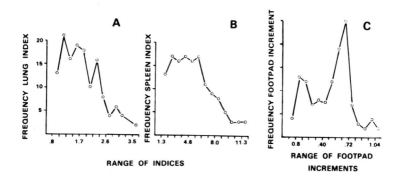

**Figure 1.** Frequency of lung index (A), spleen index (B), or footpad increment (C) in $F_2$ progeny of (B6 x CBA)$F_1$ mice.

To further analyze the inheritance of responsiveness to BCG-E, we examined $F_2$ progeny from (CBA/J x B6)$F_1$ mice. The frequency distribution of lung and spleen indices for $F_2$ progeny is shown in Fig. 1A and 1B. As expected for polygenic responses, there was not a distinct segregation into two populations. However, as discussed later, when the frequency distribution of footpad increments (DH to SRBC) were plotted, two discrete populations (suppressed and non-suppressed) were observed (Fig. 1C).

Additional analysis of linkage to the Igh allotype was performed using BALB/cJ and BALB/c.$Igh^b$ mice (Table 2). The results indicate that BALB/c mice are low responders compared to B6 mice and that CGI both in the lungs and spleen is substantially and significantly increased in BALB/c.-$Igh^b$ compared to BALB/c mice (P<0.005, P<0.02, respectively). Note that BALB/c.$Igh^b$ mice did not respond as well as B6 mice, presumably because they do not possess other Igh unrelated responder genes. Data in Table 2 also show that responsiveness to BCG-E is dominant since the lung and spleen indices of (B6 x CBA)F$_1$ mice are quantitatively similar to those of B6 high responder mice.

Table 2. Development of BCG-Induced Chronic Granulomatous Inflammation in Various Inbred and Congenic Mice*

| Strain | Genotype H-2 | Igh | Lung Index†† | Spleen Index†† |
|---|---|---|---|---|
| C57BL/6J | b | b | 3.3 (0.13)† | 10.1 (0.41) |
| CBA/J | k | a | 1.2 (0.12) | 2.2 (0.18) |
| (C57BL/6J x CBA/J)F$_1$ | b/k | b/a | 2.8 (0.11) | 9.9 (0.49) |
| BALB/cJ | d | a | 1.3 (0.20) | 4.3 (0.10) |
| BALB/c.Igh$^{b++}$ | d | b | 2.3 (0.05) | 5.8 (0.45) |

*Mice were injected with 300 µg of killed BCG in an oil-in-saline emulsion and evaluated 28 to 33 days later.
++Kindly provided by Dr. Noel Warner. BALB/c.Igh$^b$ mice were produced after the seventh backcross.
††Organ indices are organ weight/body weight experimental animal ÷ organ weight/body weight of normal animal. These values provide an approximation of the fold increase in organ, e.g., a lung index of 2 indicates that the organ has doubled weight.
†Data are expressed as arithmetic mean ± S.E. A minimum of 5 animals were used for each experiment.

We have also reported that B6 mice which develop BCG-E induced CGI are suppressed in their ability to develop several immunologic responses (2,15): (i) their spleen cells display minimal proliferation to both T and B cell mitogens as well as to the specific antigen, PPD, (ii) they develop a minimal primary antibody response to SRBC, and (iii) they are markedly suppressed in the development of DH to SRBC. In marked contrast, CBA mice which develop only minimal CGI in response to BCG-E were not anergic in any of the above parameters. The mechanisms responsible for anergy have been further characterized using the development of DH to SRBC as the test system. First, it is apparent that the spleen is an important source of factors responsible for suppression since splenectomized BCG-E-treated B6 mice were no longer suppressed in their response to SRBC (Group 1, Table 3). It should also be noted that splenectomized B6 mice not treated with BCG did not develop DH to SRBC indicating that when

SRBC are given i.v. at this dose, the spleen is both a source of suppressor factors (BCG-treated) and of cells which mediate DH. Data in Group 2, Table 3 also show that BCG-E treated CBA mice were not suppressed in their ability to develop DH to SRBC. Thus, the development of anergy is associated with intense CGI in the lungs and spleen.

Table 3. BCG Induced Suppression of DH to SRBC. Reversal by Splenectomy and Linkage to Immunoglobulin Allotype*

| Group | Strain | BCG-E | Sp$^{X\dagger}$ | Genotype H-2 | Igh | Footpad Increment$^{++}$ |
|-------|--------|-------|------|-----|-----|-------------------|
| 1 | C57BL/6 | - | - | b | b | 0.60 (0.06) |
|   |         | + | - |   |   | 0.16 (0.02) |
|   |         | - | + |   |   | 0.08 (0.04) |
|   |         | + | + |   |   | 0.62 (0.14) |
| 2 | CBA | - | - | k | a | 0.57 (0.06) |
|   |     | + | - |   |   | 0.77 (0.06) |
| 3 | (B6 x CBA)F$_1$ | - | - | b/k | b/a | 0.47 (0.03) |
|   |                 | + | - |     |     | 0.79 (0.04) |
| 4 | BALB/c | - | - | d | a | 0.46 (0.05) |
|   |        | + | - |   |   | 0.51 (0.08) |
|   | BALB/c.Igh$^b$ | - | - | d | b | 0.60 (0.06) |
|   |                | + | - |   |   | 0.18 (0.02) |
|   | B10.BR | - | - | k | b | 0.59 (0.08) |
|   |        | + | - |   |   | 0.14 (0.03) |
|   | C3H.SW | - | - | b | a | 0.41 (0.04) |
|   |        | + | - |   |   | 0.48 (0.06) |

*Mice were injected i.v. with 300 μg of killed BCG in an oil-in-saline emulsion. 28 days later they were immunized i.v. with 5 x 10$^5$ SRBC; 4 days later they were challenged in one hind footpad with 10$^8$ SRBC and in the other rear footpad with an equal volume of saline. The increase in footpad thickness was measured 24 hr later with a pressure-sensitive gauge.
†Three weeks prior to injection with BCG.
++Increase in footpad thickness to mm. Data are expressed as arithmetic mean and S.E. of at least 5 determinations.

The genetic basis for BCG-E-induced anergy was examined. Data in Groups 3 and 4, Table 3 show that the development of anergy is recessive since BCG-E-treated (B6 x CBA)F$_1$ mice were not anergic. In addition, a single gene (or gene complex) is responsible for anergy since approximately 50 percent of $F_1$ x B6 backcross and 25 percent of $F_2$ mice were anergic (data not shown). The unigenic nature of BCG-E-induced anergy is depicted in Fig. 1C which is a frequency distribution of footpad increments in $F_2$ mice. Two discrete peaks, characteristics of a unigenic response, are observed. Moreover, the minority of mice were low responders which is typical for a recessive trait. Data in Group 4, Table 3 shows that BCG-E-induced anergy is linked to the Igh complex since BALB/c mice ($Igh^a$) were not anergic but their congenic partners (BALB/c.$Igh^b$) were suppressed. In data not shown using BXD RI mice, there is also a significant correlation between the Igh allotype and the development of BCG-E-induced anergy. The results in Group 4, Table 3 also indicate that BCG-E-induced anergy is not influenced by genes in the H-2 complex since B10.BR mice develop anergy even though they are $H-2^k$ and C3H.SW mice ($H-2^b$)did not display anergy.

Table 4. Properties of Spleen Cells Which Transfer BCG-Induced Suppression of Delayed Hypersensitivity to SRBC in C57BL/6 Mice

| Group | Spleen Cells Transferred[*] | Killed BCG[+] | Footpad Increment[++] |
|-------|------------------------------|----------------|------------------------|
| 1 | None | + | 0.14 (0.05) |
| 2 | None | − | 0.61 (0.08) |
| 3 | BCG | − | 0.06 (0.02) |
| 4 | Normal | − | 0.56 (0.08) |
| 5 | BCG-adherent | − | 0.14 (0.04) |
| 6 | Normal adherent | − | 0.65 (0.06) |
| 7 | Carbonyl iron-treated BCG | − | 0.68 (0.05) |
| 8 | BCG-nonadherent | − | 0.56 (0.02) |
| 9 | Anti-Thy1-treated BCG | − | 0.21 (0.03) |
| 10 | Anti-mouse Ig-treated BCG | − | 0.09 (0.03) |

[*]Spleen cells were obtained from either BCG-injected or normal B6 mice and transferred to recipients intraperitoneally as follows: Group: 3 and 4) 1.1 x $10^8$ cells, 5 and 6) 33 x $10^6$ plastic petri plate adherent cells, 7) 63 x $10^6$ cells which did not adhere to carbonyl iron, 8) 35 x $10^6$ nylon wool nonadherent cells, 9 and 10) 80 x $10^6$ anti-Thy1 or anti-Ig+C treated cells.
[+]Mice were either injected i.v. and tested for DH 28 days later, or tested for DH 24 hr after receipt of cells.
[++]See legent to Table for evaluation of DH.

We have also investigated the properties of cells in the spleen responsible for anergy (Table 4). This was possible because anergy could be transferred from BCG-E-treated B6 mice to normal syngenic recipients (Group 1). Analysis of this phenomenon revealed that anergy was mediated by plastic petri plate-adherent, carbonyl iron-adsorbed cells (Groups 3-7). Anergy could not be transferred with T cell-enriched, nylon wool-nonadherent cells from BCG-E-treated mice and was not associated with Thy-1 or Ig bearing cells (Groups 8-10). All these data indicate that anergy is mediated by splenic macrophages from BCG-E-treated B6 mice.

The current study has shown that BCG-induced CGI in mice is multigenic, dominant and influenced by genes linked to the Igh locus. Other studies have shown that this response is not linked to the H-2 complex (1,17). The pulmonary lesions produced by the i.v. injection of killed BCG into either rabbits or mice resemble those in several human diseases, e.g., sarcoidosis, HP. Both of these diseases are likely to be mediated by immunological mechanisms and may be influenced by variably inherited traits (10). Therefore, definition of the immunogenetics of BCG-induced CGI in mice is likely to provide information related to pulmonary disease in man. One mechanism involved in low responsiveness in CBA mice has recently been uncovered in our laboratory (Moore et al. submitted). We observed that cyclophosphamide (Cy) given two days prior to BCG augments the response of these normally low responder mice to this agent. Furthermore, the potentiating effects of Cy can be reversed with Thy-1$^+$ spleen cells from BCG-E-treated mice not treated with Cy. This indicates that Cy-sensitive suppressor T cells are involved in the control of BCG-E-induced CGI in mice and implies that a similar mechanism occurs in pulmonary inflammation in man.

The meaning of linkage of BCG-E-induced inflammation to the Igh complex is not clear at the present time. However, as stated previously, BCG-E-induced CGI is probably T-cell-mediated DH. It is possible therefore that linkage to the Igh complex is somehow associated with $V_H$ receptors on T lymphocytes. For example, the interaction of Lyt-1$^+$ inducer and Lyt-123$^+$ lymphocytes in the feedback inhibition loop is restricted by genes linked to the Igh complex (4), and the development of cross-reactive DH in a hapten antigen system is also influenced by genes in the Igh complex (16). The reality of this concept with respect to pulmonary inflammation requires further studies.

The present study has also shown that the development of anergy in association with BCG-induced CGI is under genetic control. It is recessive, unigenic, and also linked to

genes in the Igh complex. The implications of linkage to
the Igh complex are not clear at the present time since
anergy is mediated by macrophages. However, in some cases,
macrophages serve as intracellular messengers for T cell
products (3). We are presently testing this concept. Cells
which mediate anergy are found in the spleen and have properties characteristic of macrophaes by several criteria:
(i) they are adherent to plastic, nylon wool, and carbonyl
iron, and (ii) they do not bear Thy-1 or Ig surface markers.
Since they are recovered only from chronically inflammed
spleens, it is likely that they are activated; however,
this was not formally tested.

Chronic pulmonary inflammation is sometimes associated
with anergy, particularly in sarcoidosis. The mechanisms
associated with anergy are not clear. Based on the present
study, anergy could be associated with the development of
suppressor macrophages; such cells have been described in
sarcoidosis (8). The role of anergy in the inflammatory
process is also unclear; however, we have shown that suppressor factors obtained from BCG-induced splenic macrophages
can substantially reduce the intensity of chronic inflammation in both the spleen and lungs (Allen et al. submitted).
Thus, one possible role of suppressor macrophages is control
of the inflammatory response. This concept will also require further studies.

## ACKNOWLEDGEMENT

The authors appreciate the typing and editing of the
manuscript by Ms. Rita Pavelko and Ms. Sharon Olecheck, the
provision of BALB/c.Igh$^b$ mice by Dr. Noel Warner and the
help in statistical analysis by Dr. John Kalbfleisch. This
study was supported by NIH grants #HL 22301, GM 18684, HL
15389, CA 22105 and by funds from the Veterans Administration. The Jackson Laboratory is fully accredited by the
American Association for Accreditation of Laboratory Animal
Care.

## REFERENCES

1.  Allen, E.M., Moore, V.L., and Stevens, J.O.    J.
    Immunol. 119:347, 1977.
2.  Allen, E.M., and Moore, V.L.   J. Reticul.Soc. 26:349,
    1979.
3.  Cantor, H., and Gershon, R.K.   Fed.Proc. 38:2058, 1979.

4.  Eardley, D.D., Shen, F.W., Cantor, H., and Gershon, R.K. J.Exp.Med. 150:44, 1979.

5.  Galindo, B., and Myrvik, Q.U. J. Immunol. 105:227, 1970.

6.  Galindo, B., Lazdins, J., and Castillo, R. Infect.-Immun. 9:212, 1974.

7.  Galindo, B., Myrvik, Q.N., and Love, S.H. J.Reticul.-Soc. 18:295, 1975.

8.  Goodwin, J.S., DeHoratius, R., Ismel, H., Peake, G.T., and Messner, R.P. Ann.Intern.Med. 90:169, 1979.

9.  Headings, V.E., Weston, D., Young, R.D.Jr., and Hackney, R.L.Jr. Ann.N.Y.Acad.Sci. 278:377, 1976.

10. Hunninghake, G.W., Gadek, J.E., Kawanami, O., Ferrans, V.J., and Crystal, R.G. Am.J.Pathol. 97:147, 1979.

11. Moore, V.L., Myrvik, Q.N., and Leake, E.S. Infect.-Immun. 7:743, 1973.

12. Moore, V.L., and Myrvik, Q.N. J.Reticul.Soc. 16:21, 1974.

13. Moore, V.L., and Myrvik, Q.N. J.Reticul.Soc. 21:131, 1977.

14. Roberts, R.C., and Moore, V.L. Am.Rev.Respir.Dis. 116:1075, 1977.

15. Schrier, D.J., Allen, E.M., and Moore, V.L. Fed.Proc. 28:1174, 1979.

16. Weinberger, J.Z., Greene, M.I., Benacerraf, B., and Dorf, M.E. J.Exp.Med. 149:1136, 1979.

17. Yamamoto, K., and Kakinama, M. Microbiol.Immunol. 22:335, 1978.

## DISCUSSION

Cudkowicz: Has Moore ever been able to induce suppressor macrophages in vitro?

Moore: We have not been able to do that. However, we can get suppressor macrophages out of the inflamed spleen.

Nakamura: Would Moore say that in the case of BCG inducing DTH, there are any specific suppressor cells other than macrophages?

Moore: We do not have another antigenic model for assessing those suppressor cells in the case of the cyclophosphamide experiments. So we do not really know whether it is specific in this instance. We are trying to do the same thing with Nocardia asteroidis and Corynebacterium parvum, so that we will have some specificity controls.

Nakamura:    I would think Moore has macrophage suppressor
cells in the granulomatous reaction.    And this suppressor
macrophage, induced by BCG injection, might well be non-
specific.    I wonder if there could be a BCG-specific suppressor in the system; it might be a T cell rather than a
macrophage.

Moore:    In the experiments I showed, we were not able to
demonstrate any effect of specific T cells as judged by
using anti-Thy 1 antiserum.    We think this may be a macrophage doing something T cell-directed, though we do not have
any relevant information on it at present.

Nakamura:    In the system I work with, we get BCG-specific
suppressor T cells;    these inhibit the induction of DTH in
the footpad reaction.    And Moore's results with the footpad
reaction give me the impression of being very similar.

Moore:    You know what happens in cases of chronic inflammatory reactions, as typified by Mycobacterium leprimurium.
First suppressor macrophages are evident;    then, if one
follows the reaction long enough, suppressor T cells appear.
That could be what is happening in our system as well;    the
key could be the time sequence.

# MURINE LEPROSY AS A MODEL FOR THE ANALYSIS OF GENETIC FACTORS CONTROLLING RESISTANCE TO MYCOBACTERIAL INFECTION

Otto Closs and Martinus Lovik
University of Oslo
Institute for Experimental Medical Research
Ullevaal Hospital
Oslo 1, Norway

Murine leprosy is caused by the obligate intracellular parasite <u>Mycobacterium</u> <u>lepraemurium</u> (MLM). The bacillus causes a slowly progressing chronic infection in mice and rats which previously was believed to be invariably fatal. Several workers have reported that mice may show varying resistance to MLM infection (4,8,11). Various inbred strains of mice differ in their resistance to MLM infection indicating that the resistance is determined by genetic factors of the host. Some of the studies on the resistance to MLM infection in three of the most frequently used inbred mouse strains are listed in Table 1. Although there are some discrepancies, most workers have found C57BL/6 mice to be relatively resistant and BALB/c and C3H to be susceptible.

Table 1. Resistance to <u>M. lepraemurium</u> infection in three frequently studied inbred mouse strains.

| | Level of resistance | | |
|---|---|---|---|
| Strain | Resistant | Intermediate | Susceptible |
| C57BL/6 | Kawaguchi (8) Closs and Haugen (4) Lagrange et al. (9) Alexander and Curtis(1) Preston (16) | | Lefford et al. (11) |
| BALB/c | | Closs and Haugen (4) | Kawaguchi (8) Lefford et al. (11) Alexander and Curtis (1) Preston (16) |
| C3H | Lefford et al.(11) | | Kawaguchi (8) Closs and Haugen (4) Lagrange et al. (9) |

GENETIC CONTROL OF NATURAL RESISTANCE
TO INFECTION AND MALIGNANCY

201

Important aspects of murine leprosy as experimental model are illustrated by the different course of the infection after local inoculation in C57BL/6 and C3H/Tif mice. Shortly after inoculation the bacilli become located within macrophages. In the C3H mice naked granulomas, without practically any infiltration of lymphocytes, will form at the site of infection. The infection will progress slowly and disseminate gradually until, after several months, the animal dies in a cachetic state without any stage having shown signs of a cell mediated immune reaction against the bacilli. In the C57BL mice, the histological picture of the infection is almost indistinguishable from that seen in C3H mice for the first four weeks of the infection. About four weeks after inoculation, a strong cellular reaction develops at the site of infection with massive infiltration of lymphocytes and epithelioid cell formation. The granuloma that forms as a result of this reaction has the histological appearance of a delayed type hypersensitivity reaction (5,6). When the local reaction develops, the bacilli cease to multiply and unless a too large inoculum has been given ($10^8$ AFB or more), the number of acid fast bacilli (AFB) will remain constant thereafter. Thirty-two weeks after inoculation of $3 \times 10^6$ MLM into one hind foot pad, the total number of AFB that could be recovered from the foot pad, the popliteal, inguinal, and retroperitoneal lymph nodes and spleen, was about 3,000 times higher in C3H/Tif mice than in C57BL/6J mice (3). Thus, the differing susceptibility of C57BL and C3H mice to MLM infection manifests itself both as a clear qualitative difference in the local reaction to the infection, and a clear quantitative difference in the multiplication of the bacilli.

For intracellularly growing parasites, immune activation of macrophages is connected with limitation of growth in vivo, and is frequently associated with expression of certain cell mediated immune responses such as delayed type hypersensitivity (DTH) (14). The differing susceptibility of C3H and C57BL mice to MLM infection is not likely to be due to a general defect in the ability of C3H mice to mount a cell mediated immune reaction because resistance to certain other intracellular parasites such as Salmonella typhimurium and Leishmania tropica may show a reverse susceptibility pattern in these strains (2,15). A number of interactions between mononuclear phagocytes and T lymphocytes are required at various levels in order to produce an effective killing of the bacilli (Fig. 1). Genetic variation in factors operating at each level may give rise to variations in natural resistance to MLM infection. However, we do not know the protective antigen nor the exact subset of cells involved and their mechanisms of action, therefore, the presence or absence of these factors cannot be directly tested (10).

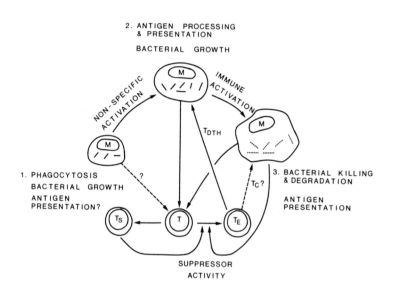

**Figure 1.** Simplified scheme of the proposed cellular inter-actions involved in the generation of a protective immune response to M. lepraemurium. It involves a series of steps which all may be essential in order to develop protective immunity: After phagocytosis of the bacilli the macrophages (M) may either present antigens to the T lymphocyte populat-ion (T) directly, or after non-specific activation, as in-dicated by arrows. Upon stimulation of the T lymphocyte population either suppressor cells ($T_S$) or effector cells ($T_E$) may be generated. $T_E$ may either activate the macro-phages by producing soluble mediators ($T_{DTH}$), or another subset of T cells may be produced acting directly to limit the multiplication of the bacilli by combined cytotoxic and bactericidal activity ($T_C$). The generation of $T_E$ is re-gulated by $T_S$ and M suppressor mechanisms. Each step is probably under control of one or several genetic factors.

We have studied the effect of immunization with an ultrasonicate of MLM (MLMSon) in C3H/Tif and C57BL/6 mice. A single injection of 50 µl of MLMSon (0.8 mg protein ml$^{-1}$) in Freund's incomplete adjuvant (1:1) was given subcutaneously on the thorax. Six weeks later by foot pad testing with MLMSon (0.8 µg protein per dose), a strong DTH reaction was demonstrated in C57BL mice while the C3H mice showed only weak DTH reactivity. Challenge experiments with live bacilli indicated that in C57BL mice immunization with MLMSon did not, in itself, confer protective immunity, but seemed to accelerate the development of such immunity (7). Evidence was found that the specificity of the protective immune response induced in C57BL mice by a small inoculum of live MLM was different from that of the immune response induced by MLMSon in these mice. By further immunization, a strong DTH response to MLMSon antigen could be induced in C3H mice. Such MLMSon immune C3H mice did not have any increased ability to limit the multiplication of MLM. No local reaction was observed when live MLM was injected into the foot pad. Even when a strong DTH reaction was induced repeatedly at the site of infection by injecting MLMSon into the foot pad together with the bacilli, and every two weeks thereafter, no reduction in the multiplication of bacilli was observed (12). Thus, in these experiments a clear dissociation was demonstrated between DTH to MLMSon and protective immunity to MLM infection.

Information about the factor(s) responsible for the differing susceptibility of C3H and C57BL/6 mice to MLM infection is likely to contribute significantly to our understanding of the mechanisms involved in resistance to mycobacterial infections. At present genetic analysis seems to offer one of the best approaches to define factors which show association with the mechanisms of resistance. Experiments so far have indicated that the (C57BL/6 x C3H)F$_1$ hybrid is as resistant as C57BL/6, and consequently that resistance to MLM infection is inherited as a dominant trait (Closs and Lovik, unpublished observations). However, if a model is to be usable for genetic analysis, relevant markers must be available for the trait which is under investigation. In studies of MLM infection several different parameters of resistance have been used: size of the local leproma after subcutaneous inoculation (8), histological appearance of the local reaction (5), local multiplication and dissemination of the bacilli (3), time of survival after intravenous inoculation (11), and multiplication of the bacilli in the popliteal lymph node after foot pad inoculation (9).

The use of different parameters of resistance may explain some of the discrepancies regarding the susceptibility

of various inbred mouse strains to MLM infection, as exempl-
ified in Table 1. While C57BL/6 mice, as opposed to C3H
mice, are able to limit the multiplication of a small subcutaneous inoculum of MLM (3,9) the survival time of the
former strain is shorter than that of C3H after a large intravenous inoculum (9,11).

The marker most closely associated with resitance to
MLM infection certainly is the ability to inhibit multiplication of the bacilli. However, MLM is an extremely slow
growing mycobacterium with an average doubling time of two
weeks or more, and to follow the multiplication and dissemination of the bacilli is both time-consuming and labori-
ous.the differing distribution patterns of the bacilli in
various suceptible strains of mice complicate the matter
further (13). As indicated above, the ability to mount a
DTH response to MLM antigens is not a usable marker since it
does not always correlate with resistance to MLM infection.
Several reports have shown a correlation between the development of a local reaction (foot pad swelling) to the infection and ability to inhibit multiplication of MLM (3,9).
Thus, based on observations in C57BL/6 and C3H mice, the
ability to mount a strong local reaction to live MLM bacilli
appears to be a usable and convenient marker for genetic
factors involved in resistance to MLM infection. However,
unless the resistance can be shown to be controlled by a
single gene, the correlation between this marker and resistance would have to be confirmed in every instance.

## REFERENCES

1. Alexander, J., and Curtis, J. Immunology 36:563, 1979.
2. Behin, R., Mauel, J., and Sordat, B. Exp.Parasitol.
   48:81, 1979.
3. Closs, O. Infect.Immun. 12:480, 1975.
4. Closs, O., and Haugen, O.A. Acta.Path.Microbiol.Scand-
   Section A 82:459, 1974.
5. Closs, O., and Haugen, O.A. Acta Path.Microbiol.Scand-
   Section A 83:51, 1975.
6. Closs, O., and Haugen, O.A. Acta.Path.Microbiol.Scand-
   Section A 83:59, 1975.
7. Closs, O., and Lovik, M. Infect. Immun. 1980 (in
   press).
8. Kawaguchi, Y. Jap.J.Exp.Med. 29:651, 1959.
9. Lagrange, P.H., and Hurtrel, B. Clin.exp.Immunol. 38:-
   461, 1979.
10. Lagrange, P.H., and Closs, O. Scand.J.Immunol. 10:285,
    1979.

11. Lefford, M.J., Patel, P.J., Poulter, L.W., and
    Mackaness, G.B. Infect.Immun. 18:654, 1977.
12. Lovik, M., and Closs, O. Scand.J.Infect.Dis. 1980 (in
    press).
13. Lovik, M., and Closs, O. In Perspective in Immunology.
    E. Skamene, P.A.L. Kongshavn, and M. Landy (eds). New
    York, Academic Press, 1980 (in press).
14. Mackaness, G.B. J.exp.Med. 129:973, 1969.
15. Plant, J., and Glynn, A.A. Nature 248:345, 1974.
16. Preston, P.M. Transactions R.Soc.Trop.Med.Hyg. 73:212,
    1979.

DISCUSSION

Poulter: A while back I was also working on MLM. I can
confirm Closs' results in a totally different manner. We
found that in animals exhibiting resistance to MLM by restricting multiplication of the bacteria in the liver and
spleen, they lost completely the ability to mount a DTH reaction. So I would certainly agree that the DTH response,
particularly to sonicated antigen, is not a particularly
good marker of resistance to this organism. Also, I wonder
what Closs can tell us about the utilization of sonicates.
When he sonicates his mycobacteria, he is releasing components from within the cells which the host may not experience
at all in reacting to live microorganisms. I rather think
the response to some of these intracellular particles is a
quite different one and may be irrelevant to protection, in
contrast to those antigens on the external cell wall of
Mycobacteria.

Closs: I would certainly agree that the antigens active in
the sonicate do not seem to be relevant to protective immunity.

Poulter: My comment relates to the whole of this session.
As an immunologist who has been working on the acquired
phase of the response for a number of years, I am very
pleased to see the increasing interest in the natural noninduced responses. But one thing that has not been mentioned at all in this session is the native or acquired responses to endogenous flora of the host. I cannot help wondering
whether any cross-reacting immunity or defense mechanisms
against such flora in the animal would have any effect on
the varied phenomena reported here. Has anyone worked with
these mouse strains in the germ-free state where this sort

of issue can be controlled? I guess not. Does anyone here think it is worth doing? I know I would be interested in doing it myself.

Participant: The only data that comes readily to mind is the sort of thing that has been done via oral challenge. And a search of the literature, on susceptibility of animals to a Salmonella infection, would show that the general experience is that sterilizing an animal's gut with antibiotics renders it more susceptible.

Collins: Responding to Closs' comment, I would say that in leprosy one does not use a sonicate to skin test; whole cells of leprum are employed and they give a reaction which peaks at about 4 weeks. In M. lepremurium, he has been footpad-testing with whole organisms, whether live or dead probably does not matter, and he was assessing the reaction at 48 hours. My query is whether Closs assessed the response at 4 to 6 weeks, so that the test was comparable to the Matsuda-response. In that event did he find suppression?

Closs: Well, we certainly have looked at 4 weeks, and we do not get a response unless we are dealing with a resistant strain, and unless the bacilli are viable.

# GENETIC CONTROL OF RESISTANCE TO BACTERIAL INFECTIONS

## Chairman's Summary

Emil Skamene

Montreal General Hospital Research Institute
Montreal, Quebec H3G 1A4, Canada

Genetic influences on the outcome of interactions between the host and pathogenic bacteria have long been suspected and explored. However, the precise knowledge of such
genetic systems and the way they govern the host's responses
have, until very recently, eluded understanding despite continued investigative efforts over the last four decades.
Given the complexity of bacterial microorganisms and the
multitude of host defense mechanisms that have evolved in
mammals during evolution, it was judged rather improbable
that a gene controlling the overall level of resistance
would be operative. Improbable they may be, but such events
have nonetheless in these past few years occurred independently in many laboratories due mainly to the availability
and widespread use of genetically well defined mouse
strains: inbred, mutant and recombinant. It has become
evident that the genetic systems controlling resistance are
definitely less complex than originally conceived and that
they are in fact available to analysis.

## MAPPING OF RESISTANCE GENES

This Symposium marshalled the evidence for many recent-
ly-discovered genes that singly, or in concert, control resistance to a wide variety of microbial pathogens: Salmonella
typhimurium, Listeria monocytogenes, Rickettsia tsutsugamushi, Mycobacterium tuberculosis, Mycobacterium lepraemurium to name only the most actively considered. The evidence for their operation was provided by studies ranging
from the rather preliminary dealing mainly with differences
in strain distribution of resistant and susceptible animals,
to formal Mendelian-type experiments on segregating hybrid
and backcross populations, to finally, elegant mapping
studies employing either classic linkage analysis or the
newer techniques based on the strain distribution pattern
studies of selected resistance traits among the recombinant
inbred mice. Of major importance in the quest for understanding of genetic resistance are the polymorphic alleles
of widely-distributed genes (e.g. Ity, Lr, Ric) although

discovery of deficiencies in host resistance based on the action of mutant genes (e.g. $Lps^d$, xid) have also contributed to our present knowledge of host defense mechanisms. Genetic analysis of any trait, in general, and of the trait of resistance in particular, has its own intrinsic elegance and it provides the student of host defenses with a essential definitive quality. Mapping the resistance genes also serves well the mouse geneticists in their efforts to fill the blanks on the chromosome map. It may be asked, however, whether our knowledge of the mechanisms of anti-bacterial defences is advanced thereby? The answer is, albeit somewhat hesitantly, yes. By mapping the resistance genes we may, first of all, discover a clustering of genetic resistance systems governing responses to unrelated infections, something which should be helpful in our deductions as to what the common defense mechanisms might be. Already, this early in the game, there is an example of such clustering, i.e., the Ity and Lsh genes that control resistance to Salmonella typhimurium and protozoa Leishmania donovani in mice map close in the vicinity on the first chromosome. Whether this is a case of gene identity, or rather of close linkage of two unrelated genes is presently under active investigation in several laboratories.

Another important aspect of resistance gene mapping lies in providing insight as to the persistence of sensitive alleles among polymorphic genes present in broad populations: it is logical to expect that the sensitive alleles must have some survival value to have been preserved in evolution. It is theoretically possible that susceptibility to one organism may be linked with resistance to another thus making the locus relatively neutral. The strain distribution of Salmonella-susceptibile (Ity-s) and Listeria-resistant (Lr-r) mouse strains for example, proves to be almost identical, thus raising the possibility of such a balancing selection. Unfortunately, formal linkage studies thus far have not supported the hypothesis of Ity-s and Lr-r linkage.

The mapping of resistance genes could, moreover, lead to possible identification of the mechanism of a resistant phenotype by, for example, linking it to gene(s) coding for enzymes or other proteins that play a role in host defense. Beyond that, one could, expect to discover markers (cellular, serological etc.) for specific resistance genes which could serve to identify the resistant and susceptible individuals in a random population without the need for typing by destructive infection. Presence of such marker(s) would also be invaluable in creating co-isogenic lines that differ only in the resistance gene. Several such lines are

presently being bred, using the trait or resistance to infection itself as a typing method. Existence of these congenic lines will surely facilitate greatly studies on the
phenotypic expression of resistance genes.

## PHENOTYPIC EXPRESSION OF RESISTANCE GENES

The mechanism of resistance gene action is properly
the central concern of most investigators in this newly
evolving field. Operational definition is needed for processes controlled by the genetic systems under consideration. However, the closest approach thus far achieved is a
sort of negative definition, one of exclusion: most of us
are studying processes which do not fulfill the criteria of
classical antigen-induced specific immune responsiveness.
The Symposium incorporated the term "natural resistance" in
its' title as it seems a realistic expectation that at least
empirical criteria for this term in antibacterial defenses
would soon emerge. Perhaps we should now take a lesson from
the "hybrid resistance" and "NK" story and define the processes controlled by resistance genes in terms of (a) their
temporal appearance in ontogeny, (b) the time sequence
before the emergence of specific immune response, (c) the
time sequence for the inactivation of the bacterial invader
from the moment of its introduction in the body, (d) bone
marrow dependence, (e) radiation sensitivity, etc.     This
approach has been used successfully for unravelling the cellular mechanisms of genetic resistance to Listeria and, in
part, to those related to Salmonella. Following the NK cell
analogy we immediately have to realize a handicap:  most of
us in this field work, by necessity, with in vivo models
using only the crudest, all or none criteria such as host
survival or death, or an estimation of the total bacterial
burden (which by itself is the result of at least 3 unrelated processes) as our measure for defining resistance or
sensitivity. There is a broad  consensus that at least one
group of natural resistance genes is expressed in the macrophage response to infection; but there is felt an urgent
need for additional in vitro correlates of antibacterial
defenses.

## MACROPHAGE BACTERICIDAL FUNCTION

Considering that macrophage is the major effector cell
of defense against intracellular bacterial parasites, and
that host resistance genes controlling the response to
several such infections in vivo appear to be expressed at
the level of the macrophage, it would be logical to expect,

that macrophage populations derived from sensitive hosts
would be inferior in handling appropriate bacteria in vitro
as compared with those derived from resistant hosts.

Surprisingly, this is not the case as judged by con-
census of Symposium participants, though there are occasional published reports to the contrary. Technical problems
of macrophage bactericidal assays thus far evade resolution
and several newer approaches need trial and refinement to
advance progress in this field. One of these approaches is
to use temperature-sensitive (TS) mutants of bacterial
strains which fail to multiply at 37°C. Using TS mutants
one should be able to eliminate the problem of bacterial
overgrowth a situation which often complicates the perfor-
mance and interpretation of bactericidal assays. The main
stumbling block in defining the cellular level of resistance
gene action, where macrophage is concerned, would appear to
be macrophage heterogeneity. Until now the only "specificity" allowed referred to T cells; the term "nonspecific" as
when applied to macrophages is clearly a misnomer, as mounting in vitro evidence indicates. As methods for growing and
cloning macrophages in vitro rapidly become available, one
should use the advantages of cloning methods to seek segregation of cell subtypes with distinct functional qualities.
Whether this approach in the search for cellular expression
of resistance gene action will take us in the direction of
macrophage receptor heterogeneity for different bacteria, or
in the direction of heterogeneity with respect to intracellular bacterial killing (or both) only time will tell.

## "RESISTANCE GENES" MAY NOT BE TRUE RESISTANCE GENES AFTER ALL

Our failure to translate the impressive in vivo traits
of genetic antibacterial resistance into in vitro cellular
correlates may have a basis other than the purely technical
one. The "resistance genes" may have ben discovered as such
only because of our methods of detection (i.e. in vivo resistance or sensitivity). There are, of course, precedents
for this view: the Fv-2 resistance gene was named after the
virus resistance it seemed to control but, the fact is, it
is now recognized as being a gene controlling erythroid
differentiation, independently of any infection. One cannot
escape the feeling that the story of at least one of the
genes we now consider - Lr (Listeria-resistance) will turn
out to be analogous, especially as its product seems to control the tempo and magnitude of macrophage proliferation and
differentiation rather than cellular macrophage bactericidal
processes per se. In this context it should be mentioned

that _Listeria_ _monocytogenes_, for the past 2 decades the favourite target for assessing the bactericidal power of activated macrophage turns out to be the less than ideal as the organism for such assays: it proves to be  extremely easy to kill, by both the normal, resident macrophages and by non-immunologically stimulated inflammatory macrophages as well and can easily trigger the genetic system of natural resistance towards rapid production of young metabolically active listericidal macrophages.

## RELATIONSHIP BETWEEN NATURAL RESISTANCE GENES AND OTHER ASPECTS OF HOST DEFENSE

It seems that a defect in natural resistance may result in a deficiency in the specific immune response and even preclude successful specific vaccination (e.g. in the case of salmonellosis). If generally applicable, this is of considerable importance, since alternative prophylactic and therapeutic strategies would be required to handle such infections in genetically deficient individuals.  It has, furthermore, become obvious that animals genetically sensitive to BCG infection first of all, have a higher incidence of spontaneous tumors and, moreover fail to respond to BCG-induced tumor immunotherapy.  This is an extremely important aspect of genetic resistance that has significant practical consequences.  It should be noted here that a conceptually similar finding was reported  in connection with genetic resistance to protozoa, where only animals genetically resistant to Leishmania infection responded to appropriate chemotherapy.

Finally, another aspect of the interrelationship between genetic resistance and overall host defenses deserves comment.  It is the concept that a defect in genetic resistance may, in fact, be the result of the development of a specific immune response such as in anti-BCG response. Evidence was given that BCG-specific suppressor T cells are responsible for genetically-determined sensitivity to BCG of certain mouse strains.  It should remind us that separate genetic systems operate at different stages or levels of "natural" resistance to various infections and the overall susceptibility may be due to different genetic defects (or effects) occurring at different stages of infection.

## CONCLUSION

The field of genetic resistance to bacteria has now attained the phase of rapid continuous growth.  It is

evident that the genetic handle is an extremely powerful
tool in probing for an understanding of cellular mechanisms
of body defenses, their defects and the possible ways for
their manipulation to benefit the host.

# IS GENETIC RESISTANCE TO MOUSE HEPATITIS BASED ON IMMUNOLOGICAL REACTIONS?

Frederik B. Bang and Thornton S. Cody
Department of Pathobiology
The Johns Hopkins University
School of Hygiene and Public Health
Baltimore, Maryland 21205

## INTRODUCTION

Driven by the eternal question, "What is the use of a discovery?" Benjamin Franklin, who was observing the ascent of a balloon, said, "What is the use of a baby?" (1). Abraham Flexner, years later, gave a lecture on "The usefulness of useless knowledge" (2).

In a school of public health where, for the past twenty years, work on mouse hepatitis, its genetics and pathogenesis has gone on, the same kinds of questions arise. We suggest that the congenic specific virus model which we have developed (as well as other models) is essential for characterizing some of the specific factors involved in resistance to disease. It may also develop into a useful model for tests of substances suspected to alter susceptibility to viruses.

In order to describe the system, we must go back to the work of plant pathologists who, in studies of genetic resistance, developed important concepts far ahead of animal pathologists. Much of this has been summarized in the excellent book by Day on "Genetics of Host-Parasite Interactions" (3). Bedeviled by the chaotic number of races of plants that presented a certain degree of resistance to a particular fungus and none to another, and by the variable virulence of one fungus for different races of plants, Flor (4), in 1942, first began to bring order into the system by discovering that there is a matching of host genes for resistance with viral genes for virulence, a so-called gene for gene concept. This idea was based on direct mendelian analysis of the virulence of the rust on different hosts and analysis of the genetics of the resistance of the host against different rusts. There was a direct matching of genes for susceptibility for those with virulence. This recognition, in turn, led to a useful simplification, that of the quadratic check, where one matches host and agent in a box and gives the name incompatible, i.e., genetically incompatible, to that situation where little or no disease is produced, <u>even though infection does take place</u>. Plant pathologists have carried this type of analysis much further

analyzing the reaction of plants to a variety of fungi, in-
sects, nematodes and viruses. Even in plant viruses which
may be expected to have fewer genes, the method has uncovered as many as eleven different combinations of host and
virus genes (5).

In 1960, when we were fortunate enough to find that
macrophages are specifically susceptible to mouse hepatitis
and that there are accompanying genetic differences in the
response of the mouse to a particular strain of virus, we
started a study of the nature of this genetic resistance.
However, there may also be a change in the virus, now established as a mutation which overcomes the genetic resistance. We were led to the necessity of putting our data in
the plant pathologists' format (Fig. 1):

<u>Figure 1</u>

|          | C3H | PRI |
|----------|-----|-----|
| MHV-PRI  | –   | +   |
| MHV-C3H  | +   | +   |

<u>Usefulness of this approach.</u> When the host and the
agent have been sufficiently "purified" (see below), this
arrangement has a number of advantages. It makes it possible to determine whether a particular one-step change in
the host gene is accompanied by a specific biochemical
change, and the check, i.e., the comparison of the two different compatible situations, gives further data on how the
host resistance may be overcome. It is our belief that such
an arrangement, in which one finally uses congenic strains
of mice, is essential for analysis of phenotypic change.

EVIDENCE FOR THE GENE FOR GENE CONCEPT IN MOUSE HEPATITIS

There is a close association between the resistance of
macrophages under optimal conditions and the resistance of
the adult mouse itself. This has allowed us to test individual mice for resistance or susceptibility to the standard
strain of virus by culturing their macrophages, testing
these, and then to breed from the appropriate animal. Thus
the gene for susceptibility, found originally in the PRI

mice, has been introduced by 20 backcrosses into the resistant C3H mouse, and this C3H$_{SS}$ mouse is just as susceptible (in terms of amount of virus to initiate a fatal infection) as is the original PRI mouse. The evidence that the mouse has one main gene for susceptibility to this virus then rests on (i) the preliminary analysis of crosses and $F_2$ generations (6), (ii) the detailed analysis of a series of backcross susceptible and resistant mice (7), and (iii) the facts that 50% of the offspring of backcrosses of susceptible mice through 20 generations to the C3H resistant mice yielded cultures that were susceptible to standard virus in tissue culture (8), and (iv) that the final C3H$_{SS}$ mouse derived by macrophage testing and subsequent breeding from "susceptible" mice, and inbreeding of these backcrosses, is a mouse that is fully susceptible (i.e., dies) when inoculated with hepatitis virus which is adapted to the susceptible PRI mouse (8).

## ONE-STEP CHANGE IN THE VIRUS

The evidence that the virus which overcomes this resistance (or incompatibility) differs from the original virus by one gene is indirect, but nevertheless strong. Originally the change in the virus from one which was avirulent for the C3H mouse to one which became virulent was seen in the occasional development of virulent strains of virus for adult C3H mice when the avirulent virus was grown in baby C3H mice which are routinely susceptible to the MHV-PRI (9). Then it was shown that inoculation of C3H macrophages in our special medium (90% horse serum and beef embryo extract) with very large amounts ($10^7$ LD$_{50}$) of virus did cause destruction of the cells and this was accompanied by the emergence of a virulent virus (10). Finally, fluctuation analysis of the appearance of this virulent strain has shown that a stable mutant emerges during the growth of the virus in susceptible cells.

## PATHOLOGY OF DISEASE

Although the virus destroys liver and probably has this effect primarily through its effect on the Kupffer cells (11), three qualifications are important. First, the virus does grow in the incompatible strain of mouse and in this produces minor lesions from which the mouse recovers often without symptoms (12); secondly, a roughly similar titer of infectious particles will produce infection in the incompatible situation (all mice surviving) and in the compatible (12); and thirdly, there is a marked destruction of lymphoid

tissue in the susceptible mice (13), just as was originally
pointed out by Ruebner in early work on mouse hepatitis in
outbred strains of mice (14).

## ONTOGENY OF RESISTANCE

A number of genetically resistant mouse models show
little or no resistance in the newborn, but acquire resistance with maturation.  The time of maturation of resistance
differs from one virus system to another (Fig.2).

**ONTOGENY OF RESISTANCE
TO THREE VIRUSES**

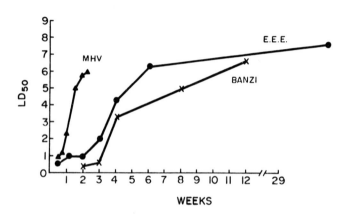

WEEKS

Fig. 2. All data in terms of the degree of resistance; i.e,
survival following peripheral inoculation of the virus in
log10 dilutions.
  1) MHV data taken from Gallily, R., Warwick, A., and
     Bang, F.B. 1967. Ontogeny of macrophage resist-
     ance to mouse hepatitis in vivo and in vitro.
  2) EEE data from Lennette, E.H., and Koprowski, H.
     1944. Influence of age on the susceptibility of
     mice to infection with certain neurotropic viruses.
     J. Immunol. 49:175-191.
  3. Banzi data - Personal communication from P. Bhatt,
     Yale University School of Medicine.

The rather striking similarity of the curves for maturation
of immune recognition systems, as measured by B cell response (15), leads us to suggest that the maturation of

genetic resistance and of antigen recognition is dependent upon a similar development of clones of lymphoid cells.

## PHENOTYPIC CHANGES IN SUSCEPTIBILITY OF MICE - CHANGE FROM INCOMPATIBILITY TO COMPATIBILITY

The interaction of environment and heredity is such a basic part of biology that there should be no surprise in the finding that a number of substances can produce phenotypic changes which override the genotypic resistance. To properly diagram this, it is necessary to add a third dimension to our square, thus creating a cube which shows the interaction of environment. Thus if the genes are maintained without change, the effect of a variety of substances and conditions may be studied.

We had recognized for some years that the administration of cortisone (9), cytoxan (16), X-ray and other so-called immunosuppressants changed the incompatible pair into a compatible one, without significant change in the virus. Indeed the treated incompatible mouse approached closely to susceptible in degree of susceptibility as measured by $LD_{50}$'s. Infection with <u>Epirythrozoon coccoides,</u> the red cell parasite discovered by Gledhill et al. (17), as an associated pathogen in the original mouse hepatitis also makes the incompatible pair into a compatible one.

## CHANGE FROM COMPATIBILITY TO INCOMPATIBILITY

Dr. W. Weiser, during her thesis work, studied the effect of Concanavalin-A (Con-A) on resistance as manifest in the incompatible pair. It had no apparent effect, but she also tested the effect of the drug on the compatible (susceptible) pair, and found that this stimulator of soluble immune response suppressor (SIRS) caused an increase of resistance; i.e., it caused the genetically compatible pair to become phenotypically incompatible. This effect was demonstrable both in the mice and in macrophage cultures from these mice. In addition, complete Freund's adjuvant and possibly endotoxin have a protective effect. Thus the arrows of phenotypic conversion can be pushed either way (Fig. 3).

### Figure 3

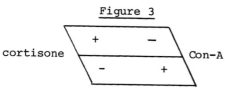

cortisone        Con-A

## MACROPHAGE CULTURES AS A REFLECTION OF PHENOTYPIC CHANGE IN SUSCEPTIBILITY

In the first work on the macrophage cultures, there was a constant association between the behavior of the virus in the mouse and its behavior on macrophages. This meant that cells from a resistant mouse were resistant in vitro, those from susceptible mice were susceptible in vitro, and finally that as the young resistant C3H mouse acquired resistance in vivo, liver cultures grown on a collagen substrate also yielded macrophages which were susceptible when derived from young mice, and resistant when derived from older mice.

However, demonstration of in vitro resistance demanded specific conditions. Lavelle early demonstrated a remarkable modifying effect of different sera (18). We had started our studies of macrophages in Chang's medium, originally developed for the growth of rat leprosy bacilli in mouse macrophages (19), and obtained the strong correlation which was the original finding upon which all later work was based. Frequently since then, we found that we had to work with a particular horse serum to avoid antibodies to ocornaviruses and that commercial horse sera were unsatisfactory. New workers frequently wished to change to media such as 20% fetal calf serum, which were free of antibodies and gave splendid-looking cultures and offered one the opportunity to compare with other work on macrophages. However, the high degree of the resistance ($10^6$ to $10^7$) manifest in the incompatible situation frequently dropped by a hundred- to a thousand-fold in these media, without changing the interaction of virus and cells in the compatible situations. Lavelle investigated these differences and found that the resistance of the incompatible cells in fetal calf sera could be almost completely restored by adding small amounts of mouse serum (18).

In order to study these factors which influence in vitro susceptibility in a more quantitative way, the original plaque studies of Shif (20) on macrophages have been refined. During the course of these, it was found that there is a marked increase in the number of plaques produced in the incompatible system not only if fetal calf serum is substituted for 90% horse serum, but also if agarose is used as an overlay instead of agar in the presence of fetal calf serum (21). These are phenotypic changes; i.e., virus recovered from these cultures remained the original wild type, producing a low titer on resistant cells in horse sera and failing to kill C3H mice. Furthermore, there was no effect of either sera or agarose on the titer of the virus in both of the compatible systems, that is, in the original PRI virus on PRI cells, or of the virulent mutant on the resistant cells. Thus the phenotypic effect was limited to infection of the resistant mouse with the avirulent agent.

If, as seems to be occurring now in the influenza studies of Haller and Lindenmann (22), the results can be explained in terms of an interferon-like substance saving the genetically resistant cells, then we would say that fetal calf serum and agarose inhibit the formation of this substance and horse sera and agar encourage it.

### IMMUNOLOGY OF GENETIC RESISTANCE

Until a few years ago, we were able to phenotypically change the outcome of the incompatible infection of the mouse, but could not change the susceptible cells in tissue culture or obtain susceptible macrophages from the phenotypically susceptible but genetically resistant mouse. However, as immunological advances pointed to the lymphocyte-macrophage interaction (23), we suddenly realized that previous work on apparent transformation of resistant cells, done by Kantoch in our laboratory (24), could be interpreted in a new light. In the original work, it had been shown that if a crude extract of cells taken from the peritoneum of a susceptible mouse was added to the resistant cells, these latter became susceptible. In some unpublished work, Huang later found that a much higher degree of susceptibility obtained if the supernatant of cultures containing living cells was used (25). Recognizing that this might be due to a mixed lymphocyte reaction, Weiser compared the effect of a supernatant from allogeneic PRI-susceptible cells with the supernatant from congenic $C3H_{SS}$ (the congenic susceptible) on the resistant C3H cells and found that the PRI cells did, as before, cause susceptibility, whereas the $C3H_{SS}$ did not (26).

Since that time, it has been shown that supernatants from both mixed lymphocyte cultures and cortisone-treated spleen cells make both the mouse and its macrophages susceptible, and Weiser has also found that the reverse, i.e., conversion of susceptible cells into resistant, may be produced by Con-A or complete Freund's adjuvant. More recently, Taylor has evidence that endotoxin will encourage resistance. Thus the change in susceptible to resistant and the reverse in the mice has been also observed in the macrophages.

Obviously we are in the midst of the problem of immune regulation, and to discuss this briefly, we turn to the work of Benacerraf and Germaine (23). In their diagrammatic

summary, it may be seen that the complex interactions which
lead to antibody response or suppression are pushed one way
or another on the basis of how the macrophage handles the
initial antigen, and that this, in turn, calls into play
greater or lesser inputs from the suppressor or helper
cells.

Our evidence that similar specific interactions occur
between the lymphocytes and the macrophage and that this interaction determines the susceptibility of the mouse rests
on the following data:

1) Extensive destruction of both macrophages and
   lymphocytes is apparent in liver, spleen and thymus
   in the compatible system (27).

2) Complete correlation between genetic resistance and
   macrophage resistance when macrophages are grown in
   media which promote resistance.

3) Correlation of resistance of macrophages as seen in
   liver and cultures and resistance of the developing
   mouse.

4) Phenotypic alteration from incompatibility to compatibility with mixed lymphocytes and cortisone,
   both in vitro and in vivo. Role of lymphokines in
   this.

5) Phenotypic alteration from compatibility to incompatibility by Con-A and Freund's adjuvant, both
   demonstrated in vivo and in vitro.

6) Phenotypic depression of resistance (suppression of
   interferon production?) by different media (fetal
   calf) and substrates (agarose).

There is a renewed interest in the effectiveness of interferon in protecting animals against virulent outcome,
stimulated by the finding by Gresser and his associates
(28,29,30) that anti-interferon makes avirulent mild infections become serious. In the original work with Warwick
(32), the presence of resistant cultures from C3H mice in
the same roller tube with the susceptible PRI cultures did
not protect the susceptible cells, and Shif (20) showed that
mixed cultures of susceptible macrophages from the two allogeneic mice yielded plaques with only half of the cells susceptible. More recently, the same experiments with the congenic mice showed a mixture of susceptible and resistant
cells developing in the plaque, roughly in proportion to the
input of susceptible and resistant cells. The interfering
substance has specificity!

Obviously much needs to be done before the idea that it
is the early warning system of the immune mechanism which is

responsible for death or survival can be proven. To come back to my original statement about the "usefulness" of the system, we may finish with the suggestion that the marvelous sytem in which the host and virus are sufficiently incompatible so that infection without severe disease takes place, is just the kind of practical system needed for tests of "immunosuppression". Preliminary work in our laboratory has now established that malnourished mice respond with a very high mortality and that even slight deviations from the optimum diet introduce mortality, which we literally never have seen in the genetically resistant mice raised on a regular mouse chow (32).

CONCLUSIONS

1) A genetically resistant mouse is one that recognizes a specific signal (the virus) and through a lymphokine turns on a non-specific intracellular mechanism.

2) Since mixtures of congenic susceptible and resistant cells remain resistant or susceptible, there is specificity to the message. This is only partly explained by the fact that the resistant cells are specially sensitive to interferon.

3) This resistance mechanism may also be turned on by non-specific stimuli such as Concanavalin-A.

4) It is suggested that the genetically defined incompatible host virus pair allows for a more accurate and sensitive test of environmental factors which cause the fatal outcome of infection. Data from a study of nutrition are presented in support of this.

REFERENCES

1. Van Doren, C. Benjamin Franklin. New York, Garden City Publishing Co.Inc.,p.700: 1938.

2. Flexner, A. Keynote address at opening of Squibb Institute for Medical Research, New Brunswick, N.J., 1938.

3. Day, P.R. Genetics of Host-Parasite Interaction. San Francisco, W.H. Freeman & Co., 1974.

4. Flor, H.H. Adv.Gen. 8:29, 1956.

5. Drijfhout, E. Agric. Res. Rep. 872. Wagenigen (Neth.): Centre for Agricultural Publication and Documentation.

6. Bang, F.B., and Warwick, A. Proc.Natl. Acad. Sci. 46:1065, 1960.

7.  Kantoch, M., Warwick, A., and Bang, F.B. J.Exp.Med. 117:781, 1963.
8.  Weiser, W., Vellisto, I., and Bang, F.B. Proc.Soc.Exp.Biol.Med. 152:499, 1976.
9.  Gallily, R., Warwick, A., and Bang, F.B. Proc.Natl.Acad.Sci. 51:1158, 1964.
10. Shif, I., and Bang, F.B. J.Exp.Med. 131:851, 1970.
11. Unpublished data.
12. Sheets, P.H., Shah, K.V., and Bang, F.B. Proc.Soc.Exp.Biol.Med. 159:34, 1978.
13. Unpublished data.
14. Ruebner, B.H., and Bramhall, J.L. Arch.Pathol. 69:190, 1960.
15. Cancro, M.P., Gerhard, W., and Klinman, J.R. J.Exp.Med. 147:776, 1978.
16. Willenborg, D.O., Shah, K.V., and Bang, F.B. Proc.Soc.Exp.Biol.Med. 141:762, 1973.
17. Gledhill, A.W., and Niven, J.S.F. Br.J.Exp.Pathol. 38:284, 1957.
18. Lavelle, G.C., and Bang, F.B. J.Gen.Virol. 12:1, 1971.
19. Chang, Y.T. Transactions of the Symposium on Resarch in Leprosy, sponsored by the Leonard Wood Memorial (American Leprosy Foundation) and The Johns Hopkins University School of Hygiene and Public Health, 1961.
20. Shif, I., and Bang, F.B. Proc.Soc.Exp.Biol.Med. 121:829, 1966.
21. Cody, T.S. Doctor of Science thesis, The Johns Hopkins University School of Hygiene and Public Health, Baltimore, Maryland, 1980.
22. Haller, O.A., Arnheiter, H., and Lindenmann, J. Inf.Imm. 13:844, 1976.
23. Benacerraf, B., and Germaine, R.N. Fed.Proc.38:2053, 1979.
24. Kantoch, M., and Bang, F.B. Proc.Natl.Acad.Sci.48:1553, 1962.
25. Huang, J.H. Unpublished data.
26. Weiser, W., and Bang, F.B. J.Exp.Med.143:690, 1976.
27. Weiser, W. Doctor of Philosophy dissertation, The Johns Hopkins University, Baltimore, Maryland, 1978.
28. Gresser, I., Tovey, M.G., Bandu,M.T., Maury, C., and Brouty-Boye, D. J.Exp.Med.144:1305, 1976.
29. Virelizier, J.L., and Gresser, I. J. Immunol.120:1616, 1978.
30. Gresser, I., Tovey, M.G., Maury, C., and Bandu, M.T. J.Exp.Med.144:1316, 1976.
31. Bang, F.B., and Warwick, A. Virology 9:715, 1959.
32. Zaman, S.N. Master of Science thesis, The Johns Hopkins University, Baltimore, Maryland, 1979.

DISCUSSION

Kirchner:   I have been intrigued by the findings which Bang
has published to the effect that MLC supernatants make resistant cells susceptible.   Under the same conditions of
such an MLC, we and others have shown that relatively large
amounts of type II interferon are produced.   MIF and other
lymphokines are also produced in such supernatants and Bang
has also shown, for example, that sea-star MIF has the same
type of effect.   My query now is whether Bang has actually
tested the MLC supernatant for the presence of MIF and
interferon.

Bang:   In dealing with the MLC we know we are working with
crude complex material in which are probably present the
different factors Kirchner has mentioned.   He is perfectly
correct in raising the matter of interferon activity, as it
would presumably produce an effect just the opposite to that
we obtained.   But these are the data.

O'Brien:   What are Bang's C3H resistant and susceptible sublines?   I seem to recall that one was the HeJ.

Bang:   We originally obtained our C3H from Dr. Andervont and
it is the Heston subline.   We have maintained it for about
20 years but have not had occasion to test it for the endotoxin part of the story.

O'Brien:   So both the resistant and susceptible sublines are
C3H Heston sublines?

Bang:   Yes.   The C3H susceptible strain was made by the introduction into them of the gene from the PRI mice through a
series of twenty back-crosses and then a creation, by inbreeding of that particular series of back-crosses.   It is
the same strain except for any possible mutation that may
have occurred in .the last few years.

Dupuy:   Can the in vitro resistance of macrophages be
abrogated by means of anti-theta antiserum and complement?

Bang:   We have not done that.   What we have done most recently is to use cortisone which has such a striking effect
on the incompatible pair, producing infection and death in
this particular situation; we have been particularly interested in the effect on macrophages.   Three doses of cortisone will change the mouse to the point where cells taken a
day or so after the third dose will remain susceptible in

tissue culture for about 4 or 5 days. This cortisone effect, demonstrable in vitro for the first time, is also neutralized by the Con A material.

Gavora: My question for Bang concerns the change of the classical four-square plan to the cube he made by adding the phenotypic change to it. Is not the phenotypic change, in fact, some kind of expression from the genotype as well? Should it be called phenotypic change since it is, or must be, genetically predetermined?

Bang: I do not know how to answer Gavora's point whether the semantics are correct or not. What I am trying to emphasize is that we are keeping the genotype as standard as we can by repeatedly cloning the virus to be sure it is the original strain, and by continuous tests on the mouse, by the use of congenic strains of mice. I think it is the kind of phenotypic change geneticists are so familiar with - the fact that one can have an Himalayan rabbit which under certain temperature conditions, will develop a black fur coat. It is the temperature that influences this on top of the genotype. So, yes, we are working on a genotype and changing it phenotypically in its manifestation.

# HOST DEFENSE MECHANISMS IN GENETIC RESISTANCE TO VIRAL INFECTIONS

O. Haller, H. Arnheiter, and J. Lindenmann
Division of Experimental Microbiology
Institute for Medical Microbiology
University of Zurich
P.O.B. 8028 Zurich, Switzerland

## INTRODUCTION

Compared with acquired immunity relatively little is known about resistance mechanisms in natural, genetically determined host defense against viruses. Inborn resistance may be caused by barriers at several points in the virus-host interaction. Depending on the system studied, the following possibilities have been considered: presence of humoral inhibitors in serum or secretions, lack of cell surface receptors, abortive infection, release of non-infectious virus, production of defective interfering particles, induction of interferon, triggering of cellular, humoral and secretory immune responses, peculiarities of macrophages and activation of natural killer (NK) cells.

In most cases, resistance to viral infections is under polygenic control and has a complex mode of inheritance. There are, however, instances where a single gene locus determines the degree of susceptibility to a virus. These simple situations should offer a practicable approach to elucidating some of the factors involved. In laboratory mice, single gene inheritance has been well documented in resistance to mouse hepatitis virus and to flaviviruses (2). Another good example is the resistance to the lethal effects of various orthomyxoviruses exhibited by mice carrying the dominant allele (26). Extensive studies, exploring some of the factors mentioned above, have been performed on the mechanisms by which the host gene Mx might confer resistance. In this review, possible host defense mechanisms will be discussed and their relevance for other instances of inherited resistance to viral infections will be considered.

## RESISTANCE TO ORTHOMYXOVIRUSES GOVERNED BY THE DOMINANT ALLELE Mx

Resistance to influenza virus was detected by chance when mice of the inbred A2G strain were infected with an otherwise lethal dose of neurotropic NWS virus (23). Resistance could be shown to be due to the presence of a single dominant allele, called Mx (24). Mx-bearing mice of various

genetic backgrounds proved to be resistant to challenge with
a variety of pneumotropic, neurotropic and hepatotropic influenza A viruses but were as sensitive as non-Mx-bearing
control mice to other, unrelated viruses such as vesicular
stomatitis virus (VSV), encephalomyocarditis virus (EMC) or
herpes simplex virus type 1 (HSV-1) (13,25). In homozygous
animals resistance became fully established within 48 to 96
h of birth, in heterozygous animals within 14 to 17 days
(24). Influenza virus replicated to 100 times higher levels
in susceptible as compared to resistant mice (13,26). Initially experiments on the resistance mechanisms indicated
that lack of virus receptors or presence of virus inhibitors
were most likely not responsible for the resistant state
(26). Further studies with a hepatotropic strain of influenza virus indicated that, whereas the livers of infected
susceptible mice revealed widespread and severe necrosis of
hepatocytes, livers from similarly infected resistant mice
showed but a few focal lesions with pronounced cellular infiltration, which were self-limiting (13). Hence, a plausible explanation postulated a particularly early or particularly efficient immune response.

IMMUNE RESPONSE AND NATURAL RESISTANCE TO INFLUENZA VIRUS

Newborn animals from genetically resistant strains are
usually fully susceptible to infection. In genetic resistance to mouse hepatitis virus, neonatal thymectomy prevents
development of resistance, and treatment with cortisone,
X-rays or cyclophosphamide all break down the established
resistance of the adult mouse (2). We have therefore tested
the effects of various immunosuppressive treatments on the
course of influenza virus infection in A2G mice. Resistance
could not be abrogated by these treatments although they
prevented inflammatory infiltration by mononuclear cells at
the site of viral replication and appeared to delay virus
clearance (7,13). We have also introduced the gene Mx into
nu/nu mice known to lack a functional T cell system. Expression of the resistance phenotype to various influenza A
viruses was unimpaired in such Mx-bearing nude mice (12,19).
However, nude mice surviving virus challenge had significantly lower antibody titers than similarly infected non-
nude controls. Furthermore, these animals being immunologically not fully competent were unable to clear the virus
from the lungs and became chronic virus carriers (unpublished observations).
    We concluded that expression of resistance in mice
carrying the allele Mx was independent of conventional T and
B cell responses. Nevertheless, acquired immunity seemed to

be indispensable to viral clearance and to recovery from disease.

## MACROPHAGES AND NK CELLS IN ANTIVIRAL RESISTANCE

There is good evidence for a protective role of macrophhages in viral infections. These cells monitor the main body compartments and are thought to represent a first line of antiviral defense. In the liver, Kupffer cells lining the sinusoids constitute an intact barrier protecting the adjacent parenchymal cells. Recruitment of mononuclear phagocytes is considered an important component of host defense. In both, genetic resistance to mouse hepatitis virus (3,30) and resistance to flaviviruses (8) macrophages from resistant but not from susceptible animals have been found to be capable of restricting virus replication in vitro. It has been proposed that the age dependent development of resistance to herpes simplex virus in mice was due to functional maturation of the macrophage population after birth (21,22). To investigate this matter in our model system we have adapted an avian influenza A virus to grow in peritoneal macrophages. This virus strain grew equally well in Kupffer cells isolated from mouse liver (Fig. 1).

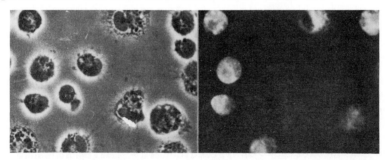

Fig. 1. Kupffer cells isolated from livers of susceptible A/J mice 6 hrs after infection with macrophage adapted influenza A virus. The same area is shown by phase contrast (left) and immunofluorescence microscopy (right). Kupffer cells exhibit an indented or oval nucleus and a vacuolated cytoplasm (4). Indirect staining of acetone fixed cells with virus specific mouse antiserum and FITC coupled rabbit anti-mouse Ig shows bright fluorescence of infected cells.

Macrophages and Kupffer cells obtained from resistant animals did not allow virus replication and showed no cytopathic effect, whereas macrophages from susceptible mice by interposing themselves between the virus and its secondary targets, might be the main factor mediating resistance in

vivo. To test this hypothesis, transfer experiments were
performed in which macrophage precursors were adoptively
transferred from resistant to lethally irradiated H-2 identical susceptible mice and vice versa (16). These experiments summarized in Table 1 showed that animals of susceptible genotype died of infection in spite of harbouring resistant macrophages, and animals of resistant genotype survived, although their macrophages were susceptible. In conclusion, the genetically determined capacity of macrophages
to restrict influenza virus multiplication was obviously not
a decisive factor in determining in vivo susceptibility or
resistance.

In hemopoietic chimeras NK cell populations are known
to be of donor genotype (14). Enhanced resistance to herpes
simplex virus type 1 (28) or to NK sensitive tumor cells

Table 1.  Resistance phenotype of chimeras repopulated with
bone marrow stem cells from resistant/(Mx/+) or susceptible
(+/+) donors.

| Type of chimeras | | Resistance phenotype[2] | |
|---|---|---|---|
| Donor | Recipient[1] | Macrophages | Intact animal |
| Mx/+ | +/+ | resistant | susceptible |
| +/+ | Mx/+ | susceptible | resistant |
| Mx/+ | Mx/+ | resistant | resistant |
| +/+ | +/+ | susceptible | susceptible |

[1] Irradiated with 850 rad and reconstituted with $3 \times 10^7$
viable bone marrow cells of sex-matched histocompatible
donors.

[2] Macrophage cultures were established from individual
chimeras 12 weeks after marrow grafting and were tested
for susceptibility to infection with macrophage-adapted
influenza virus. Two weeks later, the chimeras themselves
were tested for resistance to influenza virus infection
(16).

(15) is transferable to susceptible animals by marrow stem
cells from genetically resistant donors. The present findings would therefore argue against the possibility of NK
cells being mediators of resistance to orthomyxoviruses.
This notion is supported by the fact that various treatments
known to impair NK cell function did not affect innate resistance of A2G mice (19).

## ROLE OF INTERFERON

Recent work with potent antiserum to type I mouse interferon has clearly demonstrated the beneficial role of
interferon in the initial response of mice to different
viral infections (6,9,10). That interferon would be involved in innate resistance of A2G mice to influenza virus seemed rather unlikely. Resistance was highly selective for
orthomyxoviruses, whereas interferon is not thought to be
virus specific. Furthermore, the amount of interferon produced after infection with influenza virus was constantly
much lower in resistant mice as compared to susceptible controls (7,17). Nevertheless, treatment with anti-interferon
serum rendered resistant A2G mice fully susceptible to the
lethal action of influenza virus, and virus titers in such
mice reached levels similar to those observed in genetically
susceptible animals as evidenced in Table 2 (17). Similarly, the use of anti-interferon serum had indicated that interferon was part of the specific resistance of C3H/HeJ and
A/J mice to mouse hepatitis virus type 3 (MHV-3) (31).

Table 2. Effect of anti-mouse IF serum on inborn resistance
to hepatotropic influenza A virus[1]

| Mouse strain | Genotype | Virus titers[2] | | Mortality[3] | |
|---|---|---|---|---|---|
| | | NSG | AIFG | NSG | AIFG |
| A/J | (+/+) | 6.1 | 6.6 | 100% | 100% |
| A2G | (Mx/Mx) | 3.0 | 6.5 | 0% | 100% |
| (A/J x A2G)F[1] | (Mx/+) | 3.5 | 6.4 | 0% | 100% |

[1] Sheep anti-mouse interferon globulin (AIFG), neutralizing
titer of $1.2 \times 10^6$, or normal sheep serum globulin (NSG)
were given i.v. immediately before virus challenge as
described (17).

[2] $Log_{10}$ $EID_{50}$/ml of heparinized blood pooled from 5 mice
per group 48 h after infection.

[3] % deaths on day 7 after infection of 4 mice per group
with 100 $LD_{50}$ of TURH virus i.p.

## INTERFERON DEPENDENT RESISTANCE AS A PROPERTY OF EACH TARGET CELL

Peritoneal macrophages obtained from A2G mice pretreated with anti-interferon serum proved to be susceptible to
influenza virus infection (17). Another way for obtaining
susceptible macrophages from resistant mice was to keep mac-

rophages <u>in</u> <u>vitro</u> long enough for resistance to wane.
After 2-3 weeks of cultivation, resistant macrophages became
phenotypically susceptible and supported influenza virus
growth to the same extent as macrophages from genetically
susceptible mice. The resistance phenotype could be restored in susceptible <u>Mx</u>-bearing macrophages by treatment
with doses of interferon that left non-<u>Mx</u>-bearing cells susceptible (18). This finding is illustrated in Fig. 2.

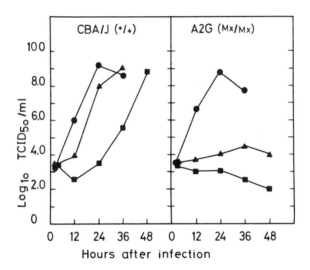

Fig. 2:
Interferon induced inhibition of influenza virus growth in
cultured macrophages from susceptible CBA/J and resistant
A2G mice
Peritoneal macrophages cultured for 2 weeks were treated for
18 hrs with 40 (▲) or 400 (■) reference units of mouse interferon type I and were then infected with macrophage-
adapted influenza A virus at a multiplicity of 5.0 together
with untreated control cultures ( ● ) as described (18).
Virus growth was measured by infectivity titrations of cell
free supernates on chick embryo fibroblast monolayers at the
times after infection indicated.

Our assumption was that endogenous interferon acted on peritoneal macrophages in vivo, and that this effect waned during prolonged cultivation in vitro. Since earlier attempts
to demonstrate resistance in monolayer cultures of fetal

brain or kidney cells had failed (29, and unpublished results) we speculated at first that phenotype expression in vitro was a peculiarity of macrophages. However, we have since been able to show the resistance phenomenon in vitro in other cell types as well, such as adult mouse hepatocytes (1) or brain cells in aggregating cultures (11). Macrophages and hepatocytes from adult animals differ from fetal cells in that they preserve a high degree of cellular differentiation in culture and may thus be quite representative for the population of adult target cells likely to be encountered by the virus during its growth in vivo.

Resistance due to the allele Mx is operative selectively against orthomyxoviruses but not against a large number of other viruses (25). If interferon were responsible for resistance of Mx-bearing cells, it should be possible to demonstrate virus specificity of interferon action in such cells. With both macrophages and hepatocytes it could be shown that influenza virus growth was but little affected by large doses of interferon in non-Mx-bearing (susceptible) cells, whereas it was very efficiently inhibited in Mx-bearing cells. In contrast, increasing doses of interferon inhibited three unrelated viruses (VSV, EMC and HSV-1) markedly and independently of Mx genotype (1,18).

These experiments revealed that interferon together with the resistance gene Mx selectively limited influenza virus replication in the actual host cell. The details of the interaction between Mx and interferon are at present not well understood. We believe, however, that in vivo a similar resistance mechanism is operative in most, if not all, cells throughout the body. Recent experiments show that newborn mice (which do not exhibit resistance) can be protected against lethal infection with influenza virus by treatment with interferon if they carry the allele Mx but not if they lack it. The interplay of interferon and host genes may well be a more general occurrence than hitherto suspected and may provide a clue to the better understanding of individual variations in susceptibility to viral diseases.

CONCLUDING REMARKS

We have presented here curent evidence for a genetic control of sensitivity to interferon action at the single cell level resulting in virus specific host resistance. We do not know at present to which extent this concept might apply to other virus-host systems. In most instances of genetically determined resistance several host defense mechanisms seem to be involved. Although the present concept has been discussed with regard to flaviviruses (20), further studies on flavivirus resistance have inferred that the inhibitory effect of interferon in resistant cells was merely superimposed on an intrinsic, cellular restriction of flavivirus replication and that the basic mechanism was likely to be enhanced production of defective interfering particles (5). A third situation where interferon appeared to be involved was inborn resistance of mice to mouse hepatitis virus, but, again, other factors seemed to be of similar importance (31). Among these, macrophages have been proposed to play a key role mainly because of the striking correlation between in vitro macrophage resistance and resistance of the intact animal. We have recently observed that cultured hepatocytes isolated from adult mice likewise expressed resistance or susceptibility to infection with MHV-3 according to their genotype. Marked polycaryon formation and production of infectious virus were seen in hepatocytes from susceptible C57BL/6J mice but not in cells from resistant A/J mice (Arnheiter and Haller, in preparation). It would thus seem that genetic resistance to acute infection with MHV-3 is expressed not only in macrophages but also in the ultimate host cell of the liver parenchyma. The possible involvement of interferon in this resistance has to be investigated. Although both resistance to orthomyxoviruses and resistance to mouse hepatitis virus are seemingly expressed in adult cells in vitro, the differences between the two systems are nevertheless obvious: whereas resistance to mouse hepatitis virus would seem to depend on many factors for its manifestation in vivo (including host cell resistance, immune mechanisms, macrophage functions and interferon, the relative roles of which await further clarification) it is now quite clear that the interaction of interferon and the host gene Mx sufficiently accounts for the resistance to influenza virus as observed in A2G mice.

ACKNOWLEDGMENT

This work was supported by grants No. 3.139.77 and 3.393.78 from the Swiss National Science Foundation.

REFERENCES

1.    Arnheiter, H., Haller, O., and Lindenmann, J. Virology (in press).
2.    Bang, F.B. Adv.Virus Res. 23:269, 1978.
3.    Bang, F.B., and Warwick, A. Proc.Natl.Acad.Sci.U.S.A. 46:1065, 1960.

4.  Crofton, R.W., Diesselhoff-den Dulk, M.M.C., and van Furth, R. J.Exp.Med. 148:1, 1978.

5.  Darnell, M.B., and Koprowski, H. J.Infect.Dis. 129:248, 1974.

6.  Fauconnier, B. C.R.Hebd.Seances Acad.Sci. 271:464, 1970.

7.  Fiske, R.A., and Klein, P.A. Infect.Immun. 11:576, 1975.

8.  Goodman, G.T., and Koprowski, H. Proc.Natl.Acad.Sci.U.S.A. 48:160, 1961.

9.  Gresser, I., Tovey, M.G., Bandu, M.-T., Maury, C., and Brouty-Boye, D. J.Exp.Med. 144:1305, 1976.

10. Gresser, I., Tovey, M.G., Maury, C., and Bandu, M.-T. J.Exp.Med. 144:1316, 1976.

11. Haller, O., and Honegger, P. 1980 (submitted).

12. Haller, O., and Lindenmann, J. Nature (Lond.). 250:679, 1974.

13. Haller, O., Arnheiter, H., and Lindenmann, J. Infect.Immun. 13:844, 1976.

14. Haller, O., Kiessling, R., Orn, A., and Wigzell, H. J.Exp.Med. 145:1411, 1977.

15. Haller, O., Hansson, M., Kiessling, R., and Wigzell, H. Nature (Lond.). 270:609, 1977.

16. Haller, O., Arnheiter, H., and Lindenmann, J. J.Exp.Med. 150:117, 1979.

17. Haller, O., Arnheiter, H., Gresser, I., and Lindenmann, J. J.Exp.Med. 149:601, 1979.

18. Haller, O., Arnheiter, H., Lindenmann, J., and Gresser, I. Nature 283:660, 1980.

19. Haller, O., Arnheiter, H., and Lindenmann, J. "Natural Cell-Mediated Immunity Against Tumors". R.B. Herberman, Ed. Academic Press, New York (in press).

20. Hanson, B., Koprowski, H., Baron, S., and Buckler, C.E. Microbios 1B:51, 1969.

21. Hirsch, M.S., Zisman, B., and Allison, A.C. J.Immunol. 104:1160, 1970.

22. Johnson, R.T. J.Exp.Med. 120:359, 1964.

23. Lindenmann, J. Virology 16:203, 1962.

24. Lindenmann, J. Proc.Soc.Exp.Biol.Med. 116:506, 1964.

25. Lindenmann, J., and Klein, P.A. Arch.ges.Virusforsch. 19:1, 1966.

26. Lindenmann, J., Lane, C.A., and Hobson, D. J.Immunol. 90:942, 1963.

27. Lindenmann, J., Deuel, E., Fanconi, S., and Haller, O. J.Exp.Med. 147:531, 1978.

28. Lopez, C. "Third International Symposium on Herpes Viruses and Oncogenesis". G. de The, W. Heule, and

F. Rapp, eds. World Health Organization, Geneva, p. 775, 1978.

29. Vallbracht, A. Ph.D. Dissertation, University of Tubingen, Tubingen, West Germany, 1977.

30. Virelizier, J.-L., and Allison, A.C. Arch.Virol. 50:279, 1976.

31. Virelizier, J.L., and Gresser, I. J.Immunol. 120:1616, 1978.

## DISCUSSION

Dupuy: Would Haller tell us whether it is possible to transfer resistance by doing co-culture between fresh and aged macrophages?

Haller: We have not tried the experiment you proposed, but have explored something similar. We have sought to determine whether it was possible, by co-cultivation of resistant and susceptible macrophages, to protect the susceptible macrophages. However, this yielded rather inconclusive results. We discerned some degree of protection, but we think that this could equally well be attributable to the fact that the resistant macrophages, which then do not exhibit the cytopathic effect, survive and phagocytize the virus in the supernatant we measure. This could give the impression that we have protection, but that was not actually the case. Rather, it was merely removal of infectious virus in the culture by the surviving macrophages. This has proved to be a very difficult issue to resolve.

Dupuy: Has Haller looked for specific binding of interferon in populations of macrophages with and without the Mx allele?

Haller: The binding of interferon, or the differential binding of interferon to cells, has also proved difficult. Up to now it is still a problem to even measure interferon binding. I have just become aware of recent work, now in press, from Gresser's laboratory where they compare binding to various cell types of iodinated highly purified interferon. We hope to do a collaborative study on that.

Bang: Haller has emphasized very nicely the difference between mouse hepatitis and his influenza system. Are the lymphocytes affected in the hepatitic variant of influenza that he has studied? Also, are there mechanisms of altering the susceptibility of the macrophage in vitro other than by mere aging?

Haller: I do not know about the role of lymphocytes, wheth-er they get infected or not. I can well imagine lymphocytes being important as interferon-producing cells. As to the other question, there are two means of obtaining susceptible macrophages from resistant animals. As I have already ex-plained, one way is by just letting them remain in culture. One could also add various drugs in vitro, something we have not yet done. Another way to get susceptible macrophages is to pre-treat the resistant mouse with anti-interferon anti-body and harvest the macrophages from such treated mice; these macophages are susceptible. So to us that indicates that somehow in our mice, which are conventionally reared of course, macrophages in the peritoneal cavity are exposed to endogenous interferon and that is why they are resistant from the very beginning. During culturing in vitro they would lose with time this resistant state.

Kirchner: With regard to his influenza studies, has Haller ever compared serum interferon levels after injection of influenza into susceptible and resistant mice or has he done this in vitro by using PE cells or spleen cells, i.e., checked for differences in interferon production?

Haller: That is, of course, an important point that has always intrigued us. The resistant mice produce less inter-feron than the susceptible ones. Interferon production in these systems proves to be merely a reflection of viral replication. If one has good viral replication in a tissue, high titers of interferon are obtained, whereas, in the re-sistant system, viral replication is inhibited and conseq-uently there is less interferon produced. These findings, which are very well established in our system, have led us to the opinion that interferon cannot be a causative agent. The difference occurs at the level of the interferon action.

Kirchner: Has Haller tried inactivated virus as an inter-feron inducer?

Haller: No, I have not.

Zisman: In his resistant cultures, did Haller check only for infectious virus, or did he determine growth of virus by lack of detecting infectious virus, or did he utilize other approaches also, such as immunofluorescence.

Haller: Of course we have done immunofluorescence studies,

but we have also checked for viral protein synthesis in macrophages from resistant and susceptible mice, by infecting the cells and then labelling the proteins with $^{35}$S-methionine. Aged macrophages, carrying the Mx gene when they are infected, produce the virus-specific proteins just as do infected macrophages from the susceptible animal. But, if one pretreats the cell with 40 units of interferon, this does not really inhibit the influenza virus replication in susceptible macrophages. However, in the presence of the Mx gene, there is no viral protein synthesis at all which says something about the molecular mechanisms of the Mx gene and interferon. Obviously, viral transcription or translation is arrested at a very early stage of viral replication in these cells.

Zisman: Does Haller discern any differences between macrophages obtained from young resistant mice as compared with adult resistant mice?

Haller: We have not studied that issue.

Massanari: Does Haller know what type of interferon is being dealt with in this work? What was the source of interferon he was using?

Haller: It was highly purified type I interferon induced by NDV in mouse C243 cells which was provided by Gresser. We have not examined type II in this regard, but plan to do that.

Dupuy: What happens if Haller treats the resistant macrophages with trypsin? Do they lose their resistance?

Haller: No, we have tested that and there is no change in regard to their phenotypic expression. We made another observation in that connection. Actually we were comparing resistant macrophages with macrophages from susceptible animals which had been immunized against influenza virus. If one takes peritoneal macrophages from animals immunized with influenza virus, puts them in culture and infects them with the same strain of influenza virus, they are also resistant. But this resistance is trypsin sensitive, and one can restore it by adding small amounts of anti-viral antibody. So we think this involves cytophilic antibodies on the macrophage surface which can be removed by trypsin treatment, whereas our resistant macrophages never become susceptible as a result of such treatment.

Kaplan: The virus specificity of this effect makes me wonder whether the interferon effect has something to do with cell surface receptors rather than a terminal metabolic process. Does Haller know whether there is a differential binding of the virus due to the interferon?

Haller: Yes, we have examined the binding of the virus - radioactively marked - and looked at the binding of aged susceptible, or aged interferon-treated resistant macrophages, as well as macrophages from susceptible animals, and there was no difference. So influenza appears to bind the same extent to macrophages of resistant and susceptible mice, independently of whether they express the resistance phenotype or not. Accordingly, we rather think that absorption of the virus is the same; now we are looking at penetration, but as yet we have no answers. But we can say there is early arrest of viral replication, probably at the level of transcription or translation.

Participant: I wondered if Haller had done any experiments looking at somatic cell hybrids, fusing these two genotypes to see what happens.

Haller: We have not done that.

GENETIC STUDY OF MHV3 INFECTION IN MICE:   IN VITRO
REPLICATION OF VIRUS IN MACROPHAGES

C. Dupuy, D. Lafforêt-Cresteil
and J.M. Dupuy


Inserum U.56, hop.Bichêtre,
France et Institut Armand-Frappier
Laval-des-Rapides,
Québec, Canada

MHV3 infection in mice displays various types of sensitivity depending on the inbred strains tested:   resistance
(A/J), fully susceptibility, leading to death in 5-7 days
(DBA/2; C57BL/6) and semi-susceptibility (2).   The latter
type, observed in some inbred strains as well as in F1 hybrids between susceptible and resistant parents, is characterized by an acute disease leading to death in 10-30% of
infected adult mice, and in animals which survived, by the
development of a chronic neurologic disease with persistent
MHV3 infection (2).
    Genetic study of acute and chronic MHV3 induced diseas-
es was carried out in segregating generations of a cross involving susceptible C57BL/6 and resistant mouse strains (4).
We found that 1 or 2 recessive genes are involved in resistance of acute and chronic disease but that the genes involved in both diseases are different.   In addition, the use
of congenic lines showed that the presence of the H-2$^f$
allele conferred to heterozygote as well as to homozygote
mice, the capacity to resist to the development of a chronic
disease (4).
    The determination of MHV3 titer in serum from F1 hy-
brids, 4 days after infection, showed a strict correlation
between virus titer and outcome of the infection (2).   Since
it was shown that MHV3 replicates in Swiss mouse embryo
cells (1), as well as in liver cells from newborn mice (6)
and in macrophages (5), we assumed that the capacity of
cells to restrict or not viral replication was playing a
major role in controlling the yield of virus and that intracellular control mechanisms might be under genetic influence.   In vitro studies were, therefore, undertaken in order
to assess viral replication according to strain sensitivity.

RESULTS

Peritoneal exudate cells (PEC) were obtained from susceptible (DBA/2,B6), resistant (A/J) and semi-susceptible
(B6 x A/J)F1 hybrids) mice. After 3 days in culture, adherent cells were shown to have morphological, functional
(98% phagocytosis of yeast particles) and biochemical
(esterase positive cells) criteria of macrophages. MHV3 infection of cultures was followed by the development of foci
which are giant multinucleated cells surrounded by a zone of
lysis (Fig. 1).

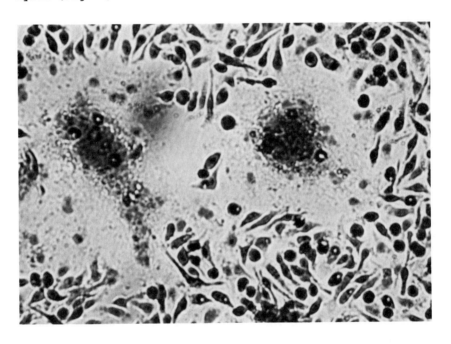

Figure 1. Focus formation in culture of mouse macrophages
12 hours after infection with MHV3. Safranine coloration.
(Magnification: x 200).

As shown in Fig. 2, when macrophages from susceptible DBA/2
or B6 mice were infected in vitro with increasing doses of
MHV3 the number of foci enumerated in culture 24 hours later, displayed a linear relation with the infection dose.
Kinetics experiments showed that foci appeared in culture 6
hours after in vitro infection, regularly increased and, depending on the infective dose, reached a plateau at 24 or 48

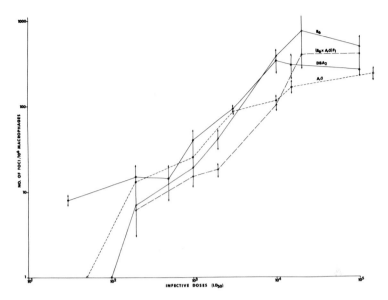

Figure 2. Number of foci in relation to increasing doses of MHV3. Foci were enumerated 24 hours after _in vitro_ infection in cultures of macrophages originating from A/J (resistant), DBA/2 and B6 (susceptible), and (B6 x A/J)F1 hybrids (semi-susceptible) mouse strains.

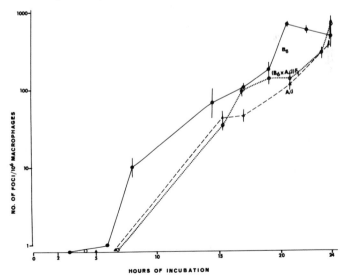

Figure 3. Kinetics of focus formation in cultures of macrophages obtained from B6, A/J and (B6 x A/J)F1 hybrids. Infective dose of MHV3 was $10^4$ LD50.

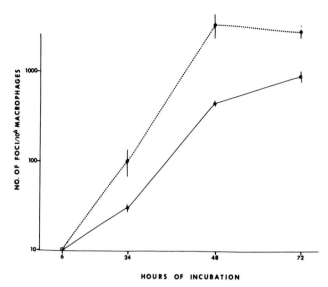

Figure 4.  MHV3 replication in culture of mouse macrophages from A/J mice in relation to time.  No. of foci observed in A/J macrophages after <u>in vitro</u> infection with 3 x 10$^3$ LD50 of MHV3 (●——●); no. of foci observed in DBA/2 macrophages, 24 hours after 1 hour incubation with 1 ml of supernatant obtained at different times, from A/J cell cultures (●---●).

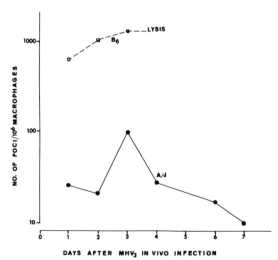

Figure 5.  No. of foci observed in macrophages cultured <u>in vitro</u> for 24 hours and obtained either from susceptible B6 (□-----□) or from resistant A/J (●——●) mice, 1 to 7 days following <u>in vivo</u> infection..

hours (Fig. 3). Twenty four hours after the plateau of foci has been reached, cells are totally lysed.

When macrophages from resistant A/J or from semi-susceptible F1 hybrids mice were infected in vitro, they showed no capacity to restrict viral infection, even when infected with low doses of virus (Fig. 2). The increase of focus number according to time after in vitro infection showed a similar pattern as that observed in susceptible macrophages.

Focus formation and increase in macrophage cultures reflected viral replication since supernatants of such cultures were infective as tested in vivo and in vitro (Fig. 4).In vitro titration of supernatants from A/J macrophage culture taken at 6, 24 and 48 hours after infection showed a regular increase of viral replication of more than 2 logs within 48 hours (Fig. 4).

Experiments were done in order to assess the ability of macrophages to support or not viral replication in vitro, when infected in vivo. In the experiment shown in Fig. 5, $10^3$ LD50 of MHV3 was injected i.p. in B6 and A/J mice. Various times after infection, PEC were obtained and adherent cells were cultured in vitro for 24 hours. When taken 1 to 3 days after in vivo infection, macrophages from B6 mice developed 24 hours later high number of foci and important lysis. The pattern showed by A/J macrophages was different: viral replication was observed up to day 3 after in vivo infection, but the numbers of foci was significantly lower than the one observed in B6 mice. After day 3, the number of foci diminished and no focus was seen after day 7 (Fig. 5).

## DISCUSSION

In vitro infection of macrophages with MHV3 was followed by replication of virus as demonstrated by increasing number of foci and increasing infectivity of culture medium according to time. The cytopathic effects of MHV3 led to foci formation and lysis as already shown (5). When macrophages of various mouse strain sensitivity were tested in vitro to assay their capacity to support or not MHV3 replication, no difference between macrophages from resistant or susceptible animals was seen.

However, daily MHV3 titrations performed in serum, brain and liver of infected mice, revealed a regular virus increase in susceptible DBA/2 mice whereas no or little viral replication was found in A/J resistant animals (3). Since A/J macrophages after in vitro infection did not show any restriction of viral replication (Fig. 2), we studied the capacity of such cells to support viral replication in vitro, after in vivo infection. When such experiments were performed, a significant difference in replication of virus was observed in A/J as compared to B6 macrophages. In A/J macrophages, MHV3 titers remained lower than in B6 cells, total lysis never occurred and no focus was observed after day 7.

Although a similar capacity of virus replication was seen in vitro in macrophages from different mouse strains suggesting an absence of genetic control of intra-cellular MHV3 replication, it was extremely important to observe that macrophages obtained from in vivo infected mice displayed a restriction of viral replication in resistant mice. Such a restriction was already present when peritoneal cells were taken as soon as one hour post infection (to be published). This indicates the existence of an innate resistance, present in A/J mice and absent in susceptible strains. Such a mechanism is different from that operative in resistant mice 4 days or more after infection which is of immune nature (to be published). Cells and/or factors responsible for the innate resistance against MHV3 infection, observed in A/J mice, are presently under study.

## REFERENCES

1.   Haff, R.F.   Virology 18:507, 1962.
2.   Le Prevost, C., Virelizier, J.L., and Dupuy, J.M. J.Immunol. 115:640, 1975.
3.   Le Prevost, C., Levy-Leblond, E., Virelizier, J.L., and Dupuy, J.M.   J.Immunol. 114:221, 1975.
4.   Levy-Leblond, E., Oth, D., and Dupuy, J.M.   J.Immunol. 122:1359, 1979.
5.   Mallucci, L.   Virology 25:30, 1965.
6.   Paradini, F., and Piccinino, F.   Experientia 24:373, 1968.

# GENETIC CONTROL OF RESISTANCE TO JHM, A NEUROTROPIC STRAIN OF MOUSE HEPATITIS

Jeffrey A. Frelinger and Stephen A. Stohlman

Departments of Microbiology and Neurology
University of Southern California
School of Medicine
Los Angeles
California 90033

## INTRODUCTION

The mouse has proven to be the most useful model system for studies of naturally occurring genetic resistance and has been used to test genetic control of a variety of infectious agents. Genetic resistance to viral infections has been studied using mice for over 40 years (13). Recently, the mapping of the major immune response genes of mice to certain loci has spurred attempts to correlate naturally occurring host resistance with the various immunological effector mechanisms that are believed to determine the outcome of viral infections. Genetic models of mouse resistance to viral infection have been described which are single gene, H-2 linked, and polygenic (2,7,8,9).

Naturally occurring genetic resistance to MHV induced hepatitis was first described by Bang and Warwick (1). Using the strain 2 of MHV they found a single recessive gene responsible for resistance and that the phenotypic expression of the genotype was characterized by resistance of the peritoneal macrophage population. MHV strain 3 causes a spectrum of diseases from acute fatal hepatitis to chronic neurological disease. Two genes have been implicated, one H-2-linked that is responsible for the susceptibility to the chronic disease, and one responsible for resistance to the acute disease (6).

JHM is a neurotropic strain of MHV. JHM virus causes a lethal CNS infection characterized by acute encephalomyelitis and both acute and chronic demyelination (4,11,14). The role of this virus in causing demyelination is of interest since the demyelination results from a cytolytic infection of oligodendroglial cells (5) and the pathological process of the chronic disease resembles human multiple sclerosis. In our previously reported studies of resistance to MHV-JHM, we found a marked resistance of the SJL strain of mice compared to eleven other strains (10).

MATERIALS AND METHODS

Mice. The A.SW, B10.M, $F_1$, and backcross mice were bred in
the immunogenetics mouse colony, University of Southern
California School of Medicine. All other mice were purchased from Jackson Laboratory, Bar Harbor, Maine at 6-8 weeks
of age and held until tested. All animals were tested at 12
weeks of age by intracranial inoculation with 1000 $LD_{50}$ of
the JHM strain of MHV (MHV-4) in 0.032 ml. Following injection, mice were observed daily for disease and death. Mice
surviving longer than 3 weeks post challenge were considered
resistant. No deaths occurred later than 14 days following
challenge.

Virus. The virus used through was the seventh suckling
mouse brain passage of JHM obtained from Dr. Leslie Weiner.
The virus pool used consisted of a 10% brain homogenate prepared in phosphate buffered saline, pH 7.2. The $LD_{50}$ titer
was determinbed in sucking Swiss-Webster mice and the pool
adjusted to contain 1000 suckling mouse brain lethal doses
per 0.032 ml.

RESULTS

In a strain survey, only SJL mice showed significant
resistance to JHM (Table 1).

Genetic analysis of B10.S x SJL crosses suggested that
resistance is mediated by at least two genes: one dominant,
designated Rhv-1 and one recessive, designated Rhv-2. The
segregation studies were conducted to minimize H-2 linked
effects; however, the lack of obvious H-2 control of disease resistance in the strain distribution is apparent
(Table 1), since SJL mice are resistant, and both A.SW and
B10.S mice which share the same H-2$^S$ haplotype are susceptible. This argues against an effect of H-2 on resistance
to MHV-JHM encephalomyelitis, and is consistent with our inability to transfer protection with T cells from SJL to
younger susceptible SJL (11).

Since (B10.S x SJL)$F_1$ mice are susceptible, we began a
strain survey to determine a strain of the genotype Rhv-1
R/R, Rhv-2 S/S. Crosses to SJL of such a strain would be
resistant.

Table 2 shows the eight crosses thus far tested. Twenty percent of the (C3H/HeJ x SJL)$F_1$ were resistant to i.c.
challenge with MHV-JHM but insufficient animals have been
tested to reach significance. However, BALB/c x SJL showed
significant resistance. This resistance is not complete,
only 40% of the animals tested were resistant.

Table 1. Mortality of Various Strains of Inbred Mice
Following Intracerebral Inoculation with 1000 SMB $LD_{50}$ of
MHV-JHM*

| Strain | H-2 haplotype | Ig-1 | Survivors/total | Percent resistance |
|---|---|---|---|---|
| A | a | e | 0/10 | 0 |
| C57BL/6 | b | b | 0/25 | 0 |
| C57BL/10 | b | b | 0/10 | 0 |
| BALB/c | d | a | 0/50 | 0 |
| NZB | d | e | 0/10 | 0 |
| B10.M | f | b | 0/7 | 0 |
| AKR | k | d | 1/20 | 5 |
| CBA | k | a | 0/10 | 0 |
| C3H/HeJ | k | a | 0/20 | 0 |
| DBA/1 | q | c | 0/10 | 0 |
| RIII | r | c | 0/10 | 0 |
| B10.S | s | b | 0/40 | 0 |
| A.SW | s | e | 0/40 | 0 |
| SJL | s | b | 80/100 | 80 |
| SJL-Ig-1a | s | a | 2/2 | 100 |

*After Stohlman and Frelinger (10).

Table 2. Mortality of $F_1$ Mice Crossed with SJL after
Intracerebral Inoculation with MHV-JHM

| Strain | Rhv Rhv-1 | Rhv-2 | Genotypes of Inbred Mouse Strain % Survivors of Cross to SJL | |
|---|---|---|---|---|
| SJL | R | R | - | |
| BALB/cJ | S | R | 41 | (37/90) |
| A.SW | S | S | 0 | ( 0/30) |
| C57BL/10SgSn | S | S | 0 | ( 0/25) |
| C57BL/6J | S | S | 0 | ( 0/18) |
| C3H/HeJ | S(?) | S | 20 | ( 4/20) |
| DBA/2 | S | S | 2 | ( 1/57) |
| RIII/J | S | S | 11 | ( 3/27) |
| NZB | S | S | 0 | ( 0/14) |

Table 3. Backcross Analysis of Resistance to Intracerebral
Challenge with MHV-JHM

| Cross | Postulated Rhv genotypes of Progeny | Phenotype | % Resistant[1] | % Survivors Observed expected | |
|-------|-------------------------------------|-----------|----------------|----------|----------|
| (BALB/c x SJL)F₁ x SJL | Rhv-1 R/R; Rhv-2 R/R | Resistant | (80%) | 57% (8/14) | 60% |
| | Rhv-1 R/S; Rhv-2 R/R | Resistant | (40%) | | |
| (BALB/c x SJL)F₁ x BALB/c | Rhv-1 R/S; Rhv-2 R/R | Resistant | (40%) | 19% (17/89) | 20% |
| | Rhv-1 S/S; Rhv-2 R/R | susceptible | ( 0%) | | |

[1]Based on survival of: SJL = 80%, (BALB/c x SJL)F₁ = 40%.

Backcross animals were produced ([BALB/c x SJL]F₁ x
SJL, and [BALB/c x SJL]F₁ x BALB/c and tested for resistance. Table 3 shows that the survival rates of these backcrosses were in close agreement with the values predicted by
the model, that is, only the single dominant/recessive gene
from SJL is segregating in the BALB/c x SJL backcrosses.

## DISCUSSION

Analysis of the genetic control of natural resistance
to MHV-JHM shows: 1) two genes are responsible for resistance, one dominant (Rhv-1) and one recessive (Rhv-2); 2)
resistance is not associated with the major histocompatibility linked Ir genes; and 3) that BALB/c have the resistance
gene at Rhv-2 but carry the resistance gene at Rhv-1.
Our understanding of the genetic resistance to MHV-JHM
differs from the other two proposed models which have examined naturally occurring genetic resistance to other strains
of MHV (1,6). Resistance to MHV-2 and MHV-3 acute hepatitis
are controlled by a single gene, while susceptibility to
MHV-3 chronic immunopathological CNS disease is controlled
by an H-2 linked gene. In both cases where a single gene
controls resistance to acute fatal hepatitis, macrophages
from the resistant animals are refractory to viral infection
in vitro, while the macrophages from the susceptible animals
support viral replication in vitro. We have shown this mechanism does not operate in SJL mice resistant to JHM (11).
We recognize that other genetic models may also fit
these data. Such quantitative models (major genes with
modifiers, variable penetrance, etc.) all seem more complex

than the model proposed here. At this time we favor the simpler model. Definitive tests are underway of this two gene model.

## ACKNOWLEDGEMENT

This work was supported by Grants RG 1233-A-1 from the National Multiple Sclerosis Society, NS 15079, NS 12967, and CA 22662 from N.I.H.

Jeffrey A. Frelinger is a recipient of ACS Faculty Research Award FRA-174.

## REFERENCES

1.  Bang, F., and Warwick, A.   Proc.Natl.Acad.Sci. USA. 46:1065, 1960.
2.  Chalmer, J.E., Mackenzie, J.S., and Stanley, F. J.Gen.Virol. 37:107, 1977.
3.  Cheesebro, B., and Wehrly, K.   Proc.Natl.Acad.Sci.USA. 76:425, 1979.
4.  Herndon, R., Griffin, D., McCormick, U., and Weiner, L.P.  Acta Neurol. 32:32, 1975.
5.  Lampert, P., Sims, J., and Kniazeff, A.   Acta Neuropath. 24:76, 1973.
6.  Levy-Leblond, E., Oth, D., and Dupuy, J.   J.Immunol. 122:1359, 1979.
7.  Lilly, F., and Pincus, T.   Adv.Cancer Res. 17:231, 1973.
8.  Lopez, C. Nature 258:152, 1975.
9.  Martinez, D.  Infect.Immun. 23:45, 1979.
10. Stohlman, S.A., and Frelinger, J.A.   Immunogenetics 6:277, 1978.
11. Stohlman, S.A., and Weiner, L.P.   Neurol., 1980 (in press).
12. Stohlman, S.A., Frelinger, J.A., and Weiner, L.P. J.Immunol., 1980 (in press).
13. Webster, L.T.  J.Exp.Med. 65:261, 1937.
14. Weiner, L.P.  Arch.Neurol. 28:298, 1973.

# GENETIC RESISTANCE TO HERPESVIRUS INFECTIONS: ROLE OF NATURAL KILLER CELLS

Carlos Lopez
Sloan-Kettering Institute for Cancer Research
425 East 68th Street
New York, N.Y. 10021

## INTRODUCTION

The herpesviruses of man include herpes simplex viruses-type 1 and 2 (HSV-1, HSV-2), herpes zoster virus, cytomegalovirus (CMV), and Epstein-Barr virus (EBV). The herpesviruses are important human pathogens: Acute infections are a cause of significant morbidity and mortality and infections with certain of these viruses appear to be linked (perhaps etiologically) with human cancer (35). The basis for resistance against primary or reactivated herpesvirus infections has received considerable attention during the past few years. Assays have been developed to evaluate humoral and cell mediated immune capacities of patients with severe, recurrent herpesvirus infections. However, little information has been generated which clearly defines the mechanisms responsible for resistance to these viruses.

This chapter will concentrate on two approaches to the study of genetic resistance to herpesvirus infections. First, I will discuss the study of primary immunodeficiency diseases associated with severe herpesvirus infections. This approach has taught us much about resistance mechanisms to other organisms (15) and should help define defense mechanisms responsible for herpesvirus infections. Second, I will discuss three animal models of genetic resistance to herpesvirus infections. This approach is relatively new and offers great potential for the definition of the mechanisms required for resistance.

## PRIMARY IMMUNODEFICIENCY DISEASES

Although resistance to any pathogen must probably depend on several components of the defense system, an association between susceptibility to that organism and a specific deficiency would help define at least some of the systems required for resistance (1). Conversely, primary immunodeficiency diseases are rarely of a single cell type which might allow such a clear definition of function. Nevertheless, inborn errors of metabolism have been important to the study of immunobiology and that basic information can be further applied to the understanding of defense against herpesvirus infections.

GENETIC CONTROL OF NATURAL RESISTANCE
TO INFECTION AND MALIGNANCY

253

Combined immunodeficiency disease, whether severe or variable, will not be considered since these tell us little about the specific deficiencies responsible for susceptibility to infection (19).

## WISCOTT-ALDRICH SYNDROME

The Wiscott-Aldrich Syndrome (WAS) has been shown to be due to a single, X-linked recessive gene. Studies by Cooper et al. (11) and Blaese et al. (8) indicate that these patients have a defect in the appropriate initiation of specific immune responses. These studies showed that patients, especially those early in their disease, have T-cells and B-cells and that these components responded in many of the in vitro assays. The defect of the afferent limb of the immune response can be found early and appears to be responsible for the progressive immunodeficiency observed later in the disease. Severe and prolonged infections with herpesviruses (HSV and CMV), severe infections with viruses usually associated with benign disease, and life-threatening infections with bacteria and fungi are usually associated with WAS (41). Although herpesvirus infections are often life-threatening for these patients, WAS is a somewhat heterogeneous disease and some patients are more severely affected than others. Even though the specific immune deficiency has not been defined in patients with WAS, it does appear to be hematoloic in nature since bone marrow transplantation clearly reconstitutes the immune system and allows patients to live normal healthy lives (36).

## X-LINKED LYMPHOPROLIFERATIVE SYNDROME

A new syndrome has recently been described in which young male members of certain families succummed to a lymphoproliferative disease caused by Epstein-Barr virus (EBV) (4,38). The susceptibility found with this syndrome is determined by an X-linked recessive gene and is in this way similar to WAS. Patients with this syndrome demonstrated a marked susceptibility to EBV, a virus which only rarely causes life-threatening infections in man, and an increased susceptibility to other infectious agents. As with patients with WAS, an immunological surveillance mechanism responsible for recognizing and initiating a response (here to EBV infection) appears to be defective.

## ANIMAL MODELS OF GENETIC RESISTANCE TO HERPESVIRUS
## INFECTIONS

The study of herpesvirus infections has relied heavily on the use of animal models since these have allowed investigators to focus on one aspect of the virus infection or another. For example, mouse models have been used to define some of the mechanisms involved in latent infections with HSV-1 (42). When compared to the study of naturally occurring herpesvirus infections in man, animal models allow the control of many important parameters of infection such as age and sex of the mice and route and concentration of virus inocula (3). The use of inbred strains of mice for studies of resistance, in addition, offers several other advantages. These mice have a homogeneous genetic background and therefore should respond similarly to the virus infection. Inbred strains of mice also allow the use of genetic tools for the study of defense systems and, since much is known about mouse genetics (23), correlations with other systems are possible and could be helpful.

Although animal models of genetic resistance offer many advantages, certain disadvantages must also be considered. For example, these models may not resemble human disease sufficiently to teach us much about our own defense systems. Resistance to HSV-1 infection of mice might be based on mechanisms different than those found in man. This is especially true for the herpesviruses because there appears to be evidence of co-evolution of virus and host. Thus, herpesvirus infections appear to have selected natural hosts capable of controlling the infections. When inoculated into a closely related but different species, herpesviruses may cause violent, deadly infections; e.g., when accidently inoculated into humans, B-virus, an inocuous virus of Rhesus monkey's, causes an almost uniformly fatal infection (44). The co-evolution which selected resistance to this virus in Rhesus monkeys might not be reflected in a mouse model. However, one might also argue that study of this great susceptibility could more clearly indicate the specific systems which evolved to produce resistance.

Three animal models of genetic resistance will be discussed. These models have in common at least minimal evidence which suggests that natural killer (NK) cells play a role in resistance to that infection.


## GENETICS OF RESISTANCE TO HSV-1 IN THE MOUSE

Using a newly isolated strain of HSV-1, I first showed that adult inbred strains of mice differed in their resistance to infection (27). Mice were found to be resistant, moderately susceptible, or very susceptible to an intraperitoneal infection with HSV-1 (strain 2931). Susceptible mice demonstrated hind-leg paralysis and usually died 5-10 days post inoculation. When inoculated intracerebrally, all strains of mice were found to be susceptible to $10^1$ plaque forming units (PFU) of virus indicating that, if virus reaches the target organ, the infection will kill the mouse. Thus, genetic resistance appeared to determine the ability of the host to stop the virus infection from reaching the ultimate target cells, the spinal cord or brain.

Additional studies were carried out to determine whether other strains of HSV-1 also gave the same pattern of resistance when inoculated into very susceptible, moderately susceptible and resistant mice. Although each of the 8 strains of HSV-1 tested has demonstrated varying degrees of virulence, they killed susceptible (A/J) mice at a lower concentration than moderately susceptible (BALB/c) mice and none of the viruses tested killed more than 10% of the resistant (C57B1/6) mice, even when $10^6$ PFU was inoculated. All other studies were carried out with HSV-1 (strain 2931) since it demonstrated the greatest virulence and thus the greatest differences between resistant and susceptible strains of mice. For the majority of the genetic studies, a challenge dose of $10^6$ PFU of virus was used since this appeared to most clearly differentiate resistant and susceptible strains of mice. The studies by Kirchner et al. (21), using a different strain of HSV-1, have confirmed some of these observations.

A series of genetic studies have been undertaken to determine whether resistance was a dominant or recessive trait, the number of loci responsible and their mode of segregation. $F_1$ crosses between resistant and susceptible mice were found to be resistant indicating that resistance was a dominant trait. $F_1$ mice were backcrossed to susceptible or moderately susceptible parents and the progeny challenged with virus. In both cases approximately 25% of the progeny survived indicating that two, independently segregating genes were required for resistance. Further backcrosses of resistant progeny to very susceptible mice resulted in progeny, only 9% of which were resistant to the virus challenge. Further backcross of these resistant progeny resulted in mice susceptible to HSV-1. These studies suggest that, although two major genes govern resistance, other genes (or the lack thereof) on the A/J background have an adverse affect on resistance. Similar experiments with BALB/c mice suggest that minor genes on this background augment resistance slightly (Lopez, submitted for publication).

The major histocompatibility complex (MHC) of the mouse, the H-2, contains immune response (Ir) genes responsible for the capacity of the mouse to respond to certain

synthetic antigens as well as genes governing the interaction of cells in the immune response (23). Because studies
in my laboratory (28) and others (34, for example) have suggested that resistance to HSV-1 is immunologic in nature,
studies have been undertaken to determine whether genes
within the H-2 influence resistance to HSV-1. Congenic mice
with the resistant C57BL/6 or C57BL/10 background and the
MHCs of various susceptible strains of mice were challenged
with $10^6$ PFU of HSV-1 (2931). All the congenic mice were
found to be resistant indicating that the H-2 from susceptible strains of mice did not diminish resistance. Similar
experiments with congenic mice on the A/J (susceptible)
background indicated that susceptibility was not influenced
by H-2 (Lopez, submitted for publication).

Comparison of the characteristics of genetic resistance
to HSV-1 in the mouse indicate that they are strikingly
similar to those of genetic resistance to bone marrow allografts (28). Allogeneic marrow resistance has been defined
as the ability of lethally irradiated mice to reject allogeneic bone marrow grafts in a 4-5 day assay (12,13). The
similarities include (i) strain distribution of resistant
and susceptible mice, (ii) regulation of strength of resistance by two independent, dominant genes not linked to the
major histocompatibility complex, (iii) genetic resistance,
a property of hemopoietic cells as determined by transfer of
resistance from resistant to susceptible mice by bone marrow
engraftment, (iv) maturation of resistance rapidly at three
weeks of age and (v) genetic resistance in each case impaired by macrophage poisons (28). Earlier studies by Bennett
(5) had shown that allogeneic resistance was a marrow-dependent function since destroying the marrow by treating mice
with Strontium-89 ($^{89}$Sr) had abrogated resistance. In $^{89}$Sr-
treated mice the bone-seeking isotope chronically irradiates
the marrow causing aplasia. The spleen takes over stem cell
functions of the body and provides T-cells, B-cells, and
macrophages necessary fore antibody responses and cell-mediated immune responses. Although inducing susceptibility to
allogeneic marrow (5), Friend virus leukemogenesis (24) and
Listeria monocytogenes (6), such treatment is not generally
immunosuppressive since mice are still resistant to Yersinia
pestis (6), and can still reject skin grafts normally. In
our study (31), $^{89}$-Sr-treatment of resistant mice caused
them to be about as susceptible to HSV-1 as the genetically
most susceptible strains. By comparison, experiments in my
laboratory (28) as well as studies by Zawatzky et al. (43)
have shown that athymic, nude mice are no more or only
slightly more susceptible to HSV-1 infection than similar
mice with normal T-cell function.

A pathogenesis study of [89]Sr-treated, HSV-1 inoculated mice indicated that the virus persisted in the viscera and was able to travel to the spinal cord (31). Although virus replicated in visceral tissues of untreated mice, the virus had been cleared from the tissues (except kidney) by 3 days after infection and virus could not be detected in the spinal cords of untreated mice at any time. These results suggest that the genetic resistance system described here is mediated by a marrow-dependent cell and that it functions to clear the virus infection and not allow the spread of virus to the central bervous sytem.

A number of similarities between the effector cell of allogeneic marrow resistance and natural killer (NK) cells have been documented (16,20). Most importantly, NK cells were found to be marrow-dependent cells which do not require prior experience with the target antiens in order to be active. Because of these observations, attempts were made to develop an NK assay using HSV-1 infected target cells NK-(HSV-1) in order to determine whether such an assay might reflect resistance of mice to HSV-1. In preliminary experiments, effector cells from resistant C57BL/6 mice killed HSV-1 infected fibroblast target cells better than the effector cells from moderately susceptibile BALB/c mice (29). More importantly, NK(HSV-1) was not dependent on the H-2 of the target cells so that an NK(HSV-1) assay could be developed for man without concern that autologous target cells would be required.

Our observation that NK(HSV-1) appears to reflect the capacity of inbred mice to resist this virus infection is compatible with the recent data of Kirchner et al. (22) which has demonstrated that resistance can be reflected in the capacity of effector cells from inbred mice to produce interferon when exposed to killed HSV-1 antigen. Since interferon has been shown by others (18) and us (unpublished data) to augment NK, interferon may be the mechanism by which NK is induced.

Because NK(HSV-1) appeared to correlate with genetic resistance in mice, an NK(HSV-1) assay was developed to study the correlation with resistance to the herpesvirus infections in man (10). Our results with the NK(HSV-1) assay indicate that the cell that does the killing is neither a T-cell, B-cell, nor an adherent cell and antibody is not required for the response. Since the NK(HSV-1) cell activity was not found with effector cells from two patients with osteopetrosis, our NK(HSV-1) cell appears to be a marrow-dependent cell (30). Finally, the lack of this function in patients with aplastic anemia and patients with WAS suggests that it is more closely related to the neutrophil/monocyte series than any other (unpublished results).

Although very preliminary, results obtained by the study of effector cells from 9/12 cord bloods, 3 patients with severe herpesvirus infections, and 3/4 patients with WAS suggests that NK(HSV-1) may reflect their marked susceptibility to herpesvirus infections. In each case, NK(HSV-1) was found to be 2-3 standard deviations below the normal mean suggesting that low NK(HSV-1) might be a prerequisite for susceptibility.

GENETIC RESISTANCE TO MURINE CYTOMEGALOVIRUS INFECTION

Unlike genetic resistance to HSV-1, the studies of genetic resistance to murine cytomegalovirus (MCMV) have been carried out with a virus indigenous to the host. All studies carried out to date have been with the Smith strain of MCMV and comparisons have not been made with other strains.

Selgrade and Osborn (39) first showed that certain inbred strains of mice were more resistant than others. More recently, a study by Chalmer et al. (9) has evaluated the susceptibility of a larger series of inbred strains of mice. The differences found between resistant and susceptible strains of mice were much smaller than those found with HSV-1. The amount of virus required to kill resistant versus susceptible mice differed by 4- to 10-fold as compared to the $10^5$ difference found with HSV-1. An $F_1$ cross between a resistant and a susceptible strain was prepared and challenged with MCMV. Resistance was intermediate, indicating that the genes responsible were at least partly dominant. Experiments were also undertaken to determine whether H-2 genes played a role in resistance. Unlike resistance to HSV-1, resistance to MCMV is clearly governed by genes, two of which reside within the H-2 (9). In addition to loci within the H-2, genes segregating independently of the H-2 also influence resistance to MCMV. With the relatively large number of genes governing resistance to MCMV, the complexity of the system multiplies rapidly. This was also observed in the form of genetic interactions which could not be predicted. Thus, $F_1$ crosses between two susceptible inbred strains resulted in mice more resistant than the parents (9).

The genetic complexity is also mirrored by the apparent complex interactions demonstrated between MCMV and host. Studies of the pathogenesis of virus infection in resistant and susceptible strains of mice indicated that H-2 associated susceptibility correlated with massive necrosis in many target organs (39). For example, although virus-infected cells were found in the livers of both resistant and susceptible strains of mice, only susceptible mice also demonstrated an inflammatory response and necrosis of the tissue. This observation suggests that an immunopathology causes much of the damage and an ability to respond is actually deleterious.

Studies to be presented at this conference by Bancroft et al. (2) suggest that, in 10/11 inbred strains of mice studies, NK correlated with resistance. These studies and those of Quinnan and Manischewitz (45) suggest that NK cells may play an important role in defense against MCMV infections.

## GENETICS OF RESISTANCE TO MAREK'S DISEASE IN CHICKENS

Marek's disease virus (MDV) causes lymphomas in susceptible chickens. It has been found to be present in all populations of chickens which have been tested (7,32). Although most lines of chickens are infected, demonstrate viremia, and disseminate the virus, the incidence of lymphoma and death due to the virus infection varies markedly among breeds (33). Earlier experiments had associated a specific MHC allel, $B^{21}$, with resistance to MDV (37). Formal genetic studies were carried out using chickens homozyhgous for the $B^{21}$ allel and chickens homozygous for $B^2$ (found in susceptible chickens). Exposure of $F_2$ progeny to MDV-infected chickens clearly demonstrated an association between $B^{21}$ and resistance and showed that resistance was a dominant trait. A more recent study using resistant lines of chickens ($B^{21}$ and non-$B^{21}$ lines) and susceptible chickens showed that resistance to a transplantable tumor cell line, RPL-1 (induced by JMV, a strain of MDV), correlated, for the most part, with resistance to MDV (32). The correlations found were not perfect and suggested that resistnce to the tumor was mediated by B locus associated genes while another locus appears to mediate resistance to viral transformation.

Studies of the mechanism responsible for resistance to MDV indicate that the capacity to produce antibody was not required for resistance (40). However, a recent set of experiments (25,26) suggest that resistance to MDV can be transferred from resistant, mature to susceptible, newborn chicks by a non-T, non-B, non-macrophage cell and the transferred cells were not active when transferred to an irradiated newborn recipient. More recently, these investigators showed that a population of cells from the adult chicken, similar to the population which transferred resistance to chicks, were capable of killing Marek's disease tumor cells in vitro (25). These studies suggest that an NK cell is responsible for resistance to MDV of adult versus newborn

chicks.  In addition, earlier studies might also be interpreted to indicate that NK-like cytotoxic cell function
correlated with genetic resistance to MDV (14).

## CONCLUSIONS

Preliminary data with the three animal models of genetic resistance suggest that NK cells may play an important
role in resistance to herpesvirus infections.  Although very
preliminary, our study of patients susceptible to severe
herpesvirus infections also suggest that low NK(HSV-1) might
be associated with increased susceptibility.  The study of
these animal models of genetic resistance has given us the
rationale to pursue the study of NK and its role in the defense against herpesvirus infections.

Supported in part by NIH Grants CA-08748, CA-23766, and
AI-14832, and ACS Faculty Research Award #193.

## REFERENCES

1.   Allison A.C.  Transplant Rev. 19:3, 1974.
2.   Bancroft, G.J., Shellam, G.R., and Chalmer, J.E.
     "Genetic Control of Natural Resistance to Infection and
     Malignancy".  E. Skamene (ed).  Academic Press, New
     York, (in press).
3.   Bang, F.B.  Adv.VirusRes. 23:269, 1978.
4.   Br, R.S., DeLor, C.J., Clausen, K.P., Hurtubise, P.,
     Henle, W., and Hewetson, J.F.  New Engl.J.Med. 290:363,
     1974.
5.   Bennett, M.  J.Immunol. 110:510, 1973.
6.   Bennett, M., Baker, E.E., Eastcott, J.W., Kumar, V.,
     and Yonkosky, D.  J.Reticul.Soc. 20:71, 1976.
7.   Biggs, P.M.  "The Herpesviruses".  A.S. Kaplan (ed.).
     Academic Press, New York, p.448, 1973.
8.   Blaese, R.M., Strober, W., and Waldmann, T.A.
     "Immunodeficiency in Man and Animals".  D. Bergsma,
     R.A. Good, J. Finstad (eds).  Sinauer Associates, Inc.
     pp.250, 1975.
9.   Chalmer, J.E., Mackenzie, J.S., and Stanley, N.F.
     J.Gen.Virol. 37:107, 1977.
10.  Ching, C., and Lopez, C.  Infect.Immun. 26:49, 1979.
11.  Cooper, M., Chase, H.P., Lowman, J.T., Krivit, W., and
     Good, R.A.  "Immunologic Deficiency Diseases in Man".
     D. Bergsma, (ed.).  The National Foundation.  pp.378,
     1968.

12. Cudkowicz, G. J.Exp.Med. 134:281, 1971.

13. Cudkowicz, G., and Bennett, M. J.Exp.Med. 134:83, 1971.

14. Dambrine, G., Coudert, F., and Cauchy, L. "Oncogenesis and Herpesviruses III". G. de The, F. Rapp, W. Henle (eds). International Agency for Research on Cancer, Lyon, pp.857, 1978.

15. Good, R.A., and Zak, S.J. Pediatrics 18:109, 1956.

16. Haller, O., Kiessling, R., Orn, A., and Wigzell, H. J.Exp.Med. 145:1411, 1977.

17. Haller, O., and Wigzell, H. J.Immunol. 118:1503, 1977.

18. Herberman, R.B., and Holden, H.T. Adv.Cancer Res. 27:305, 1978.

19. Hoyer, J.R., Cooper, M.D., Gabrielsen, A.E., and Good, R.A. "Immunologic Deficiency Diseases in Man". D. Bergsma (ed). The National Foundation, pp.91, 1968.

20. Kiessling, R., Hochman, P.S., Haller, O., Shearer, G.M., Wigzell, H., and Cudkowicz, G. Eur.J.Immunol. 7:663, 1977.

21. Kirchner, H., Kochen, M., Munk, K., Hirt, H.M., Mergenhagen, S.E., and Rosenstreich, D.L. "Oncogenesis and Herpesviruses III". G. de The, F. Rapp, W. Henle (eds). International Agency for Research on Cancer, Lyon, pp.793, 1978.

22. Kirchner, H., Zawatzky, R., and Hirt, H.M. Cell.Immunol. 40:204, 1978.

23. Klein, J. "Biology of the Mouse Histocompatibility - 2 Complex". Springer-Verlag, New York, 1975.

24. Kumar, V., and Bennett, M. J.Exp.Med. 143:713, 1976.

25. Lam, K.M., and Linna, T.J. Fed.Proc. 38:1278, 1979.

26. Lam, K.M., Pasternak, R.D., and Linna, T.J. Fed.Proc. 36:1247, 1977.

27. Lopez, C. Nature 258:152, 1975.

28. Lopez, C. "Oncogenesis and Herpesviruses III". G. de The, F. Rapp, W. Henle (eds). International Agency for Research on Cancer, Lyon, pp.775, 1978.

29. Lopez, C., and Bennett, M. Inter.Virol. 4:82, 1978.

30. Lopez, C., Kirkpatrick, D., Sorell, M., O'Reilly, R.V., and Ching, C. Lancet ii:1103, 1979.

31. Lopez, C., Ryshke, R., and Bennett, M. Infect.Immun. (in press).

32. Longenecker, B.M., and Gallatin, W.M. "Oncogenesis and Herpesviruses III". G. de The, F. Rapp, Henle W. (eds). International Agency for Research on Cancer, Lyon, pp.845, 1978.

33. Longenecker, B.M., Pazderka, F., Gavora, J.S., Spencer, J.L., and Ruth, R.F. Immunog. 3:401, 1976.

34. Nahmias, A.J., Hirsch, M.S., Kramer, J.H., and Murphy,

F.A. Proc.Soc.Exp.Biol.Med. 132:696, 1969.

35. Nahmias, A.J., and Roizman, B. N.Engl.J.Med. 289:667, 1973.

36. Pahwa, R., Pahwa, S., O'Reilly, R., and ood, R.A. Springer Semin Immunopathol 1:355, 1978.

37. Pazderka, F., Longenecker, B.M., Law, G.R.J., Stone, H.A. and Ruth, R.F. Immunogen. 2:93, 1975.

38. Purtilo, D.T., Hutt, L., Bhawan, J., Yang, J.P.S., Cassel, C., Allegra, S., and Rosen, F.S. Clin.-Immunol.Immunopath. 9:147, 1978.

39. Selgrade, M.K., and Osborn, J.E. Infect.Immun. 10:-1383, 1974.

40. Sharma, J.M. Nature 247:117, 1974.

41. St. Geme, J.W., Prince, J.T., Burke, B.A., Good, R.A., and Krivit, W. New.Engl.J.Med. 273:229, 1965.

42. Stevens, J.G. Curr.Top.Microbial.Immunol. 70:31, 1975.

43 Zawatzky, R., Hilfenhaus, J., and Kirchner, H. Cell.-Immunol. 47:424, 1979.

44. Hull, R.N. In The Herpesviruses. A.S. Kaplan (ed). New York: Academic Press, p.389, 1973.

45. Quinnan, G.V. and Manischewitz, J.E. J.Exp.Med. 150:-1549, 1979.

## DISCUSSION

Kirchner: I am wondering about the relevance of interferon produced in the course of the NK cell assay itself. The question is the duration of the assay. We have found a cell with all the characteristics Lopez has shown which, in the human system, is totally indistinguishable from the NK cells, and is the cell that produces high levels of type I interferon in response to HSV. So conceivably, by exposing these cells to the virus-infected cells, one induces interferon in the reaction, and then obtains good killing. Or conversely poor killing if the respective cell is missing.

Lopez: That is in fact the case. The cord bloods, for example, that do not produce NK, also do not produce interferon. So it is pretty much as Kirchner says. Our assay takes 14-15 hours. We do get induction of interferon and it is not by the target cells, but rather by the effector cells in the assay. I think that the observations Kirchner has made with interferon are quite compatible with the observations that we have made with NK cells.

Anderson: Would Lopez identify what sort of cells he is using for target cells? He maintained that they were fibroblasts.  Are they transformed?

Lopez:   No, they are not.  We use a strain of fibroblasts called FS4;  we have also used WI38, and Vero cells, which yield comparable results.

Anderson:   Has Lopez ever used primary fibroblasts?

Lopez:   If Anderson is referring to first passage cells, the answer is that we have not done this.

Anderson:   My point is that, if one is postulating that NK cells could be important in resistance to or recovery from a virus infection, then it is also important that they are able to react against normal body cell types rather than tissue culture adapted cells, as the latter may well be different in ways that we are not aware of.

Lopez:   Yes, I surely agree with that.  I think that one of the reasons that we chose the fibroblast rather than a tumor cell line, is that we wanted as comparable a system as we could have.  We have studied FS4 cells and another fibroblast cell line as early as their 3rd or 4th passage.  But it is very difficult to get enough fibroblasts to set up good comparative studies using them in the very first passage.

Cudkowicz:   I have a comment to interject on this exchange. I think Trinchieri would say that one really should not even try hard to use primary fibroblasts because interferon, while it produced during the long assay, and thus boosts the lytic activity of the effector cell, also decreases the sensitivity of the target cells, and particularly of normal, non-transformed target cells.  There is thus a built in mechanism to avoid NK lysis of "normal" cells.

My query now to Lopez is:  He mentioned briefly the osteopetrotic patient, or patients, that were treated with bone marrow grafts;  and then he stated that the host marrow regenerated, and also NK activity returned.   Is that correct?

Lopez:   What I meant was that iron and calcium studies would indicate that the marrow was regenerating from what had been mostly fibrous tissue, to something that contained osteoclasts, etc.  And at that time we were picking up higher NK (within the normal range) which had not been there before.

Amos: It seems to me that the question whether this is host or donor activity was not an issue in this instance.

Cudkowicz: Well, the reason I am asking the question is: if this is host marrow that is generating the NK cells, that would indicate to me that there is no deletion of the NK cell line in that particular type of patient. On the other hand, if there is a repopulation by foreign marrow, then of course that would not hold true. This all has importance with respect to some other issues about the origin of NK cells and how they are regulated. So I gather that Lopez does not have a clear answer to this.

Lopez: We would like very much to be able to describe whose cells those are, in the marrow transplant recipient. We have got other studies, where NK is associated with GVH in the 3rd or 4th week post transplant. They have become very important studies with respect to the virus infections which these individuals have afterwards. I do not know whether these cells are of host or donor origin.

Cudkowicz: My comment is on the two discrepancies which Lopez mentioned. One, as he certainly anticipated, radio-resistance, is apparent rather than real, in the sense that if one waits long enough, of course, there is an absolute radioresistance. The second difference that he listed, the selectivity or specificity of the effectors, I would not really count as a difference since he is using a virus, essentially, as a target, as opposed to a stem cell. If we like to think of NK cells as selective, that is exactly what one would expect.

Mogensen: Lopez clearly showed that at least two genes were involved in his resistance phenomenon, which is death from encephalitis. Would he consider it possible that one of these genes is expressed in the ability of macrophages to restrict viral replication? That gene might be X-linked, for I have seen some data from Lopez himself that in his $F_1$ generation the male mice produce susceptible macrophages.

Lopez: Mogensen's point is well taken. I think the macro-phage experiments that we have done have not defined that. We would like very much to know whether or not they co-segregate.

# STUDIES OF RESISTANCE OF MICE AGAINST HERPES SIMPLEX VIRUS

H. Kirchner, H. Engler, R. Zawatzky, and
C.H. Schroder
Institute of Virus Research
German Cancer Research Center
Heidelberg,
Fed.Rep.Germany

The mouse widely has been used as an experimental animal to study infections with Herpes Simplex Virus (HSV) (3,-4,10,14,16). Two features of HSV infection in mice have been established many years ago: First, newborn mice are considerably more susceptible to peripheral infection with HSV than adult mice. Secondly, certain strains of HSV are apathogenic for mice after peripheral infection, but may be lethal after intracerebral infection. Other virus strains, however, are pathogenic after intracerebral and peripheral injection. Two examples of such different strains of HSV-1, HSV (WAL) and HSV (ANG) are investigated in our laboratory (see below).

Lopez recently has shown that adult mice of certain inbred strains are highly susceptible to intraperitoneal (i.p.) infection with HSV, whereas other inbred strains are relatively resistant (11). Resistance against HSV was not caused by lack of susceptibility of target cells (i.e. brain cells) to viral infection but by differences in the antiviral defense system (12). This observation has been confirmed in our laboratory (7) but the mechanisms, that cause resistance of mice against HSV infection remain to be elucidated.

In the following we summarize some of the data that have been performed in our laboratory during the past years. Some of this information has been published (5,6,7,8,9,18) whereas other data will be published in detail elsewhere (Kirchner, H., Engler, H., Schroder, C.H., and Marcucci, F., manuscript in preparation). The experimental details of our experiments have been given in the aforementioned references.

As previously published (7) C57BL/6(B6) mice are at least a thousandfold more resistant to i.p. infection with HSV-1 (WAL) than AKR,A/J,BALB/c and DBA/2(D2) mice. However, resistance of B6 mice can be broken by immunosuppression with cyclophosphamide. Resistance is dominant and B6D2F1 hybrids are at least as resistant as B6 mice.

In the first series of experiments we have tested the levels of serum interferon in mice. As shown in Table 1 measurable titers of interferon were detected in both B6 and

D2 mice after i.p. infection with HSV-1 (WAL). Two aspects of these experiments are noteworthy: First, serum interferon could be demonstrated only after injection of virus concentrations high enough to even kill C57BL/6. There seems to exist a certain paradox in that measurable amounts of serum interferon could be detected only after injection of a virus dose ($10^6$ or $10^7$ PFU) which would eventually kill the mice. Secondly, there was a significant difference observed

Table 1. Serum interferon in mice after i.p. injection of HSV(WAL)

| Virus dose | Time after injection | Mouse strain | |
|---|---|---|---|
| | | B6 | D2 |
| $10^7$ PFU | 6 hr | 1040* | 140 |
| $10^5$ PFU | 6 hr | 10 | 10 |
| $10^7$ PFU | 24 hr | 230 | 250 |

*IU/ml, means of 10 individual sera

between B6 and D2 mice but only if the early titers of interferon were compared at 6 hr after infection. There was no difference when interferon titers were compared at 24 hr. The difference observed at 4 hr may be quite meaningful. If endogenous interferon plays a role in the antiviral defense, it may be the rapidly produced interferon which is of importance. The same also holds true for the newer concept according to which interferon in addition to its direct antiviral effect may play a role in the antiviral defense by activating certain effector systems such as natural killer cells (17).

That NK cell activation plays a role in antiviral defense is suggested by recent studies from our laboratory. We have teted NK cell killing of YAC-1 cells by spleen cells of mice after injection of HSV(WAL). YAC-1 cells were killed to a significantly higher degree by B6 spleen cells than by

Table 2. HSV-induced interferon production in spleen cell cultures.

| Mouse Strain | Interferon titer(IU/ml) |
|---|---|
| A/J | 30 |
| AKR | 25 |
| BALB/c | 5 |
| D2 | 15 |
| B6 | 200 |
| B6D2F1 | 400 |

D2 spleen cells.

Our data have shown significant difference in HSV-induced interferon production between B6 and D2 mice when tested 6 hr after injection of high virus doses.  One may speculate that the same difference exists in the tissue also after injection of lower doses of HSV at which a clearcut difference in the $LD_{50}$ exists.  We have therefore tested interferon production in tissue culture.  HSV-induced (Type 1) interferon production in mouse spleen cells was determined.  Spleen cells of B6 mice produced significantly higher amounts of interferon than spleen cells of D2 mice (Table 2).  B6D2F1 spleen cells also produced high levels of interferon whereas low titers were produced by A/J and AKR spleen cells.  Thus, a correlation appears to exist between resistance and in vitro capacity of spleen cells to reproduce interferon.

The genetic analysis of HSV-induced interferon production yet has to be performed.  DeMaeyer and DeMaeyer-Guignard (1) have mapped the gene that is responsible for interferon production in response to Newcastle Disease Virus.  Subsequently, this group has shown that interferon production in response to mouse mammary tumor virus is controlled by another gene (2).  Probably HSV-induced interferon production may be controlled by yet a different gene.

In further experiments we have analyzed the cell type that produces (type 1) interferon in response to HSV in spleen cell cultures.  This cell was not a T cell since it was present in spleen cell cultures of nu/nu mice and in it was not sensitive to treatment with anti-theta serum plus complement.  Initially, we have speculated that the producer cell of interferon may be a cell type related to the NK cell (9).However, our recent data indicate that the producer cell of interferon is sensitive to 500 R of X-irradiation and that it is present in spleens of newborn mice.  Both observations are incompatible with the assumption that the producer cells are NK cells.  Furthermore, passage through nylon wool removed the producer cell of interferon.  Collectively our data suggest that HSV-induced interferon production in spleen cell cultures is a function of B cells.

In view of the finding mentioned above that spleen cells of nude mice produced normal levels of interferon in vitro, we were interested to test the $LD_{50}$ of nude mice after i.p. infection with HSV.  Nu/nu mice were at least as resistant ot HSV-1 infection as their heterozygous littermates (18).  These results are in accordance with data of Mogensen and Andersen (13) who have studied infection with HSV-2 in mice.

Recently we also have started to work with HSV(ANG), a

type 1 strain of HSV (15). This virus strain is apathogenic
for adult B6 and D2 mice (or any other mouse strain tested
so far) after i.p. infection. However, HSV-ANG kills mice
after intracerebral infection or by i.p. infection if mice
are immunosuppressed by cyclophosphamide. We have observed
a phenomenon which we believe to be quite noteworthy, although we do not understand its significance.: HSV-ANG when
given simultaneously with or prior to (4 hr) pathogenic HSV-
WAL protected mice against lethal encephalitis (Table 3).
UV-inactivated HSV-ANG protected as well as infectious
virus.

Preliminary data suggest that HSV(ANG) is not a better
inducer of interferon than HSV(WAL) and that defective interfering particles do not play a role in protection. Further studies will be aimed at defining the role macrophages
and natural killer cells might have in this protection.

Table 3. Protection of D2 mice against pathogenic
HSV-1(WAL) by injection of HSV-1(ANG)

| Virus Injected | Dead Mice/Group |
|---|---|
| $10^3$ PFU HSV(WAL) | 10/10 |
| $10^7$ PFU HSV(ANG) | 0/10 |
| $10^3$ PFU HSV(WAL) + $10^6$ PFU HSV(ANG) | 0/10 |

HSV(ANG) was given 4 hrs before HSV(WAL). Both viruses were
injected i.p.

## CONCLUSIONS

Previously it has been established that there are differences in the susceptibility of inbred mouse strains to infection with HSV, but the reasons for these differences were
not know. Our data have shown a striking correlation between resistance and interferon production. Higher titers of
interferon were produced by resistant mice than by susceptible mice, both in vivo and in vitro. Higher titers of NK
cell activity were observed when HSV was injected in resistant mice than were observed after injection of HSV into susceptible mice.

## REFERENCES

1. DeMaeyer, E., DeMaeyer-Guignard, J. J.Virol. 3:506, 1969.
2. DeMaeyer, E., DeMaeyer-Guignard, J., Hall, W.T., and Bailey, D.W. J.Gen.Virol. 23:209, 1974.
3. Ennis, F.A. Infect.Immun. 7:898, 1973.
4. Johnson, R.T. J.Exp.Med. 119:343, 1964.
5. Kirchner, H., Hirt, H.M., Becker, H., and Munk, K. Infect.Immun. 16:9, 1977.
6. Kirchner, H., Hirt, H.M., Rosenstreich, D.L., and Mergenhagen, S.E. Proc.Soc.Exp.Biol.Med. 157:29, 1978.
7. Kirchner, H., Kochen, M., Hirt, H.M., and Munk, K. Z. Immunforsch. 154:147, 1978.
8. Kirchner, H., Scott, M.T., Kirt, H.M., and Munk, K. J.Gen.Virol. 41:97, 1978.
9. Kirchner, H., Peter, H.H., and Hilfenhaus, J. In "Virus-Lymphocyte Interactions. Implications for Disease". M. Proffitt (ed.). Elseviers North holland Inc. p.259, 1979.
10. Lodmell, D.L., and Notkins, A.L. J.Exp.Med. 140:764, 1974.
11. Lopez, C. Nature (Lond) 258:152, 1975.
12. Lopez, C. In "Oncogenesis and Herpes viruses III." G. de Thé, W. Henle, and F. Rapp (eds). IARC Scientific Publications 24 International Agency for Research on Cancer Lyon, 1978.
13. Mogensen, S.C., and Andersen, H.K. Infect.Immun. 19:792, 1978.
14. Rager-Zisman, B., and Allison, A.C. J.Immunol. 116:35, 1976.
15. Stegmann, B., Zentgraf, H., Ott, A., and Schroder, C.H. Intervirology 10:228, 1978.
16. Stevens, J.C., and Cook, M.L. J.Exp.Med. 133:19, 1971.
17. Welsh, R.M.Jr. J.Immunol. 121:1631, 1978.
18. Zawatzky, R., Hilfenhaus, J., and Kirchner, H. Cell.Immunol. 47:424, 1979.

## DISCUSSION

Lopez: I am impressed with the in vivo interferon data. We, too, tripped up over not using enough virus and not looking at the right time. But I would like to ask a question with respect to Kirchiner's newborn animals making interferon, and making a lot of interferon at that. This finding does not seem to correlate with their marked susceptibility to virus infection. Would Kirchner comment on that discrepancy?

Kirchner: Actually I wanted to ask Lopez about this very point. You see, the old data of Zisman, for example, have shown that newborn mice are much more susceptible to certain strains of Herpes virus than adult mice which are in fact resistant. Since then, the model has been used the way Lopez uses it and I think it has been more a question of the mouse strain rather than the age. It also depends very much on the virus strain. So the question is: are C57BL, with a given type of virus, really more resistant when they are young? We have not investigated this issue as yet.

Lopez: Working with 2931 the virus we work with routinely, and with (B6xA)F$_1$, I can say that they gain their resistance very abruptly at 3 weeks of age.

Kiessling: I am a little bit reluctant to accept Kirchner's interferon-producing cells as being B cells because the only difference from ordinary NK cells is the fact that they are somewhat adherent. But it has been shown recently that following activation the NK cell, in fact, becomes adherent. I think he may well be dealing with an NK cell that is producing interferon.

Kirchner: Well, I would agree. I rather rushed through those data. In the human system, for example, we believe that the producer cell is pretty similar to the NK cell. In this system we have long speculated that it is a cell related to the NK cell. What argues against it, is that it is present in newborn spleens, that it is radiosensitive, and it is removed by nylon. But I fully agree. What we are presently doing is to utilize anti-NK cell serum to really settle this problem. Kiessling's concern is very well taken.

Amos: I would agree. It seems rather abrupt to jump to the conclusion that it is a B cell.

Kirchner: Actually we have been very worried about this all the time. Certainly our main conclusion was that it is a cell which does not share properties with most T cells, and does not share properties of most macrophages. But, for example, if we do (under strictly controlled conditions) anti--theta treatment by monoclonal antibody, we can reduce NK cell activity against YAC cells by 60%, like many laboratories, and we do not affect interferon production at all. But again this point is well taken.

**Kiessling:** Maybe I could add a comment about a collaborative study using NK-deficient beige (bg/bg) mice. We have, at the moment, some rather preliminary data showing that beige mice have a much higher mortality than the bg/+ when inoculated with HSV virus.

**Kirchner:** I, too, have one more point. Based on this observation that one gets high interferon titers at 6 hours, we have also done NK cell assays against YAC cells and find there is a clear-cut, significant difference between resistant and susceptible mice.

**Rosenstreich:** This is obviously a very complex infection, but now I am confused. Would Kirchner comment on the relationship between (1) these observations, and (2) his previous observation that endotoxin-unresponsive mice were _more_ resistant to HSV infection, and (3) his observation that activation of some spleen cells, under conditions which would give interferon production, enhances the growth of HSV.

**Kirchner:** We have observed, as has Rosenstreich, that LPS-resistant mice are also much more resistant to HSV infection. Now, subsequently, we do not see differences with respect to interferon between the two sub-strains. So, in contrast to the situation where we compare B6 and other strains, there is no difference in the present situation. But, since it is known that this infection is under the control of more than one gene, it may very well be that the interferon gene (which we are presently mapping, together with De Maeyer) is only one of several involved.

**Karre:** I have a general question as to what other speakers have referred to as the association between resistance to virus infections and NK cells. How does Kirchner envision the role of NK cells in _in vivo_ resistance to virus infections? Are the NK cells synthesizing interferon which protects other cells? Or are the NK cells actually swimming around and killing infected cells? Or are they doing both?

**Kirchner:** Well, I would speculate (and this is supported by Lopez's work) that NK cells can also kill virus-infected cells, early, at a time before they release infectious virus. I would envision the role of interferon as an activator of NK cells, besides its direct antiviral effect. Maybe it is more important that it activates NK cells that kill virus infected target cells.

**Karre:** The reason I ask is that, by definition, we tend to

think of NK cells as killer cells but, analogous to macrophages and to T cells, they may well have several independent functions. For instance, if they are present from
birth,some of the other functions may be present from birth
whereas the killer function does not develop until 3 or 4
weeks. I would just like to remind Kirchner that there is
at least one model now whereby one can study only the killer
function of NK cells, and that is the beige model, which
will be discussed later on by Roder.

Kirchner: I would agree with Karre. The NK cells has been
defined as a cell which lyses certain lymphoma cells. Although Lopez and many others would think that it also kills
virus infected cells, I think this point has to be very
carefully evaluated before we accept that the very same cell
that kills the lymphoma cell is the one that also kills the
virus infected target cell.

Amos: That is a point well made. To me it is rather paradoxical that some cells are very good targets for ADCC but
poor for NK, while others are the reverse, and very few indeed are good targets for both.

Kirchner: Yes. Well I would counter that by also stressing
that interferon not only activates NK cells but also activates macrophages. It is really quite conceivable that
other mechanisms play a more important role than do NK
cells.

Haller: I have a comment to contribute to this discussion.
One could be very cynical and say that interferon is the
major antiviral factor which actually protects the animal
directly but at the same time interferon also induces NK
activity that one can measure. This induction of NK activity is not really relevant but simply a parameter of interferon production. I do not think that it is clear in any of
these systems whether interferon acts directly or via NK
cells, and I think that the role of NK cells in vivo is
still very unsettled.

Kirchner: I would agree with Haller.

Zisman: This is all very well, but it has been shown that
in many virus infections, there is a correlation between interferon and the magnitude of viral titers. I do not see
how one can doubt a protective role in vivo for interferon.
People have been looking into this since 1956.

**Kirchner:** Yes, but the point is that it is now well known that interferon can be genetically mapped to certain genes, and this has been done for various non-pathogenic viruses. On the other hand, it is well known that there is genetic resistance against viruses. I think there are very few situations where the amount of interferon induced in the system has clearly been correlated with resistance or susceptibility.

**Zisman:** I want to make comment, and this is directed to Kirchner and maybe to Lopez as well. In the resistance to Herpes virus, the systems mentioned are route-dependent. What happens if mice are injected intracerebrally?

**Kirchner:** Well, they die of course, of encephalitis.

**Zisman:** Yes, but is there any genetic restriction?

**Kirchner:** One can demonstrate a difference, though it is quite small, but statistically significant. The point is, since we are studying a model where we infect peripherally in order to study defense mechanisms, we use a model that expands the genetically-determined differences.

**Zisman:** There is one more comment which I would like to make on NK cells and their role vis-a-vis virus-infected cells. It has been shown by Bloom et al. that persistently infected viral cells are preferentially killed by NK cells. There are some studies which show that NK cells have some specificity. Amos inquired about what makes a given lymphoid cells suceptible or resistant to NK cells. Herberman's group have shown that there are structures which NK cells will recognize preferentially.

**Kirchner:** I think that is a very important point and Cudkowicz has also done very important studies on this as well. But, as Kiessling has already pointed out, at the moment the target structure is not really known, and everyone is hesitant to accept killing that is directed against targets other than lymphoma cells as "natural killing".

**Anderson:** I would like to make two points. Firstly, with reference to Haller's comment about interferon being the thing which cures or not, in a viral infection. In our own model which is not a Herpes virus model, we have very strong evidence to suggest that, even where one has very good production of interferon, one can still produce a lethal infection, when mice are treated with cyclophosphamide. But

it does knock out virtually every cell type. So, in the
absence of cell types known and unknown, interferon alone is
not able to resolve a virus infection in vivo, whatever it
may be able to do in vitro. The second point I would like
to pick Kirchner up on is the data he presented where an
apathogenic and a pathogenic strain of Herpes simplex, given
simultaneously, results in protection. I wonder whether he
has done the reverse experiment, i.e., given irradiated or
inactivated lethal virus to see if that would protect
against a lethal dose of his apathogenic virus.

Kirchner:  I think your latter point deals with a very important experiment;  we are just about ready to do it.  As
to the first question.  We do not want to overstress the
role of interferon.  All we are saying is that after three
years of search, we have found one thing that correlates
very well.  Obviously, the cytomegalovirus sytem has yielded
the same type of data.  So I think these are data which do
show a correlation.  Most certainly they are not saying that
interferon is really doing the entire job in defense.

Lopez:  In defense of natural killing, I think there is one
situation that Haller and Kirchner pointed out.  In the one
week old mouse which does produce a lot of interferon, we
have shown it to be very susceptible to infection, which
would argue against the interferon by itself playing a role.
We have not done the parallel experiment:  does a one week
old animal have NK?  However, other studies working with
other targets would indicate that they do not.  Our own
studies with newborn cord bloods, indicating that there is a
very low incidence of normal NK in those, would again make a
better correlation between NK and resistance at that time,
than interferon.

# ASSOCIATION OF HOST GENOTYPE WITH THE AUGMENTATION OF NATURAL KILLER CELLS AND RESISTANCE TO MURINE CYTOMEGALOVIRUS

Gregory J. Bancroft, Geoffrey R. Shellam
and Jane E. Chalmer

Department of Microbiology
University of Western Australia
Perth, Western Australia

The outcome of infection with MCMV is strongly influenced by the genetic constitution of the host (1,7), and accordingly various mouse strains may be classified as relatively resistant or susceptible. However, whilst the mechanisms of resistance are not known, they must act early in the infection since susceptible animals can die within 3 days after virus administration.

Whilst a variety of host responses such as cytotoxic T-cell and neutralising antibody have the potential to influence infection, it is unlikely that they can entirely account for such early genotype-related difference, since their peak responses occur later in the infection (2,4). This suggests that naturally-occurring defence mechanisms may be important and we have therefore investigated levels of natural killer (NK) cell activity in resistant and susceptible strains during MCMV infection. The cytotoxicity of spleen cells from control or infected male mice aged 12-15 weeks was measured in a 4 hr $^{51}$Cr release assay against the NK-susceptible target cell, RBL-5. Activity was assayed at various times after the i.p. administration of the Smith strain of salivary gland-passaged MCMV.

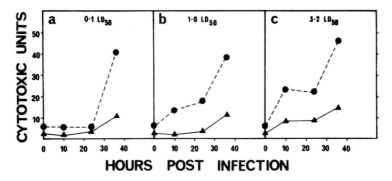

Figure 1. Augmentation of cytotoxicity in BALB/c (▲——▲) and C3H (●--●) mice during infection with MCMV.

Stimulation of cytotoxicity was observed in the spleens of BALB/c and C3H/HeJ (C3H) mice in the first 36 hours after infection with MCMV (Figure 1). However the resistant C3H strain (relative $LD_{50}$ = 26) showed greater boosting than the more susceptible BALB/c (rel. $LD_{50}$ = 1) at all doses examined. The time of augmentation was dose dependent, being present as early as 12 hours after injection of 1.0 or 3.2 $LD_{50}$. Stimulation was virus related and was not due to an effect of constituents of salivary gland tissue.

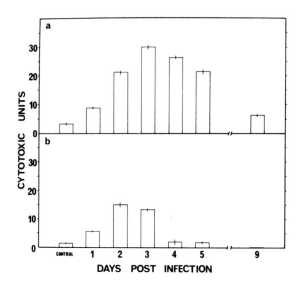

Figure 2. Kinetics of augmentation during sub-lethal infection of BALB/c and C3H mice.

During a sublethal infection with 0.5 $LD_{50}$ MCMV (Figure 2) augmented cytotoxicity was observed in C3H mice (panel a) for 8 days, with maximum levels at day 3. In contrast, boosting was observed for only 3 days in BALB/c mice (panel b) and peak levels of cytotoxicity were lower than in C3H. Spleen cell numbers did not decrease during infection of C3H mice, but began to fall rapidly at day 3 in BALB/c. Cytotoxicity per unit cell number also declined after this time in BALB/c mice. Examination of CBA and A/WySn mice, which

also differ in their resistance to MCMV, again showed an
apparent association between resistance to infection and
augmentation of cytotoxicity (Figure 3). Thus following injection of 1.0 $LD_{50}$ MCMV, cytotoxicity was not augmented in
A/WySn mice (rel. $LD_{50}$ = 0.5) whereas in the resistant CBA
strain (rel. $LD_{50}$ = 26) a marked boost was observed within
12 hours.

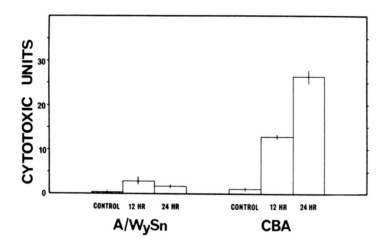

Figure 3. Augmentation of cytotoxicity in CBA and A/WySn
mice after infection with 1.0 $LD_{50}$ MCMV.

Figure 4 summarises data obtained on the association
between resistance and the augmentation of cytotoxicity by
MCMV against RBL-5 target cells. Examination of cytotoxicity 24 hours after 3.0 $LD_{50}$ MCMV demonstrated a significant
correlation (r = 0.68 p<0.02) between augmentation of
splenic cytotoxicity and resistance to infection in 10 of 11
mouse strains examined; the exception being the highly resistant B10.BR strain. Of particular interest was that
"beige" mutant C57BL/6J mice, previously reported as having
impaired NK cell function (5,6) did not show augmented cytotoxicity and were more susceptible to infection (rel. $LD_{50}$ =
0.5) than their NK competent heterozygous littermates (rel.
$LD_{50}$ = 4.0).

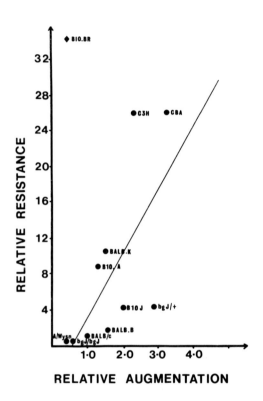

**Figure 4.** Correlation between resistance to MCMV and NK augmentation during infection.

In characterising the cytotoxic cells induced in the spleen early in infection, BALB/c athymic (nu/nu) mutants and heterozygotes (nu/+) were tested for cytotoxicity after injection with 3.0 $LD_{50}$ MCMV (Figure 5). Stimulation of lysis with similar target specificity was observed in both nude and intact mice, suggesting that augmentation and target cell killing are not dependent upon the thymus or thymus derived cells. Additional studies in CBA mice demonstrated that 85% of induced cytotoxicity was mediated by plastic non-adherent cells and that treatment with anti-Thy 1.2 serum and C' did not significantly reduce lytic activity.

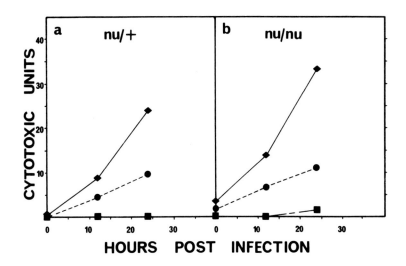

Figure 5. Augmentation in BALB/c nu/nu and nu/+ mice. Cytotoxic activity was assayed against RBL-5 (◆———◆), W/FuG-1 (●--●) and P815 (■---■) target cells.

Thus cytotoxic cells closely resembling the NK cells of normal mice are stimulated early in MCMV infection and this augmentation is dependent upon the virus dose and the genetic constitution of the host. In addition, a significant correlation was observed between the genetic patterns of resistance to MCMV and the stimulation of NK activity. However, whilst both H-2 and non H-2 associated genes are important in determining resistance to infection with this virus (2), in the present study the effect of the H-2 complex on the augmentation of NK cytotoxicity was not clear, whereas the influence of non H-2 genes was more pronounced. Thus for the H-$2^a$ haplotype, B.10A mice were more responsive than A/WySn, and for the H-$2^k$ haplotype, CBA showed greater stimulation than BALB.K mice. The mechanism of genetic control of stimulation is as yet unknown, however interferon, shown to be responsible for NK stimulation by many other viral and non-viral agents, is present early in

MCMV infection (3) and is likely to be involved in this system. If this is so, strain-related differences could be due to the genetic control of interferon production and/or the regulation of NK responses to this stimulating agent.

Since cytotoxicity was augmented early in infection and was generally greatest in resistant strains, natural killer cells may contribute to the early genotypic differences seen in MCMV resistance. This hypothesis is strongly supported by the observed susceptibility and lack of induced cytotoxicity in the NK defective C57BL/6J "beige" mutant strain and in A/WySn and BALB/c mice. An exception was the highly resistant B10.BR strain which exhibited only slight NK cell augmentation. This suggests that other natural mechanisms may also be important. However, in establishing a casual relationship between NK activity and resistance evidence of lysis of MCMV-infected target cells is required, and we are currently re-examining the observed genetic patterns of NK augmentation against targets expressing cytomegalovirus antigens.

## REFERENCES

1.  Chalmer, J.E., Mackenzie, J.S., and Stanley, N.F. J.Gen.Virol. 37:107, 1977.
2.  Chalmer, J.E. Ph.D. Thesis, University of Western Australia.
3.  Kelsey, D.K., Olsen, G.A., Overall, J.C., and Glasgow, L.A. Infect.Immun. 18:754, 1977.
4.  Quinnan, G.V., Manischewitz, J.R., and Ennis, F.A. Nature (Lond) 273:541, 1978.
5.  Roder, J.C. J.Immunol. 123:2168, 1979.
6.  Roder, J.C., and Duwe, A. Nature (Lond) 278:451, 1979.
7.  Selgrade, M.K., and Osborn, J.E. Infect.Immun. 19:1383, 1974.

GENETIC RESISTANCE TO MURINE CYTOMEGALOVIRUS INFECTION

Jane E. Chalmer

Department of Microbiology
University of Western Australia
Perth, Western Australia

The first indication of genetic control of resistance
to murine cytomegalovirus (MCMV) came as early as 1936 when
McCordock and Smith reported variation among the susceptibilities of Swiss, Buffalo and C57BL strains of mice (2).
Selgrade and Osborn (4) later observed that CBA mice were
more resistant to MCMV than were C57BL or Swiss mice, resistance being dominantly expressed.   Previous studies in our
laboratory (1) have shown that resistance is controlled by
genes linked to the H-2 complex.   In congenic strains of
mice with the BALB/c genetic background relative resistance
was found to be associated with the $H-2^k$ haplotype, whilst
the $H-2^b$ and $H-2^d$ haplotypes were susceptible (see Table
1).   However in our study $F_1$ hybrids between resistant (C3H)
and susceptible (BALB/c) mice were relatively susceptible, a
result conflicting with the dominance of resistance described by Selgrade and Osborn (4).   In the present study recombinant strains of mice were used to try to map the genes
controlling resistance to MCMV within the H-2 complex.   In
addition the resistance of various $F_1$ hybrids was tested in
order to determine whether such genes were expressed in a
dominant or recessive manner.
The effect of H-2 haplotype on resistance to MCMV can
be seen in Table 1 which depicts the relative resistance of
various congenic strains of mice with the BALB/c genetic
background.   In all experiments adult mice were inoculated
intraperitoneally with twofold dilutions of virulent, salivary gland-passaged virus of the Smith strain.   The $LD_{50}$ was
calculated by the Kaerber method and statistical analyses
performed using the $\chi^2$ test.   The resistance of BALB/c mice
was arbitrarily assigned to be 1.0 and another $LD_{50}$ values
were compared to it.

Table 1:

| Strain | \multicolumn{9}{c}{H-2 Map} | Relative $LD_{50}$ |
|--------|---|----|----|----|----|----|---|---|---|---|
| | K | IA | IB | IE | IJ | IC | G | S | D | |
| BALB.K | k | k | k | k | k | k | k | k | k | 10.2 |
| BALB.B | b | b | b | b | b | b | b | b | b | 1.3 |
| BALB.G | d | d | d | d | d | d | d | d | d | 1.2 |
| BALB/c | d | d | d | d | d | d | d | d | d | 1.0 |

GENETIC CONTROL OF NATURAL RESISTANCE
TO INFECTION AND MALIGNANCY

283

It can be seen that the k haplotype is approximately ten times more resistant than the b or d haplotypes (p <0.02), which are equally susceptible.

In order to determine the location within H-2 of the genes controlling resistance, a series of recombinant strains were examined. Due to the effect of background genes (discussed subsequently) these will only be directly compared when on the same genetic background. The resistance of recombinants with the B10 background is seen in Table 2.

Table 2:

| Strain | K | IA | IB | IE | IJ | IC | G | S | D | Relative $LD_{50}$ |
|---|---|---|---|---|---|---|---|---|---|---|
| B10.BR | k | k | k | k | k | k | k | k | k | 10 |
| B10.A(4R) | k | k | b | b | b | b | b | b | b | >5 |
| B10.A(2R) | k | k | k | k | k | d | d | d | b | >5 |
| B10.A | k | k | k | k | k | d | d | d | d | 2.1 |
| B10.A(5R) | b | b | b | k | k | d | d | d | d | 1.8 |
| B10. | b | b | b | b | b | b | b | b | b | 1.0 |

Column header spanning: H-2 Map

As on the BALB/c background, on the B10 background the k haplotype (B10.BR) was associated with a tenfold greater resistance than that of the b haplotype (B10). B10.BR,B10.-A(4R) and B10.A(2R) were all significantly more resistant that B10 (p<0.001), B10.A (p<0.01) or B10.A(5R) (p<0.01). The highest available dose of virus failed to kill any B10.-A(4R) or B10.A(2R) mice; thus the extent of their resistance cannot be calculated. It is apparent that whilst replacement of b alleles at all loci (in B10) by k alleles in (B10-.BR) results in a tenfold increase in resistance, most (if not all) of this effect can be achieved by substitution of k alleles at the K and IA subregions only [in B10.A(4R)]. Thus a gene(s) in the K/IA subregion of the H-2 complex appears to control resistance to MCMV. However in the case of B10.A, a similar substitution of k for b alleles at K, IA and IB loci [compare B10.A(5R)] failed to increase resistance. In this situation the D end of H-2 comprised d alleles, in contrast to the former situation with B10 and B10.A-(4R), where the D end had b alleles. This suggests that the D end of H-2 is also influencing resistance to the virus, and a comparison between the resistance of B10.A and B10.BR supports this suggestion. Here, substitution at the D end of H-2 of d alleles (in B10.A) by k alleles (in B10.BR) resulted in a fivefold increase in resistance. Furthermore a substitution at the D subregion alone [compare B10.A with B10.A(2R)] was sufficient to significantly alter resistance.

Thus these data strongly suggest that a gene(s) mapping close to the D locus controls resistance to MCMV.

It is not clear why the substitutions at the D locus of the d allele of B10.A for the b allele in B10.A(2R) should alter resistance, since on the BALB/c background both b and d haplotypes are equally susceptible (see Table 1). Furthermore, a similar substitution in the BALB.G recombinant (Table 1) did not alter resistance, although in this instance the K end of H-2 comprised d rather than k alleles. These data suggest that interactions might occur between the proposed K end and D end genes controlling resistance to MCMV. In the case of a $K^k$-$D^b$ interaction the outcome favours resistance, whilst in the case of $K^k$-$D^d$ susceptibility dominates. An alternative explanation is that non H-2 genes present in C57BL mice might interact with the $D^b$ gene product (and not the $D^d$ gene product) to increase resistance, whilst this does not occur in the presence of $K^b$ or in mice with the BALB/c genetic background. Such an interaction has been observed to affect the resitance of mice to ectromelia virus (R.V. Blanden personal communication).

Table 3 shows the relative resistance of recombinant strains with the C3H genetic background, compared to the resistance of BALB/c mice (relative $LD_{50}$ = 1.0).

Table 3:

| Strain | K | IA | IB | IE | IJ | IC | G | S | D | Relative $LD_{50}$ |
|---|---|---|---|---|---|---|---|---|---|---|
|        |   |    |    | H-2 Map |  |  |   |   |   |              |
| C3H    | k | k  | k  | k  | k  | k  | k | k | k | 25.8         |
| C3H.OH | d | d  | d  | d  | d  | d  | d | d | k | 5.1          |
| C3H.OL | d | d  | d  | d  | d  | d  | k | k | k | 3.3          |

The difference between the resistance of C3H and both C3H.OH and C3H.OL is significant with p <0.05 and p <0.01 respectively, whereas that between C3H.OH and C3H.OL is not significant ($\chi^2$ <1). These results support the existence of a gene(s) in the K end of H-2 which controls resistance to MCMV. The involvement of a D end gene could not be examined on this background since there is no C3H congenic strain with the d allele at all loci.

The relative resistance of various $F_1$ hybrids between C3H, C57BL and BALB/c mice is shown in Figure 1. As previously reported (1) the C3H x BALB/c (k x d) $F_1$ hybrid is relatively susceptible, although slightly (and significantly) more resistant than the susceptible BALB/c parent. In contrast the C3H x C57BL (k x b) $F_1$ hybrid is relatively resistant; indeed there is no significant difference between

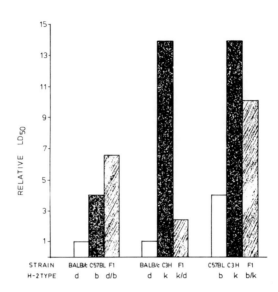

Figure 1.   Resistance of various $F_1$ hybrids between BALB/c, C57BL and C3H mice to MCMV.

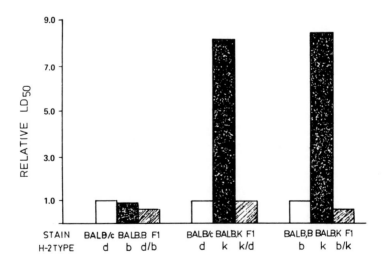

Figure 2.   Resistance of various $F_1$ hybrids between BALB/c, BALB.B and BALB.K mice to MCMV.

the resitance of this $F_1$ hybrid and its resistant C3H parent. This is in agreement with the earlier finding of Selgrade and Osborn (4) that the CBA x C57BL (k x b)$F_1$ hybrid was resistant. Of interest is the increased resistance of the b x d $F_1$ hybrid between C57BL and BALB/c compared to the susceptible parent strains. This suggests that the reasons for susceptibility of the two strains might be different, and that some sort of complementation might be occurring in vivo. It is likely that the results shown in Figure 1 were affected by non H-2 linked genes, hence to determine the relative dominance of the H-2 associated resistance, these crosses were repeated amongst congenic strains of mice with the BALB/c genetic background. The results, presented in Figure 2, contrast markedly with those just discussed. Both the k x d (BALB.K x BALB/c) and the k x b (BALB.K x BALB.B) and the k x b (BALB.K x BALB.B)$F_1$ hybrids were equally as susceptible as the susceptible parent. Thus with the H-2 associated resistance to MCMV, susceptibility is expressed as a completely dominant trait. It should be noted that the b x d (BALB.B x BALB/c)$F_1$ hybrid is slightly more susceptible than either parent, in contrast to the increased resistance of the b x d (C57BL x BALB/c)$F_1$ hybrid seen in Figure 1.

The effect of non H-2 linked genes, seen on the resistance of various recombinants and $F_1$ hybrids, was further investigated. Figure 3 shows a direct comparison between the resistance of age-matched and sex-matched mice of various strains to the same virus stock measured at the same time.

It can be seen that on the same genetic background (BALB/c or B10) the b and d haplotypes are susceptible, whilst the k haplotype is approximately ten times more resistant. However, it is also apparent that for the b as well as the k haplotype, the B10 background is associated with increased resistance compared to the BALB/c background. The C3H background is intermediate in this respect. Other data (not shown) indicate that the A strain background is the most susceptible. Thus non H-2 linked genes in the C57-BL background appear to increase resistance to MCMV. The $F_1$ studies seen in Figure 1 suggest that such genes are dominantly expressed. Conversely non H-2 linked genes in the BALB/c background are associated with increased susceptibility. Pathological studies suggest that this greater susceptibility is a result of severe splenic necrosis during MCMV infection in this strain.

Thus these experiments show that at least two genes within the H-2 complex control the resistance of adult mice to lethal infection with MCMV, one mapping to the K/IA sub-

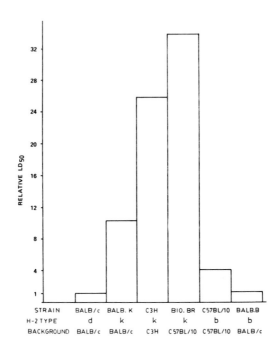

Figure 3. Effect of H-2 haplotype and genetic background on resistance to MCMV.

region and the other close to the D locus. The data suggest that between these genes, interactions may occur which affect resitance to the virus. Susceptibility is expressed as a completely dominant trait. Non H-2 linked genes, particularly in the C57BL background, also affect resistance to MCMV, however the number of such genes has yet to be determined. Susceptible mice die as early as 60 hours after virus, before the development of neutralizing antibody (data not shown) or cytotoxic T cells (3). Hence it is likely that innate or natural resistance mechanisms are involved in protection of genetically resistant strains.

Present address: Central Laboratory of the Netherlands Red Cross Blood Transfusion Service and the Laboratory of Clinical and Experimental Immunology of the University of Amsterdam, Postbus 9190, Amsterdam, The Netherlands.

REFERENCES

1.    Chalmer, J.E., Mackenzie, J.S., and Stanley, N.F.
      J.Gen.Virol. 37:107, 1977.
2.    McCordock, H.A., and Smith, M.G.   J.Exp.Med. 63:303,
      1936.
3.    Quinnan, G.V., Manischewitz, J.R., and Ennis, F.A.
      Nature (London) 273:541, 1978.
4.    Selgrade, M.K., and Osborn, J.E.   Infect.Immun. 19:-
      1383, 1974.

DISCUSSION

Amos:  Is it possible that some of the effects of H-2 that
appear to be, or could be compatible with an immunological
response may have nothing to do with that and could involve
many other factors in host resistance?

Chalmer:  I have started some studies with some of the H-2
mutants, and the preliminary data at the moment indicate
that one of these mutants, the MB-14, is more susceptible to
the virus than the wild type B6.  This is the line we have
continued with at the moment and, if it proves to be the
case, then I think we are looking at the structural antigens
controlled by the H-2$^k$ and the H-2$^d$ locus.  I have tested 5 mutants so far, and this is the only one that seems to
be differing in susceptibility to MCMV.

Amos:  Is it not possible that an appearance of a mutation
in itself renders the haplotype somewhat unstable?  I say
this because many of the so-called point mutations at K,
which itself is not (according to dogma) involved with MLC
or GVH reactions, do give positive GVH and MLC reactions.

Chalmer:  It maybe of interest that this same mutant, the
MB-14 has also been found deficient in its cytotoxic T cell
response to the leukemia virus and the Gross virus.

Lopez:  My question for Chalmer is about the tumor cells she
used for NK work.  What is the H-2 status of these cells and
why did she choose the RBL?

Chalmer:  Well the RBL-5 was used simply because it was a
sensitive target, and is also one used by many people.  I am
not sure what the H-2 type is, but I do not think there is
any evidence at the moment that the target cell structure

that is recognized by NK has any of this sort of specificity. So I think it really probably does not matter a great deal which one is chosen; a sensitive target should perhaps yield bigger differences. We have not looked at anything but RBL-5 at the moment.

Anderson: I would like to ask about the last part of the data presented, which seemed to suggest that interferon might be important in susceptibility or resistance. Has Chalmer looked at the lymphocytes from her susceptible mice to see whether they can be stimulated to high NK cell activity exogenously via interferon?

Chalmer: We have not done that.

Anderson: Has Chalmer tried introducing exogenous interferon into susceptible mice to see what effect that has?

Chalmer: Well, we are doing those studies at the moment and also using anti-interferon serum to see if we can make the resistant mice more susceptible, but the results are not in yet.

Williams: I think Chalmer's statement about the mutant is very important. My argument is with Amos. To say the possibility is that the mutants are telling us the dogma is incorrect about GVH and MLC. Along those lines, we are very lucky to have mutants at histocompatibility loci, so we will be able to make pretty definitive statements in the future. The problem comes up when we are dealing with genes that do not show histocompatibility effects and no one is searching for mutants to CMV in otherwise susceptible strains. I think eventually that sort of thing will have to be done.

Karre: Is susceptibility inherited as a dominant trait in all combinations between resistant and susceptible strains?

Chalmer: The H-2 linked susceptibility is inherited as a dominant trait but, as I showed, if one is testing the $F_1$ combination between resistant and susceptible strains which are not congenic, the (C57BL x C3H) $F_1$ is fairly resistant, whereas the (C3H x Balb/c) $F_1$ is fairly susceptible. So certainly on the non-congenic $F_1$ hosts it is not the case but, if one is looking only at the transmission of the H-2 linked control, then susceptibility is completely dominant.

GENETICS OF MACROPHAGE-CONTROLLED NATURAL RESISTANCE TO
HEPATITIS INDUCED BY HERPES SIMPLEX VIRUS TYPE 2 IN MICE

Soren C. Mogensen

Institute of Medical Microbiology
University of Aarhus
Aarhus, Denmark

INTRODUCTION

Herpes simplex virus type 2 (HSV-2) has previously been
shown to cause progressive focal necrotizing hepatitis in
most strains of mice on intraperitoneal inoculation (7).
However, a great variation in the resistance of various inbred mouse strains was noticed, making it likely that genetic factors of the mice play a role in the observed differences in resistance. The variations in resistance were manifest during the first 4 days of infection, pointing to
nonspecific, natural defense mechanisms as being instrumental in the phenomenon. Among these, macrophages take up a
prominent position and the role of macrophages in natural
resistance to virus infections is well documented (2,9).
The present study describes the inheritance of resistance to HSV-2 induced hepatitis in mice and points to the
macrophages as playing a key role as effectors of this genetically determined trait.

MATERIAL AND METHODS

The details of the materials and methods used have been
described previously (8,10). Specific points are referred
to in the results section.

Inheritance of resistance to HSV-2 hepatitis

For these studies 8-week-old specific-pathogen-free
BALB/c, GR, (GR♂ x BALB/c♀)$F_1$ and (BALB/c♂ x (GR x BALB/c)♀)
$BC_1$ mice of both sexes were inoculated intraperitoneally
with $10^6$ PFU of HSV-2. Four days later the mice were examined for macroscopic liver lesion. In Table 1, the summary
of a series of such experiments is shown. Both male and
female BALB/c mice were susceptible with many focal necrotic
lesions in all animals, whereas all GR mice of both sexes
were resistant. The characters for susceptibility and resistance segregated between male and female offspring of the
$F_1$ generation (all males susceptible, all females resist-

Table 1. Liver Lesions and Virus Titers in Mice Infected
with HSV-2

| Mouse strain | Male mice | | Female mice | |
|---|---|---|---|---|
| | No. mice with lesions / No. inoculated | Virus titer (log 10 PFU/gram) | No. mice with lesions / No. inoculated | Virus titer (log 10 PFU/gram) |
| BALB/c | 10/10 | 3.6 ± 0.5 | 33/33 | 3.1 ± 0.5 |
| GR | 0/14 | 1.3 ± 0.7 | 0/27 | 1.2 ± 1.1 |
| $F_1$ | 26/26 | 3.9 ± 0.4 | 0/40 | 1.3 ± 1.1 |
| $BC_1$ | 17/29 | [a]3.7 ± 0.8<br>[b]1.4 ± 0.6 | 10/22 | [a]3.5 ± 0.6<br>[b]1.6 ± 1.0 |

[a]Mice with lesions
[b]Mice without lesions

ant). This shows that resistance is the dominant feature, and that the resistance gene(s) is located on the X-chromosome. In the $BC_1$ generation of resistant $F_1$ females to susceptible BALB/c males the traits segregated in ratios of about 1:1 in mice of both sexes, which suggests that resistance is controlled by one major gene or a complex of closely linked genes.

The virus titers of the livers from the mice are also shown in Table 1. Virus could be isolated in titers around $10^3$ - $10^4$ PUF/gram from all mice showing liver lesions, whereas virus titers in the livers of mice without macroscopic lesions were about 100 times less. The virus titers thus reflected the macroscopic appearance of the livers.

Replication of HSV-2 in mouse peritoneal macrophages

The replication of HSV-2 in peritoneal macrophages from female BALB/c, GR, $F_1$ and $B_1$ mice was assessed by an infectious center assay, because the yield of virus from HSV-infected macrophages is too low for direct assay. Briefly, 5 x $10^5$ unstimulated peritoneal macrophages from individual mice were grown overnight in plastic petri dishes and infected with 5 x $10^5$ PFU of HSV-2. After 60 min of adsorption, the nonadsorbed virus was removed by washing and HSV hyperimmune serum treatment, and the cultures were overlaid with a target cell overlay of mouse embryonic fibroblasts for detection of virus growth in the macrophages.

The replication of HSV-2 in peritoneal macrophages from individual female mice is shown in Table 2.

Table 2.  Growth of HSV-2 in Mouse Peritoneal Macrophages

| Mouse strain | No. mice | No. infectious centers |
|---|---|---|
| BALB/c ♀ | 7 | 114 ± 10 |
| GR ♀ | 8 | 32 ± 13 |
| $F_1$ ♀ | 10 | 39 ± 14 |
| $BC_1$♀ "high" | 6 | 130 ± 23 |
| "low" | 8 | 38 ± 20 |

The number of infectious centers showed a distribution reflecting the in vivo resistance patterns:  GR and $F_1$ macrophage cultures had lower plaque counts than BALB/c macrophage cultures, and a clear-cut segregation in "high" and "low" restriction close to a 1:1 ratio was found in the $BC_1$ generation.  No difference in the adsorption rate of virus to macrophages between BALB/c and GR mice was seen (data not shown).

## Growth of HSV-2 in mouse embryonic fibroblasts

The growth of HSV-2 in embryonic fibroblast cultures prepared from individual BALB/c and GR embryos was compared. No difference could be detected in either plaquing efficiency or plaque area of HSV-2 in these cells, and the yield of infectious virus into the supernatant was also identical.

## Effect of silica on resistance to HSV-2 hepatitis

Groups of 8-week-old female BALB/c and GR mice and $F_1$ mice of both sexes were inoculated intravenously with 3 mg of silica 2 hours before intraperitoneal inoculation of $10^6$ PFU of HSV-2.  The mice were sacrificed on day 4 of infection, and the livers were examined for lesions and virus content.  As seen from Table 4, the selective blockade of the macrophage function of the mice with silica rendered resistant GR mice and $F_1$ female mice just as susceptible to the infection as BALB/c mice and $F_1$ male mice, further supporting the participation of macrophages in the natural resistance to the infection.

Table 3.   Growth of HSV-2 in Mouse Embryonic Fibroblasts

| Mouse strain | No. plaques[a] | Area[b] (mm$^2$) | Virus titer[c] (log 10 PFU/ml) | | |
|---|---|---|---|---|---|
| | | | 24 h | 48 h | 72 h |
| BALB/c | 63 ± 8 | 2.2 ± 0.7 | 3.0 ± 0.3 | 4.2 ± 0.3 | 5.1 ± 0.2 |
| GR | 62 ± 9 | 2.1 ± 0.7 | 3.1 ± 0.3 | 4.1 ± 0.2 | 5.0 ± 0.3 |

[a]Mean of plaque count in cultures from seven individual BALB/c or GR embryos.
[b]Mean area of 84 and 58 plaques, respectively.
[c]Virus titers in supernatants of cultures from seven individual BALB/c or GR embryos infected with 10$^3$ PFU of HSV-2.

Table 4.   Effect of Silica on Resistance to HSV-2 Hepatitis

| Mouse strain | Treatment | No. mice with lesions / No. inoculated | Virus titer (log 10 PFU/gram) |
|---|---|---|---|
| BALB/c ♀ | - | 10/10 | 3.4 ± 0.6 |
| | Silica | 10/10 | 4.7 ± 0.8 |
| GR ♀ | - | 0/10 | 1.5 ± 0.7 |
| | Silica | 10/10 | 4.2 ± 0.4 |
| F$_1$ ♂ | - | 10/10 | 3.2 ± 0.7 |
| | Silica | 10/10 | 4.6 ± 0.5 |
| F$_1$ ♀ | - | 0/10 | 1.4 ± 0.6 |
| | Silica | 10/10 | 4.0 ± 0.7 |

## DISCUSSION

In some animal-virus sytems, macrophages have been found to express at the cellular level the genetic resistance seen in vivo. The best clarified examples of this are the resistance of mice to flaviviruses (4) and the susceptibility of mice to mouse hepatitis virus type 2 (3) both of which are inherited as monogenic autosomal dominant characters.

This study presents evidence that the resistance of mice to the induction of focal necrotic hepatitis by HSV-2 is determined by one dominant gene (or a complex of closely linked genes) located on the X-chromosome. This unique feature of sex linkage of resistance to a virus infection appeared in the $F_1$ generation, where the characters for susceptibility and resistance segregated between male and female mice.

A cellular expression of the resistance pattern seen in vivo was found in the ability of unstimulated peritoneal macrophages to restrict the replication of the virus. Further evidence in support of the participation of macrophages in the resistance was obtained by the abolition of the resistance of GR and $F_1$ female mice with silica, which is thought to be selectively toxic for macrophages (1).

Lopez has presented evidence that the resistance of mice to HSV-1 infection is also a dominant trait, but that it is governed by at least two genes (5). The marker for susceptibility was, however, the death of the animals which is usually caused by central nervous system infection. This might be a much more complex pathogenic event than the degree of infection of the liver. Concerning the ability of peritoneal macrophages to restrict the replication of HSV-1, Lopez and Dudas (6) found a correlation between this parameter and the resistance of the animals. Macrophages from resistant $F_1$ mice failed, however, to restrict the replication of the virus, which might seem at variance with the results presented in this paper. However, their data were obtained in male mice, actually supporting the idea of sex linkage of the ability of macropahges to restrict virus replication, although this function did not segregate with the overall resistance of the mice. This points to other defense mechanisms, for instance NK cell activity, as being of importance for the final outcome of the infection.

## REFERENCES

1.    Allison,  A.C.,  Harington,  J.S.,  and  Birbeck,  M. J.Exp.Med. 124:141, 1966.

2.  Bang, F.B.  Adv.Virus Res. 23:269, 1978.
3.  Bang, F.B., and Warwick, A.  Proc.Natl.Acad.Sci.  USA
    46:1065, 1960.
4.  Goodman, G.T., and Koprowski, H.  J.Cell.Comp.Physiol.
    59:333, 1962.
5.  Lopez, C. Nature (Lond) 258:152, 1975.
6.  Lopez, C., and Dudas, G.  Infect.Immun. 23:432, 1979.
7.  Mogensen, S.C.  Acta  Pathol.Microbiol.Scand  Sect  B.
    84:154, 1976.
8.  Mogensen, S.C.  Infect.Immun. 17:268, 1977.
9.  Mogensen, S.C.  Microbiol.Rev. 43:1, 1979.
10. Mogensen,  S.C., and  Andersen,  H.K.   Infect.Immun.
    17:274, 1977.

GENETICALLY CONTROLLED RESISTANCE TO TOGAVIRUSES

Margo A. Brinton

The Wistar Institute
Philadelphia, PA 19104

Within inbred strains of mice susceptibility to disease
induced by two classes of togaviruses has been found to be
modulated by genes of the host. (1) A mendelian gene which
shows no H-2 linkage controls susceptibility to flavivirus-
induced encephalitis (4,11,12,13). (2) Lactate dehydrogenase-elevating virus, an unclassified togavirus, which normally produces a "silent" chronic infection in mice can induce a polioencephalitis in two susceptible strains (9).
Preliminary genetic analysis indicates that two host genes
may be involved and that one of them may be linked to the
H-2$^k$ locus (8).


Flavivirus Sytem

The allele confering resistance to flavivirus-induced
disease has been identified in the BRVR, BSVR (13) and PRI
(11,12) inbred mouse strains and also in two populations of
wild mice (1). Congenic resistant (C3H/RV) and susceptible
(C3H/He) mouse strains were developed through introduction
of the resistance allele from PRI into a C3H background (5).
The segregation of the flavivirus resistance alleles within
wild mouse populations indicates that this gene may confer a
selective advantage in the wild.
Factors such as age, nutritional status, and competence
of the immune response of resistant animals have been found
to influence the phenotypic expression of the flavivirus resistance allele (7,11). However, evidence has not been
obtained to indicate that any one of these factors is actually involved in the specific mechanism of resistance mediated by the product of the flavivirus resistance allele.
Resistant animals do support flavivirus replication, but
tissue titers are always lower and the spread of infection
is slower and usually self-limiting in resistant mice as
compared to susceptible ones (1,4). Flavivirus resistance
is expressed at the cellular level; cell cultures derived
from tissues of resistant mice produce lower yields of
flaviviruses after infection than do comparable cultures of
cells from susceptible mice (2,14) (Table 1).

Table 1.   Growth of WNV in Resistant and Susceptible
           Embryofibroblast Cultures

| Time After Infection (Hr) | Type of Culture | |
|---|---|---|
| | Resistant | Susceptible |
| 1 | 2.0 [a] | 2.0 |
| 24 | 2.0 | 2.7 |
| 48 | 2.7 | 3.17 |
| 72 | 2.9 | 3.89 |
| 96 | 3.3 | 5.85 |

[a] PFU/ml expressed as $\log_{10}$
[b] Cells were infected at a moi of 10

Biological and, recently, also biochemical data suggest
that flavivirus defective interfering (DI) virus particles
may play a role in the phenotypic expression of flavivirus
resistance.  We have previously shown that when culture
fluids from resistant and susceptible WHV-infected cell cultures are serially passaged every three days to fresh cultures of the same type, a cyclic rise and fall in virus titer is observed in both types of cultures (2).  However, although cyclic, the titer of infectious virus remained relatively high during passage in susceptible cultures, but
dropped rapidly during passage in resistant cultures.  Interferon levels were found to be higher in culture fluids
from susceptible cells, not resistant ones.  Only culture
fluid from resistant cells produced positive homologous interference when mixed with standard WNV and plaque-assayed
on monkey cells.  Lower virus titers and high interfering
activity are also generated readily by serial passage of WNV
in brains of adult resistant mice (Brinton, unpublished
data).  The RNA's contained in extracellular virions produced at various times after a high multiplicity infection
of resistant and susceptible cells are being analyzed.
Partially purified [3]H-Ur extracellular virus was lysed with
detergent and virion RNA was extracted with phenol and analyzed on agarose slab gels.  Virion RNA from susceptible
cultures was predominantly full-sized 42S RNA.  Substantial
amounts of 42S RNA was also found in virions from resistant
cultures even though infectivity titers of these samples was
2 to 3 logs lower than from the susceptible culture samples.
A second peak of faster migrating RNA was visible in preparations of WN virions extracted from resistant cell fluids by
48 hr after infection (Figure 1a).  By 96 hr the relative
amount of this RNA had increased and a third peak of RNA was

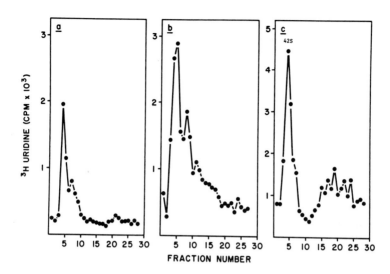

<u>Figure 1</u>. WNV RNA extracted from virions synthesized in re-sistant cells at 48 hr (a) and 96 hr (b) and susceptible cells at 96 hr (c) after infection.

also visible (Figure 1b). The WN virions from susceptible cell cultures did not appear to contain these species of RNA in detectable amounts, although a shoulder was observed on the 42S RNA peak extracted from WN virions from susceptible culture fluids 96 hr after infection (Figure 1c). It is not presently known whether or not the faster migrating RNA's isolated from WN virions grown in resistant cells are actua-lly deleted genomes, if so, they may be RNA's from DI parti-cles. The above data indicates that flavivirus DI particles are formed more rapidly and in greater numbers in resistant cells and that the homologous interference produced by these particles may also be more efficient in resistant cells than in susceptible ones.

We have previously shown that interferon-mediated in-hibition in resistant cells is more pronounced against fla-viviruses (2,6). The interaction of the interferon-induced antiviral state with the expression of the resistance gene is not currently understood on the molecular level. Recent experiments indicate that resistant animals are not rendered susceptible to flavivirus-induced disease by the injection of anti-interferon antibody (AIF) and that AIF-treated resistant embryofibroblast cultures produce lower yields of virus than comparably treated susceptible cell cultures. These experiments are being carried out in collaboration with Drs. H. Arnheiter, O. Haller, and J. Lindemann using anti-interferon Ab prepared by Dr. I. Gresser. This preliminary data suggests the possibility that the antiviral state and the flavivirus resistance allele may act in a non-specific but synergistic manner. However, more information about the molecular interactions are necessary before this phenomenon can be fully understood.

Lactate Dehydrogenase Virus Sytem

A syngeneic line of Ib leukemia cells which had been maintained in C58 mice for about 20 years was observed to spontaneously develop the capacity to produce a paralytic disease in old C58 mice (10). C58 mice are known to spontaneously lose their immune competence during aging (3). Subsequently, young C58 and AKR mice were found to be susceptible to this disease if they were experimentally immunosuppressed prior to infection of Ib leukemia cells or cell extracts. The factor in these tumor cell preparations which is responsible for its paralytogenic activity has recently been identified as a strain of lactate dehydrogenase-elevating virus (LDV), on the basis of its morphology, physiochemical and antigenic properties, and its growth characteristics (9). Histopathologically, the disease, an age-dependent polioencephalitis (ADPE) is characterized by neuronal degeneration and by mononuclear cell infiltration of the gray matter of the spinal cord and brain stem.

Infection of mice with LDV normally results in a "silent" persistent infection which is characterized by elevated levels of certain serum enzymes, such as lactate dehydrogenase and isocitrate dehydrogenase, and by continued circulation of infectious immune complexes. Infected animals display no overt disease symptoms. However, previously isolated strains of LDV were found to possess a low level of paralytogenic activity. Four isolates of LDV, designated LDV-1 through LDV-4 were tested for their ability to induce paralysis in 6 or 12 month old C58 mice which had been given a single injection of cyclophosphamide (150 mg/kg) one day prior to virus inoculation (Table 2). The LDV strain obtained from C58 mice (ADPE agent) readily induced paralysis in 100% of both the 6 and 12 month old immunosuppressed C58 mice. In contrast, the four LDV isolates induced paralysis in only 50-60% of the 12 month old mice. Although an immuno-

Table 2. Test for Paralytogenicity of LDV Isolates in C58 mice

| Virus injected[a] | Incidence of paralysis in | | | |
|---|---|---|---|---|
| | 6-month-old mice | | 12-month-old mice | |
| | Proportion | Mean Day ± SD | Proportion | Mean Day ± SD |
| LDV-1 [b] | 0/10 | | 9/11 | 16.9 ± 5.1 |
| LDV-2 | 1/10 | 18 | 6/10 | 15.2 ± 5.2 |
| LDV-3 | 0/10 | | 8/9 | 17.1 ± 5.2 |
| LDV-4 | 0/18 | | 6/19 | 19.0 ± 5.0 |
| ADPE agent | 10/10 | 12.1 ± 2.3 | 10/10 | 10.0 ± 0.5 |

[a]Mice were given cyclophosphamide 1 day before challenge with $10^7$ $ID_{50}$ of the indicated virus (as determined by enzyme elevation assay).
[b]The four samples of LDV were isolated by the following investigators: LDV-1, M.A. Brinton and P.G.W. Plagemann; LDV-2, A. Notkins; LDV-3, S. Schlesinger; and LDV-4, V. Riley.
(Used with permission from Martinez et al. 1980).


suppressed state is required during the initial infection for the induction of paralysis, host genes are also involved, since immunosuppression of all other mouse strains did not render them susceptible (9). Apparently, the inadvertent passage off LDV in C58 mice as a contaminant of the Ib leukemia preparations led to the selection of a variant LDV which has an enhanced capacity to induce paralysis in susceptible mice.

Preliminary analysis of host genes involved in controlling susceptibility to LDV-induced polioencephalitis indicates that susceptibility may in part be H-$2^k$ linked. Also, it is not yet clear whether more than one gene is involved (9). Breeding studies to determine the number of genes are in progress.

Recently, we have begun to analyze infected C58 mice and a number of interesting observations have been made. C58 mice which were to become paralyzed maintained higher levels of infectivity in their blood than infected resistant mice. This could reflect a decreased production of antibodies able to complex the virus or, alternatively, a larger population of target cells in C58 mice. Previously, LDV was found to replicate only in macrophage-like cells. Electron microscopic investigation of spinal cords of infected C58 mice revealed the replication of virus in neurons. Virions were observed budding through cytoplasmic membranes within neurons. However, no obvious cytopathic effect was obvious in virus-containing neurons. To date virus has not been found in spinal cord neurons of resistant mice. The susceptibility of isolated neurons in culture is now being investigated. Virus infectivity titers were measured in spinal fluid at various times after infection. Surprisingly, virus was found in spinal fluid by 3 days after infection in both resistant and susceptible mice (Table 3).

Table 3. Titer of ADPE-LDV in CSF

| | | DAYS AFTER INFECTION | | |
|---|---|---|---|---|
| MOUSE STRAIN | TREATMENT | 3 | 6 | 9 |
| SWISS (r) | ----- | $6.5^a$ | 6.0 | 6.0 |
| SWISS (r) | CYCLO | 7.0 | 6.1 | 5.5 |
| C58 (s) | ----- | 7.65 | 7.0 | 7.0 |
| C58 (s) | CYCLO | 7.58 | 7.5 | 6.0 |

[a] $LOG_{10} ID_{50}/ML$

LDV apparently can readily cross the blood brain barrier even during an infection which does not induce polioencephalitis. Although these findings provide clues to the mechanism by which LDV can induce paralysis in a genetically susceptible immunosuppressed mouse, the exact sequence of events leading to the induction of this disease are not yet known.

# REFERENCES

1. Darnell, M.B., Koprowski, H., and Lagerspetz, H. J. Infect. Dis. 129:240, 1974.
2. Darnell, M.B., and Koprowski, H. J.Infect.Dis. 129:248, 1974.
3. Duffey, P.S., Martinez, D., Abrams, G.D., and Murphy, W.H. J.Immunol. 116:475, 1976.
4. Goodman, G.T., and Koprowski, H. J.Cell.Comp.Physiol. 59:333, 1962.
5. Groshel, D., and Koprowski, H. Arch. fur Ges.Virus Forsch. 18:379, 1965.
6. Hanson, B., and Koprowski, H. Microbios. 1B:51, 1969.
7. Jacoby, R.O., and Bhatt, P.N. J.Infect.Dis. 134:166, 1976.
8. Martinez, D. Infect. Immun. 23:45, 1979.
9. Martinez, D., Brinton, M.A., Tachovsky, T.G., and Phelps, A.H. Infect.Immun. 27:979, 1980.
10. Murphy, W.H., Tam, M.R., Lanzi, R.L., Abell, M.R., and Kauffman, C. Can.Res. 30:1612, 1970.
11. Sabin, A.B. Ann.NY Acad.Sci. 54:936, 1952.
12. Sabin, A.B. Proc.Nat.Acad.Sci. 38:540, 1952.
13. Webster, L.T. J.Exp.Med. 65:261, 1937.
14. Webster, L.T., and Johnson, M.S. J.Exp.Med. 74:489, 1941.

GENETIC RESISTANCE TO LETHAL FLAVIVIRUS INFECTION:
DETECTION OF INTERFERING VIRUS PRODUCED IN VIVO

Abigail L. Smith, Robert O. Jacoby
and Pravin N. Bhatt

Section of Comparative Medicine
Yale University School of Medicine
New Haven, CT 06510

Resistance of nonimmune mice to lethal flavivirus encephalitis is inherited as a simple autosomal dominant trait
(12,19). Mechanisms proposed to explain phenotypic expression of resistance include 1) innate resistance of target
cells to viral replication, e.g., reduced number or affinity
of cellular receptors for virus attachment, 2) production of
defective interfering particles by cells of resistant mice
and 3) enhanced immune responsiveness of resistant mice.
   Previous reports from this laboratory have shown that
genetic resistance of C3H/RV mice to Banzi virus infection
is severely compromised by immunosuppression with cyclophosphamide, sublethal x-irradiation or T cell depletion by thymectomy (2,7). In addition, transfer of a primed T-enriched
cell population confers protection upon challenged susceptible mice (8). Consistently significant differences in the
ability of immune cells derived from susceptible or resistant mice to lyse Banzi virus-infected target cells in in
vitro cytotoxicity assays have not been detected (13).
Darnell and Koprowski (3) implicated defective interfering
virus as one factor responsible for resistance to West Nile
virus, another flavivirus. For this reason, we are currently investigating the possible contributions of non-immuno-
logic factors to survival of resistant mice.

MATERIALS AND METHODS

Mice. Congenic mice, susceptible C3H/He (He) or resistant
C3H/RV (RV) to lethal flavivirus encephalitis, were bred and
housed at Yale University as previously described (6). Male
and female mice at 7-9 weeks of age were used in all experiments.
Viruses. Banzi virus (15) was used at the 9th passage level
in suckling ICR mice. Western equine encephalitis (WEE)
virus, strain SP 72-666 (10), was used at the 2nd passage in
suckling ICR mice.
Quantitation of virus in mouse brains. Tissue suspensions
(25%) were made in Dulbecco's modified Eagle medium contain-

ing 50% heat-inactivated fetal bovine serum (DMEM 50/50).
Brains from three to six animals were pooled for each assay.
Suspensions were centrifuged at 10,000g for 30 minutes, and
supernatants were titrated for quantitation of infectious
virus in CER cell cultures (14) grown in Linbro 24-well
plates (Flow Laboratories, Hamden, CT).

Interference Assays. A modification of the method described
by Holland and Villarreal (4) was used, using 25% brain suspensions as the pre-absorption preparations. Cultures were
then challenged with stock Banzi virus at a multiplicity of
infection of 0.01-0.1. Pre-absorption controls included uninfected RV or He brain suspensions (25%) and DMEM 50/50.
Assays were performed with CER cell substrates. All experiments were repeated at least once, and each titration was
performed three times with six replicate wells per dilution.

In vivo passage experiment. He and RV mice were inoculated
intraperitoneally (i.p.) with 500,000 $TCID_{50}$ (0.1 ml) of
stock Banzi virus. Six days later, 25% pooled brain suspensions were made and 0.1 ml was inoculated into new He and RV
mice. This procedure was repeated every 6 days for six passages. Virus in the brain suspensions was quantitated at
each passage and was used in interference assays.

Interferon Assays. Brain suspensions (25%) from Banzi
virus-infected He and RV mice (6th passage), brain suspensions from uninfected He and RV mice, and DMEM 50/50 were
assayed as described by Baron (1). A control preparation
containing 60 units of mouse interferon per ml, a gift of
Dr. G.H. Tignor, Yale University, was also included. CER
(non-mouse) and neuroblastoma clone N18 (mouse) cultures
challenged with WEE virus were used as substrates.

Statistical Methods. Calculations of standard errors are
based on mean titers from 3 independent infectivity assays,
and statistical significance was determined by student's T
test as previously reported (17).

## RESULTS

Virus content in brain and Interference assays. As previously reported (6), the brain is the only organ in which
titers differ significantly between He and RV mice after
i.p. inoculation of Banzi virus (Table 1).

Cytopathic effect (CPE) was often observed earlier with
high dilutions of virus from RV mice than with the more concentrated dilutions. This was not true of virus from He
mice. This result suggested that RV mice were producing interfering virus. He and RV brain suspensions were assayed
for their ability to interfere with the in vitro replication
of a low dose of stock Banzi virus (Tables 2 and 3).

Table 1.  Titers of Banzi Virus in Brains of C3H/He and
C3H/RV Mice after Intraperitoneal Inoculation of 250 or
500,000 TCID$_{50}$ of Virus

| | 250 TCID$_{50}$ Inoculated | | 500,000 TCID$_{50}$ Inoculated | |
| | Log$_{10}$ TCID$_{50}$/Gram | | | |
| Day Post-Infection | He | RV | He | RV |
|---|---|---|---|---|
| 2 | trace | <2.1 | trace | 2.3±0.3 |
| 3 | not done | not done | <1.3 | 2.2±0.3 |
| 4 | 2.2±0.3 | <2.1 | 4.8±0.3 | 4.3±0.3 |
| 5 | not done | not done | 6.2±0.4 | 3.2±0.3 |
| 6 | 7.5±0.4 | 5.5±0.3 | 7.2±0.4 | 5.3±0.4 |
| 8 | 7.5±0.3 | 4.5±0.4 | * | 4.8±0.3 |
| 10 | * | 3.5±0.3 | * | trace |

* all animals dead

Table 2.  Mean Titers of Banzi Progeny After Pre-Absorption
of CER cells with Brain Suspensions from C3H Mice Inoculated
Intraperitoneally with 250 TCID$_{50}$ of Banzi Virus

| Day Post-Infection of Brain Harvest | Log$_{10}$ TCID$_{50}$/0.2 ml | |
| | C3H/He | C3H/RV |
|---|---|---|
| Control * | 6.2±0.6 | |
| 2 | 5.8±0.5 | 5.8±0.5 |
| 4 | 6.3±0.4 | 6.0±0.5 |
| 6 | 6.5±0.5 | 5.3±0.4** |
| 8 | 5.8±0.5 | 5.6±0.5 |
| 10 | | 5.9±0.3 |

*Mean of progeny titers after pre-absorption with normal RV
brain, normal He brain or DMEM 50/50 ± standard error.
**significantly different from control titer, p<0.05.
- all animals dead.

Table 3.  Mean Titers of Banzi Progeny After Pre-Absorption
of CER cells with Brain Suspensions from C3H Mice Inoculated
Intraperitoneally with 500,000 TCID$_{50}$ of Banzi Virus

| Day Post-Infection of Brain Harvest | Log$_{10}$ TCID$_{50}$/0.2 ml | |
| | C3H/He | C3H/RV |
|---|---|---|
| Control* | 5.7±0.5 | |
| 2 | 6.0±0.5 | 5.3±0.4 |
| 3 | 5.7±0.5 | 5.2±0.5 |
| 4 | 5.7±0.4 | 5.3±0.4 |
| 5 | 5.7±0.3 | 4.7±0.5** |
| 6 | 6.0±0.4 | 4.3±0.4** |
| 8 | - | 4.6±0.4** |
| 10 | - | 5.6±0.4 |

*Mean of progeny titers after pre-absorption with normal RV
brain, normal He brain or DMEM 50/50 ± standard error.
**significantly different from control titer, p<0.05.
- all animals dead.

Interference by infected RV brain was greater and of longer duration after infection of the mice with a high dose of virus, an observation compatible with previous reports of interfering virus production in vivo and in vitro by other viruses (5), and interference by infected RV brain was significantly greater than that by infected He brain on day 5 and 6.

In Vivo Passage. Since interference activity was most marked on the 6th day post-infection after receipt of a high virus dose, serial i.p. passage of Banzi virus was conducted every six days after an initial inoculation of 500,000 $TCID_{50}$ of stock Banzi virus. Virus titers and results of interference assays are given in Tables 4 and 5.

Table 4. Mean Titers of Banzi Virus in Brains of C3H/He and C3H/RV Mice Passaged on the Sixth Day after Intraperitoneal Incoulation

| Passage Number | $Log_{10}TCID_{50}$/Gram | | |
| --- | --- | --- | --- |
| | C3H/He | C3H/RV | Difference |
| 1 | 7.2±0.4 | 3.4±0.3 | -3.8 |
| 2 | 6.8±0.4 | 3.0±0.3 | -3.8 |
| 3 | 7.4±0.3 | 2.8±0.4 | -4.6 |
| 4 | 7.1±0.3 | 2.8±0.4 | -4.3 |
| 5 | 7.3±0.3 | 4.4±0.3 | -2.9 |
| 6 | 7.3±0.4 | 4.6±0.3 | -2.7 |

Table 5. Titers of Banzi Virus Progeny after Pre-Absorption of CER Cells with Passaged Brain Suspensions from C3H Mice

| Passage Level of Brain Virus Used for Pre-Absorption | $Log_{10}$ $TCID_{50}$/0.2 ml | |
| --- | --- | --- |
| | C3H/He | C3H/RV |
| Control* | 5.9±0.5 | |
| 1 | 5.5±0.6 | 4.7±0.2** |
| 2 | 5.5±0.4 | 5.9±0.1 |
| 3 | 5.4±0.2 | 5.1±0.6 |
| 4 | 5.7±0.6 | 5.1±0.2** |
| 5 | 5.5±0.4 | 3.0±0.1** |
| 6 | 5.4±0.5 | 3.6±0.1** |

*Mean of progeny titers after pre-absorption with normal RV brain, normal He brain or DMEM 50/50 ± standard error.
**Significantly different from control titer, p<0.05.

There is an apparent cyclical variation in the appearance of an interfering component in the brains of Banzi virus-infected RV mice, a result again compatible with those from in vitro serial passage and persistent infections using other viruses which produce defective-interfering particles (9,11-16).

Interferon Assays. Heterologous interference was not observed (data not shown), and the interference assays were performed using a non-mouse cell culture system, thus making it unlikely that interferon was responsible for the results. Despite this, assays to detect interferon production by Banzi virus-infected He and RV mice were performed. None of the preparations, including control mouse interferon, interfered with plaque formation of WEE virus in CER (non-mouse) cells. The results of interferon assays in N18 (mouse) cells are given in Table 6.

Table 6. Titers of Interferon in Infected or Uninfected C3H (RV and He) Mouse Brain Assayed in N18 Cells.

| Preparation | Infected | Titers of Interferon |
|---|---|---|
| C3H/RV mouse brain | + | 5 |
| C3H/He mouse brain | + | >50 |
| C3H/RV mouse brain | - | <5 |
| C3H/He mouse brain | - | <5 |
| DMEM 50/50 diluent | | 0 |
| Control mouse interferon (60 units/ml) | | >20 |

*based on ability to inhibit CPE after challenge of N18 (mouse) cells with 50 $TCID_{50}$ of WEE virus; results given as reciprocal of dilution completely inhibiting CPE (starting dilution for brain preparations was 1:5).

The interferon titer in brains of susceptible mice was significantly higher than that in brains of resistant mice, a result similar to that of Vainio et al. (18) with West Nile Virus. These results are probably due to the higher levels of virus in the brains of susceptible mice.

## DISCUSSION

The important findings reported here are 1) an interfering component is detectable in the brains of Banzi virus-infected C3H/RV (resistant) mice and not in the brains of C3H/He (susceptible) mice, and 2) C3H/He mice infected with Banzi virus produce significantly higher levels of brain

interferon than do C3H/RV mice. Our findings support the
idea that interfering Banzi virus helps resistant mice to
survive infection. Proof that <u>defective</u>-interfering particles are produced requires biochemical analysis of virus from
the brains of RV mice.

With other virus groups, defective-interfering virus
may be produced during serial high multiplicity passage in
or persistent infection of several cell culture systems. In
contrast, we have been unable to detect production of interfering Banzi virus during seven high multiplicity passages
of virus in murine neuroblastoma (clone N18) cells and during eighteen serial passages of infected, undiluted fluid
from either He or RV macrophage cultures (unpublished observations). The results with macrophage culutres are in contrast to those of Darnell and Koprowski (3) with West Nile
virus in primary embryonic cultures from resistant and susceptible mice. Thus, detection of interfering flavivirus
may be dependent on several factors, including the specific
virus and host chosen for analysis. The potential contribution of interfering flavivirus production to survival of
genetically resistant mice is not clear. We believe that
survival is mediated by more than one factor. For example,
the cell-mediated immune responses of both He and RV mice
infected with a high dose of Banzi virus are well developed
by the sixth day post-infection. He mice produce more brain
interferon after Banzi virus infection than do RV mice.
However, since infected He mice die, cell-mediated immunity
combined with interferon production are apparently not adequate to confer protection. Interfering virus production by
RV mice peaks on the sixth day after inoculation. Therefore
it seems reasonable to hypothesize that interfering virus
production by resistant mice, together with developing cell-
mediated immunity and interferon, may convert a lethal infection to a non-lethal infection.


ACKNOWLEDGEMENT


The authors wish to express their gratitude to Mr.
Robert Connell for excellent technical assistance and to
Ms. Katie White for preparation of the manuscript. This
work was supported by grant number 5R01A1 14712 from the
National Institutes of Health.

## REFERENCES

1.  Baron, S.  In Fundamental Techniques in Virology.  K. Habel and N.P., Salzman (eds).  New York: Academic Press, p399, 1969.
2.  Bhatt, P.N., and Jacoby, R.O.  J.Infect.Dis. 134:166, 1976.
3.  Darnell, M.B., and Koprowski, H.  J.Infect.Dis. 129:- 248, 1974.
4.  Holland, J.J., and Villarreal, L.P.  Virology 67:438, 1975.
5.  Huang, A.S., Greenawalt, J.W., and Wagner, R.R. Virology 30:161, 1966.
6.  Jacoby, R.O., and Bhatt, P.N.  J.Infect.Dis. 134:158, 1976.
7.  Jacoby, R.O., and Bhatt, P.N.  Bull.Soc.Pharmacol.- Environ.Pathol. 5:18, 1977.
8.  Jacoby, R.O., Bhatt, P.N., and Schwartz, A.  J.Infect.- Dis. (in press).
9.  Kawai, A., Matsumoto, S., and Tanabke, K.  Virology 67:520, 1975.
10. Main, A.J., Smith, A.L., Wallis, R.C., and Elston, J. Mosq News 39:544, 1979.
11. Palma, E., and Huang, A.S.  J.Infect.Dis. 129:402, 1974.
12. Sabin, A.B.  Proc.Nat.Acad.Sci.USA. 38:540, 1952.
13. Sheets, P., Schwartz, A., Jacoby, R.O., and Bhatt, P. J.Infect.Dis. 140:384, 1979.
14. Smith, A.L., Tignor, G.H., Mifune, K., and Motohashi, T.  Intervirology 8:92, 1979.
15. Smithburn, K.C., Paterson, H.E., Heyman, C.S., and Winter, P.A.D.  S.Afr.Med.J. 33:959, 1959.
16. Tignor, G.H., Mifune, K., and Smith, A.L.  In Symposium on Advances in Rabies Research.  Center for Disease Control, Atlanta, GA. p13, 1976.
17. Tignor, G.H., Smith, A.L., Casals, J., Ezeokoli, C.D., and Okoli, J.  Amer.J.Trop.Med.Hyg. (in press).
18. Vainio, T., Gwatkin, R., and Koprowski, H.  Virology 14:385, 1961.
19. Webster, L.T.  J.Exp.Med. 57:793, 1933.

## DISCUSSION

Wainberg:  Did Smith try taking the viral progeny of the RV mouse brian and inoculating it into the susceptible strain?

Smith:  We have done that;  there is no difference in the

ability of the virus to kill - that is, susceptible mice die.

**Wainberg:** So the susceptible mouse will die even if inoculated with particles that are presumably interfering for the resistant cells.

**Smith:** There is obviously a proportion of virus which is interfering, and a proportion of virus which is "standard". Apparently the susceptible mice either do not perceive the interfering virus that is present, or are unable to replicate to amplify that population.

**Wainberg:** Could it be that Smith may not have diluted out the preparation sufficiently so as to detect the differential effect in that experiment?

**Smith:** That is possible.

**Amos:** I cannot help wondering what would happen if Smith were to test varying proportion mixtures of the C3H/He and the C3H/RV brains? Could she then show a dose dependency type of effect, as I would expect. I do not understand the mechanism of the interference. She is not, I hope, implying it is another virus that is coming in from the C3H/RVs is she?

**Smith:** I am implying that RV mice have an ability, somehow, to amplify defective interfering particles in the brain, whereas He mice do not possess that ability. And the ability to produce defective interfering virus with other virus groups, specifically rhabdo viruses, has been shown to be very much host dependent.

**Darnell:** As the one who did these original studies and has been pursuing them recently, I can say that we have found the same kind of effect in the brains. I have been more interested in looking at the cell cultures, and we do find defective particles produced in susceptible mouse cells in culture. It is just that the interference is not as extensive. So, in the case of the animal, where the virus can keep escaping, one would probably need a lot more defective particles in order to see an interference.

# THE ROLE OF H-2 IN RESISTANCE AND SUSCEPTIBILITY TO MEASLES VIRUS INFECTION

Bracha Rager-Zisman, P. Andrew Neighbour,
Grace Ju*, and Barry R. Bloom
Department of Microbiology and Immunology
Albert Einstein College of Medicine
Bronx, New York 10461

*Department of Cell Biology
Roche Institute of Molecular Biology
Nutley, New Jersey 07110

## SUMMARY

Resistance and susceptibility of mice to measles virus infection was studied. Intracerebral inoculation of measles virus produced an acute lethal encephalitis in susceptible mice. There was an age related development of resistance to infection. The strains that showed the highest susceptibility to measles virus were CBA; C3H/HeJ; C3HeB/HeJ and C3H/HeSn. Balb/c; C57B1/6 and DBA/2 exhibited intermediate susceptibility. SJL were totally resistant. Studies on the genetic basis for resistance using hybrid mice, $F_1$ (C3H x SJL) and backcross mice C3H x $F_1$ (C3H x SJL) revealed that the principal determinant of host resistance to acute infection was a dominant gene or gene(s) which segregated independently of the H-2 complex.

In the last two decades it has become apparent that in a number of viral infections host genes determine the inherent resistance or susceptibility to disease (1). In the mouse, cellular immune recognition of viral antigens by cytotoxic T-cells have been shown to be associated with gene products coded by the major histocompatibility complex (MHC) (2). Helper T-cells must also recognize the antigen on the cell surface in association with the appropriate Ia antigen, a product of the Ir genes associated with the MHC (9).

There are a number of human diseases of putative persistent viral etiology which have strong MHC linkage (8). One important case is the marked HLA-D association with Multiple Sclerosis (MS) which indicates a possible genetic predisposition to this disease. The etiologic agents for MS has not yet been identified but paramyxoviruses and particularly measles have been most frequently associated with this disease (4). One of the problems in understanding the pathogenesis of MS is the lack of a suitable animal model. In an attempt to develop an animal model relevant to MS, we have studied acute measles virus infection in mice (5).

This experimental model enabled us to investigate the pathogenesis of measles virus in different strains of mice, and
to analyze the influence of H-2 on resistance to this infection.

### AGE AND STRAIN-RELATED SUSCEPTIBILITY OF INBRED MICE TO ACUTE INFECTION

Measles virus, after intracerebral (I.C.) inoculation,
produces an acute lethal disease in 1-2 days old neonatal
mice. The clinical signs of the disease which became apparent 5-7 days after inoculation were growth retardation,
hyperactivity followed by ataxia, paralysis and death (5).

Mice from 8 inbred strains (C3H/HeJ; CBA; AKR; BALB/c;
DBA/2; C57B1/6; SJL; A/J) were examined and all were found
to be highly susceptible to acute infection when inoculated
with a high dose of measles (4.5 x $10^4$ PFU) within 2 days of
birth.

When mice from some of these strains were inoculated
with measles at different ages, there was an age-dependent
variation between strains in susceptibility to infection
(Table 1). In addition, the duration of the acute disease
and the day of death varied according to the relative
susceptibility of each mouse strain (Fig. 1).

Table 1. Mortality rates (5) in neonatal mice of various
inbred strains after intracerebral inoculation with measles
virus at different ages.

| Strain | H-2 haplotype | Age (days) at inoculation[a] | | | | | | |
|--------|---------------|------|------|------|-----|------|-------|-------|
|        |               | 1/2  | 3/4  | 5/6  | 7/8 | 9/10 | 11/12 | 18/20 |
| C3H/HeJ | k | 100[b] | 100 | 92.3 | 85.7 | 44.4 | 22.7 | 0 |
| BALB/c | d | 100 | 40.0 | 14.8 | 0 | ND[c] | ND | ND |
| C57B1/6 | b | 91.7 | 57.1 | 0 | 0 | 0 | ND | 0 |
| SJL | s | 100 | 0 | 0 | ND | ND | ND | ND |

[a]4.5 x $10^4$ PFU per mouse.    [b]mortality rate with no. dead/no. inoculated.    [c]ND, not done.

from Neighbour et al. (5).

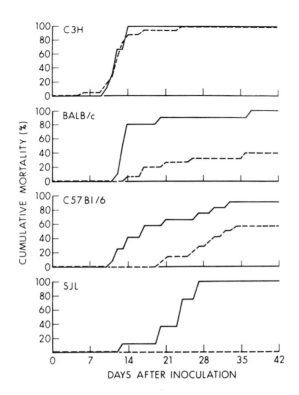

Fig. 1. Cumulative mortality rates in four inbred mouse
strains after intracerebral inoculation with measles virus
at 1-2 days (solid line) and 3-4 days (dotted line) of age
from Neighbour et al. (5).


GENETIC BASIS OF RESISTANCE

Since mice with the $H-2^k$ haplotype (C3H) were susceptible to lethal measles infection, and those with the $H-2^s$
haplotype (SJL) were resistant, experiments were performed
to determine whether the MHC controlled host susceptibility
to this disease. $F_1$ (C3H x SJL) hybrid mice, heterozygous
for the 's' and 'k' alleles were 100% resistant (Table 2),
indicating that susceptibility was a recessive trait. Progeny derived from the backcross generation of $F_1$ (C3H x SJL)
hybrids with the susceptible C3H parent exhibited an intermediate susceptibility. Surviving mice were typed for their
H-2 haplotype, and there was found to be an equal distribut-

Table 2. Relationship between H-2 and susceptibility to lethal measles infection

| Strain[a] | No. of mice inoculated | Mortality rate(%) | H-2 haplotype frequency[b] of inoculated mice | | | H-2 haplotype frequency[b] of surviving mice | | |
|---|---|---|---|---|---|---|---|---|
| | | | s/s | s/k | k/k | s/s | s/k | k/k |
| C3H | 52 | 92.3 | 0 | 0 | 100 | 0 | 0 | 100 |
| SJL | 15 | 0.0 | 100 | 0 | 0 | 100 | 0 | 0 |
| F1 (C3H x SJL) | 18 | 0.0 | 0 | 100 | 0 | 0 | 100 | 0 |
| C3H x F1 (C3H x SJL) | 74 | 56.8 | 0 | 51[c] | 49[d] | 0 | 54[c] | 46[d] |

a5-6 day old mice inoculated intracerebrally with 4.5 x 10[4] PFU of measles virus.

ball frequencies are theoretical unless indicated.

cfrequency determined by sera typing

dfrequency determined by subtraction.

[from Neighbour et al. (5).]

**Table 3.** Susceptibility of various congenic strains to lethal measles infection

| Strain[a] | H-2 haplotype | No. of mice inoculated | Mortality rate(%) |
|---|---|---|---|
| BALB/c | d | 27 | 14.8 |
| BALB.B | b | 23 | 17.4 |
| BALB.K | k | 12 | 16.7 |
| C3H | k | 52 | 92.3 |
| C3H.Sw | b | 20 | 40.0 |
| B10 | b | 19 | 47.4 |
| B10.Br | k | 70 | 70.0 |

[a]5-6 day old mice inoculated intracerebrally with 4.5 × 10⁴ PFU of measles virus.
[from Neighbour et al. (5)].

317

ion of mice with H-2$^{s/k}$ and H-2$^{k/k}$ (Table 2), indicating independent segregation of the genes controlling expression of H-2 antigens and resistance to measles virus.

To further investigate the role played by the major histocompatibility gene complex in controlling susceptibility to lethal measles infection, various congenic strains were inoculated with this virus (Table 3). The results obtained in these experiments suggested that in some strains of mice the H-2 might modify expression of the gene or gene(s) which determine resistance.

INTERACTION OF MEASLES VIRUS AND H-2D AND H-2K ANTIGENS

MHC restriction on T-cell killing requires associative recognition of virus and H-2 antigens. In most viral systems, infection by virus affects the expression of H-2 antigens (3,7). In an in vitro system we have examined the effects of measles virus infection on the expression of native H-2 determinants of the host cells. Acute infection of the mouse neuroblastoma cell line N$_2$A (H-2$^a$), with measles virus caused a selective decrease in the expression of H-2K$^a$ determinants, as measured by quantitative absorption (Table 4).

Table 4.  Expression of H-2 in measles infected N$_2$A cells.

| Time of infection (hours) | #LN cells (x10$^6$)[a] required to remove 50% of anti-H-2K$^k$ | | %decrease in expression of H-2K$^k$ | #LN cells x 10$^6$ required to remove 50% of anti-H-2D$^d$ | | %decrease in expression of H-2D$^d$ |
|---|---|---|---|---|---|---|
| | N$_2$A | MS-N$_2$A | | N$_2$A | MS-N$_2$A | |
| 24 | 0.5 | 0.5 | 0 | 1 | 1 | 0 |
| 48 | 2.5 | 5 | 50 | 1 | 1 | 0 |
| 72 | 1 | 6 | 80 | 1 | 1 | 0 |

[a] A known number of uninfected N$_2$A cells and measles virus (MS) infected N$_2$A cells were incubated with a predetermined amount of anti-H-2 sera.  Unabsorbed antibody was tested for the ability to lyse $^{51}$Cr labeled indicator lymph node (LN) cells.  The number of cells required to absorb 50% of cytotoxic activity was determined (6).

After 72 hours 80% reduction in H-2K expression was detected.  In contrast the expression of the H-2D determinants were not affected.  Treatment of N$_2$A with cycloheximide reduced expression in both H-2K and H-2D determinants.  Therefore the suppression of expression of the H-2K determinants by measles virus is selective and not simply a result of virus induced shutdown of host cell protein synthesis. The diminution by measles virus of expression of H-2K determinants was confirmed by the increased resistance of measles infected $N_2A$ cells to lysis by cytotoxic lymphocytes sensitized against the H-$2^a$ antigens (Table 5).

Table 5. Cell mediated cytotoxicity against uninfected and measles infected $N_2A$ cells.

| Effector cells | % specific $^{51}$Cr release | |
|---|---|---|
| | $N_2A$ | MS-$N_2A^c$ |
| control spleen[a] | 4.3 | 0 |
| anti-H-$2^a$ immune spleen[a] | 30.4 | 8.2 |
| anti-measles immune spleen[b] | NT | -1.8 |

[a]Effector cells were taken from C57B1/6 age-matched mice or from C57B1/6 mice immunized and boosted with A/J(H-$2^a$) spleen cells. [b]Effector cells were taken from A/J mice 9 days after immunization with measles virus. [c]$N_2A$ cells were infected with measles virus at an MOI of 1 for 72 hours.

Nevertheless, using a variety of sensitization regimens it was not possible to detect cytotoxic T lymphocytes (CTL) in this system (Table 5).

Thus it is clear that alteration of H-2 antigens by virus infection may be necessary for recognition by CTL, it is not a sufficient condition for cytotoxicity. Unlike in many other virus infections the relative role of host immune response in resistance to measles virus infection appears to be small and difficult to define. Immunosuppression with cyclophosphamide or injection of silica did not render resistant mice susceptible. There was no difference in the magnitude of antibody production against measles virus between susceptible and resistant strains. On the basis of these experiments it seemed that resistance of mice to measles virus infection is determined in the most part by gene-(s) which segregate independently of the H-2 complex, and it remains unclear whether this gene(s) regulates any immunological function. It seems possible that the H-2 locus might modify expression of the gene or genes involved in resistance or serves as a secondary determinant of resistance.

## REFERENCES

1. Allison, A.C. Prog.Med.Virol. 18:15, 1974.
2. Doherty, P.C., Blanden, R.V., and Zinkernagel, R.M. Transplant. Rev. 29:89, 1976.
3. Hecht, T.T., and Summers, D.F. J. Virol. 19:833, 1976.
4. Johnson, R.T. Adv.Neurol. 13:1, 1975.
5. Neighbour, P.A., Rager-Zisman, B., and Bloom, B.R. Infect. and Immun. 21:764, 1978.
6. Rajan, T.V., Nathenson, S.C., and Scharff, M.D. J. Natl. Cancer Inst. 56:1221, 1976.
7. Senik, A., and Neauport-Saules, C. J. Immunol. 122:1461, 1979.
8. Svejgaard, A., Platz, P., and Ryder, L.P. Clinics in Rheum. Dis. 3:239, 1977.
9. Waldman, H. Immunol. Rev. 35:121, 1977.

## DISCUSSION

Shearer:  The $F_1$ used, which was a cross between C3H and SJL, was resistant.  Has Zisman tried other $F_1$'s;  say B6 x C3H?  I ask because SJL is a very strange experimental animal and it was the most resistant one that she showed.

Zisman:  No, we went only to the extremes.

Shearer:  In Zisman's studies with the target cells which have been infected with measles, she indicated that by cytotoxicity they were less readily lysed than allogeneic targets.

Zisman:  That is correct.

Shearer:  The fact that Zisman had an apparent diminution of the K antigen and not of the D, she could do that in a way that would test only for loss in cytotoxicity for K and not for D.  The question is, can Zisman be sure her measles-infected targets are not merely less susceptible to lysis as a target, rather than that the effect is specific for that antigen?

Zisman:  We were thinking about that;  there were actually very few controls that we could do.  We tried it with different methods, but from our experience with other viruses, the virally-infected cells would not become more susceptible to lysis than uninfected cells.  But in this respect measles is certainly a peculiar virus.

Ir GENE REGULATION OF SENSITIVITY TO LEUKEMOGENESIS BY RadLV
VARIANTS AND ITS RELATIONSHIP TO PRELEUKEMIC CELLS

Peter Lonai, Emil Katz and Nechama Haran-Ghera
Department of Chemical Immunology
The Weizmann Institute of Science
Rehovot, Israel

For already several years one of us has been investigating the in vivo properties of two radiation leukemia viruses in C57BL/6 (B6) mice (1). One of these viruses A-Rad-
LV, is distinguished by its high leukemogenicity, whereas
the other, D-RadLV, causes only a low frequency of leukemia
when these viruses are injected intrathymically into young
adult B6 mice (2). Nevertheless D-RadLV injected B6 mice
after irradiation with a nonleukemic dose of X-rays (400 rad
WB), within several days following virus inoculation, develop a high frequency of leukemia (3). Thus it appears that
the leukemogenicity of D-RadLV depends on a coleukemogenic
effect. Without irradiation, however, D-RadLV was shown to
induce host resistance to the isotransplantation of D-RadLV
induced B6 leukemia cells (4). It was also found that D-
RadLV injected B6 mice harbour preleukemic cells, mainly in
their bone marrow, which have the potential to develop into
donor type leukemia in irradiated F1 recipients (5). Moreover it was shown that these preleukemic cells in normal
hosts are immunogenic, triggering resistance to RadLV induced leukemic cells (6). It follows, that D-RadLV, despite
its "low" leukemogenicity, causes the appearance of preleukemic cells which seem to be arrested from uncontrolled malignant growth unless irradiation or other coleukemogenic
effect permits their multiplication and probably differentiation.

These findings raised the question whether the difference in leukemogenicity between the two passages is due to
inherent characteristics of the viruses or to host effects.
To investigate this problem genetic experiments were performed. A large number of inbred mouse strains were infected
with A-RadLV or with D-RadLV intrathymically in young adult
age. As it was reported earlier, the leukemogenicity of
these viruses in $Fv-1^b$ type strains is linked to the H-2
complex (7). For A-RadLV $H-2^{b,d,f,j,k,p}$ and $r$ were sensitive whereas $H-2^s$ was resistant (8). On the other hand,
for D-RadLV haplotypes k, r, and s were sensitive whereas b,
d and f were resistant (9). The linkage was further demonstrated in segregating BC-1 populations and was found to be a
mendelian unigenic H-2 linked dominant trait (8). Data for
the two most characteristic strains, C57BL/10J (B10) and
B10.S, are shown in Table 1.

GENETIC CONTROL OF NATURAL RESISTANCE
TO INFECTION AND MALIGNANCY

Table 1. H-2 linked resistance to the leukemogenic effect of A-RadLV and D-RadLV

| | | A-RadLV | | | | D-RadLV | | | |
|---|---|---|---|---|---|---|---|---|---|
| H-2 | Strain | Leukemia/Total | Latency (days) | % Leukemia | Status | Leukemia/Total | Latency (days) | % Leukemia | Status |
| b | B10 | 20/21 | 89 | 95 | S | 3/20 | 296 | 15 | R |
| s | B10.S | 2/26 | 122 | 8 | R | 7/12 | 155 | 58 | S |
| b/s | (B10xB10.S)F1 | 4/20 | 267 | 20 | R | 2/20 | 198 | 10 | R |

Table 2. Effect of 400 rad whole body irradiation on H-2 and on Fv-1 associated resistance to A-RadLV and to D-RadLV

| | Strain | H-2 | Fv-1 | Virus only | | Virus + 400 rad | |
|---|---|---|---|---|---|---|---|
| | | | | Leukemia/Total | % | Leukemia/Total | % |
| A-RadLV | B10.S | s | b | 2/25 | 8 | 24/31 | 77 |
| | C3H/DiSn | k | n | 1/19 | 5 | 1/18 | 6 |
| | B10.BR | k | b | 18/20 | 90 | N.D.* | |
| D-RadLV | B10 | b | b | 0/19 | 0 | 20/20 | 100 |
| | C3H/DiSn | k | n | 3/19 | 16 | 1/18 | 6 |
| | B10.BR | h | b | 10/16 | 63 | N.D. | |

N.D. = not done.

Analysis of intra-H-2 recombinant strains have revealed that resistance to A-RadLV maps to subregions I-A and I-B and that its expression depends on complementation with a locus in the I-E/C region (7,8). Similar analysis of the effect of D-RadLV also indicated that the resistance locus maps to the H-2K - I-A interval (9). It appeared therefore that both A-RadLV and D-RadLV are highly oncogenic viruses, and that their oncogenicity in Fv-1 permissive strains is under the regulation of H-2I linked loci. Hence the low oncogenicity of D-RadLV in B/6 (H-2$^b$) mice most likely was due to the effect of H-2 linked resistance loci. Moreover it seemed to be likely that the preleukemic arrest in these mice could also be a result of H-2 linked host effects. The possibility of this suggestion was supported by the finding that H-2 linked resistant mice to A-RadLV (B10.S) are sensitive to a nonleukemogenic dose of X-rays, and, similarly to D-RadLV injected B/6 mice, when irradiated develop leukemia (Table 2). Further support was obtained when we demonstrated the presence of preleukemic cells in the bone marow of A-RadLV infected B10.S resistant mice (Table 3).

Table 3. Preleukemic cells in the bone marrow B10.S mice infected with A-RadLV

| Donor* | 1$^{st}$ recipient | Leukemia/Total (1$^{st}$ recipient) | Take of tumors transferred from 1$^{st}$ recipient to | |
|---|---|---|---|---|
| | | | B10 | B10.S |
| B10.S+A-RadLV | (B10xB10.S)F$_1$+400 rad | 13/19 | 0/13 | 13/13 |

*B10.S mice (2 1/2 month old) were infected intrathymically with A-RadLV. 30 days later their bone marrow (1 donor/1 recipient) was transferred into F1 irradiated primary recipients. Leukemia developed after 150-200 days which was transferred to parental recipients to test the origin of the tumor cells.

The mechanism of H-2 linked resistance to RadLV leukemogenesis and of the arrest of preleukemic cells was sought in genetically regulated antitumor or antivirus immunity. Table 4 demonstrates the results of a tumor transplantation test with A- or D-RadLV infected B10 and B10.S mice.

Table 4. Specific lymphoma transplantation resistance
induced by intrathymically induced A-RadLV or D-RadLV

| Strain | Immunization | Resistance status | Challenge* | Tumor bearing/ total |
|--------|--------------|-------------------|------------|----------------------|
| B10 | PBS | - | D(B10) | 6/6 |
| | D-RadLV | Resistant | " | 0/8 |
| | " | " | X(B10) | 8/8 |
| | " | " | A(B10) | 1/8 |
| | PBS | - | A(B10) | 14/14 |
| | A-RadLV | Sensitive | " | 16/16 |
| B10.S | PBS | - | A(B10.S) | 13/13 |
| | A-RadLV | Resistant | " | 3/21 |
| | " | " | X(B10.S) | 5/5 |
| | " | " | D(B10.S) | 0/6 |
| | PBS | - | D(B10.S) | 4/4 |
| | D-RadLV | Sensitive | " | 16/16 |

*Designation of the lymphoma used:   D = D-RadLV induced;   A
= A-RadLV induced;   X = fractionated X-ray induced.   Strain
of origin in brackets.

The mice were challenged 30 days after intrathymic virus infection with $5 \times 10^5$ A- or D-RadLV induced syngeneic leukemia cells.   The following results were obtained:   (a) Both
A- and D-RadLV could immunize their hosts, but this depended
on the hosts' H-2-linked resistance status;   i.e., no transplantation resistance was obtained in the sensitive combinations.   (b)   The transplantation resistance was specific,
because syngeneic X-ray induced lymphomas were not rejected.
(c)   The protection was crossreactive between A- or D-RadLV
induced lymphomas.   This suggested that whereas transplantation resistance could be induced only by that virus passage
towards which the host was H-2 linked resistant, the resulting immunity was nevertheless crossreactive, most likely due
to antigenic similarities between the lymphoma cells induced
by either one of the two viruses.

The immunological nature of this H-2 regulated transplantation resistance was further demonstrated by showing that
immunity could be transferred by spleen, thymus, or lymph
node cells of virus immune mice into naive recipients in a
Winn type assay (Table 5).

Table 5. Transfer of resistance to syngeneic lymphoma
   challenge from A-RadLV immune donors (B10.S) to naive
   recipients by lymphoid cells (Winn type assay).

| Donor | Tumor bearing/total | | |
|---|---|---|---|
| | Lymphoid cells (200:1) used for transfer | | |
| | Spleen | Thymus | Lymph node |
| Immune | 1/8 | 0/5 | 0/5 |
| Normal | 3/3 | 4/4 | 4/4 |

All these data suggest the role of H-2I linked Ir gene
like loci in resistance to virus induced leukemia. Ir gene
effects are in many cases expressed as a preferential reactivity of F1 responder cells to antigen presenting cells
of the high responder but not of the low responder H-2 type
(10). To investigate this phenomenon in our system (B10 x
B10.S)F1, (high x low responder)F1 mice were immunized with
A- or D-RadLV. These mice were then challenged with tumor
cells of both parental strains. The results (Table 6) have
shown that after A-RadLV immunization the B10.S parental
lymphoma was rejected, whereas the sensitive B10 parental
lymphoma was not. In contrast after D-RadLV immunization
the B10 lymphoma (the resistant haplotype in this case) was
rejected, whereas the B1.S lymphoma was not. This experiment clearly indicates that in the transplantation resistance induced by A- or D-RadLV lymphoma cells of the high responder, i.e. resistant haplotype are superior in presenting
the antigen involved in the reaction. It also follows that
also in this antitumor immune reaction the immunocytes seem
to recognize antigen plus high responder self H-2. This
observation is a further evidence for the role of Ir genes
in the transplantation resistance induced by A and D-RadLV.

Table 6.  RadLV-immune (B10 x B10.S)F1 hybrids can reject
lymphoma cells of the resistant but not of the sensitive
parental genotype.

| Immunizing virus | Lymphoma challenge | Status | Tumor bearing/total |
|---|---|---|---|
| A-RadLV | A(B10.S) | Resistant | 1/13 |
|  | A(B10) | Sensitive | 10/10 |
| D-RadLV | D(B10) | Resistant | 0/4 |
|  | D(B10.S) | Sensitive | 8/8 |

The above experiment tests the effect of a secondary
transplantation reaction which followed immunization with
the virus.  The H-2 restriction of the immunity, however,
strongly suggests that during the primary reaction the immune system was sensitized by virus infected F1 cells which
express the H-2 complex of the resistant (high responder)
parental haplotype.  These immunogenic cells are most likely
the preleukemic cells described previously.  More direct
evidence for this stems from earlier experiments demonstrating the induction of transplantation resistance by bone
marrow derived preleukemic prethymocytes in the D-RadLV-B/6
system (6).

These data are interpreted to suggest the following:
(1) H-2I linked Ir genes are involved in resistance to A- or
D-RadLV induced leukemia.    (2)    The effector function of
this immune reaction, however, is crossreactive between tumors induced by "high" or "low" responder viruses.  May be
that the Ir genes regulate a helper like cell, whereas the
helper dependent effector cells have no such genetic defect,
and thus the protection conferred has a broader scope.  (3)
High x low responder mice when immunized with either of the
two viruses reject only high responder H-2 type lymphoma
cells, suggesting that the Ir gene is expressed in the presentation of the relevant antigen.    (4)    It also follows that
the immunogenic signal in virus infected resistant mice is
delivered in association with H-2 products in a cell bound
form.  Since it was shown previously that preleukemic cells

can immunize resistant mice, we think that the immunogen for the high responder, resistant mice, is a preleukemic cell.

A number of authors agree that leukemogenesis in most hosts is a non single hit, multi step process (11-13). Each of these steps may be permissive or restrictive for the progression of the disease. Our data shed light to one of these steps. Accordingly RadLV variants cause the appearance of dependent preleukemic cells. These cells serve as immunogenic signals in H-2 controlled high responders. The resulting immune reaction effectively suppresses the preleukemic cells and inhibits their proliferation towards autonomous growth. In contrast, in low responders no such immune response is induced and the disease progresses in an autonomous pathway.

## REFERENCES

1.  Haran-Ghera, N. Int. J. Cancer 1:81, 1966.
2.  Haran-Ghera, N., Ben-Yaakov, M., and Peled, A. J. Immunol. 118:600, 1977.
3.  Haran-Ghera, N., and Peled, A. Adv.Cancer Res. 30:45, 1979.
4.  Haran-Ghera, N. Nature 222:992, 1969.
5.  Haran-Ghera, N. J.Natl.Cancer Inst. 60:707, 1978.
6.  Haran-Ghera, N., Rubio, N., Leef, F., and Goldstein, G. Cell. Immunol. 37:308, 1978.
7.  Lonai, P., and Haran-Ghera, N. J.Exp.Med. 146:1164, 1977.
8.  Lonai, P., Katz, E., and Haran-Ghera, N. Immunogenetics (in press).
9.  Lonai, P., and Haran-Ghera, N. Immunogenetics (in press).
10. Shevach, E.M., and Rosenthal, A.S. J.Exp.Med. 138:1213, 1973.
11. Furth, J. Cancer Res. 13:477, 1953.
12. Lilly, F. J.Natl.Cancer Inst. 49:927, 1972.
13. Kawashima, K., Ikeda, H., Stockert, E., Takahashi, T., and Old, L.J. J.Exp.Med. 144:193, 1976.

## ACKNOWLEDGEMENT

This study was supported by NCI contract NO1-CB-74151.

## DISCUSSION

<u>Kiessling</u>:    Has  Haran-Ghera  been  able  to  characterize  or
enrich  the  preleukemic  cells  by  some  separation  method?

<u>Haran-Ghera</u>:    This  was  a  serious  challenge,  but  we  succeeded
in  isolating  them  using  velocity  sedimentation  with  Ficoll
and  we  know  they  are  in  fractions  9/10.    We  would  show  that
they  were  prothymocytes  because  we  could  induce  theta  antigen  with  thymopoietin.    We  could  also  show  they  were  TL-
positive.    I  think  the  preleukemic  cells  are  prothymocytes.
They  comprise  2  to  3%  in  marrow.

<u>Winn</u>:  If  they  are  prothymocytes,  would  they  have  NK  activ-
ity?

<u>Haran-Ghera</u>:    We  will,  of  course,  test  this.    Logically  one
would  expect  this  to  be  the  case.

<u>Wainberg</u>:    Have  you  tried  to  monitor  interferon  levels  in
these  different  animals?

<u>Haran-Ghera</u>:    No.

# RECOVERY FROM FRIEND VIRUS LEUKEMIA IS DETERMINED BY THE H-2 GENOTYPE OF NONLEUKEMIC CELLS OF THE SPLEEN AND BONE MARROW

William J. Britt and Bruce Chesebro

U.S. Department of Health, Education, and Welfare
Public Health Service
National Institutes of Health
National Institute of Allergy and Infectious Diseases
Laboratory of Persistent Viral Diseases
Rocky Mountain Laboratories
Hamilton, Montana 59840

Friend virus (FV) is a murine type C oncornavirus which induces a rapidly progressive erythroleukemia in adult mice. The mouse major histocompatibility complex, H-2, influences recovery from erythroleukemia (9). At high virus doses homozygous $H-2^{b/b}$ mice have a high incidence of recovery, whereas mice of the $H-2^{a/b}$ genotype and the $H-2^{a/a}$ genotype have a low incidence of recovery (5). H-2 does not influence early events of the disease as almost all mice, regardless of H-2 genotype develop splenomegaly (2). However, in the majority of mice of the H-2 genotype associated with recovery, the spleen size returns to normal and the mice survive. Mice of the nonrecovery H-2 genotypes have persistent splenomegaly and die within 3-4 months. Thus, H-2 influences the elimination of leukemia cells rather than susceptibility to leukemia induction. Using strains of congenic mice with recombinations within H-2, we have mapped the gene which controls recovery from FV leukemia to the H-2D region (2,5).

In the present study, we investigated the organs and cell types mediating recovery from FV leukemia. Initially recovery from FV leukemia was studied in irradiation chimeras prepared by inoculating spleen and bone marrow cells of the $H-2^{b/b}$ or the $H-2^{a/b}$ genotype into lethally irradiated $H-2^{b/b}$ recipients (Table 1). The incidence of recovery correlated with the genotype of the donor spleen and bone marrow cells. Thus, a high incidence of recovery was seen when $H-2^{b/b}$ donor cells were transferred, and a low incidence of recovery was seen when $H-2^{a/b}$ donor cells were transferred. The spleen and bone marrow contain not only erythroid stem cells, which are the target cells for FV transformation, but also cells of the immune system presumably responsible for the rejection of FV leukemia cells. Therefore, it was necessary to separate the influence of the H-2 genotype of the nonleukemic cells and the leukemic cells

GENETIC CONTROL OF NATURAL RESISTANCE
TO INFECTION AND MALIGNANCY

ISBN 0-12-647680-2

Table 1. Incidence of Recovery from FV Leukemia is Associated with Cells of the Spleen and Bone Marrow

| Donor | | Irradiated recipients[1] | | Recovered mice/total[2] |
|---|---|---|---|---|
| Strain | H-2 genotype | Strain | H-2 genotype | |
| (C57BL/10 X A.BY)F$_1$ | b/b | (C57BL/10 X A.BY)F$_1$ | b/b | 41/52(79%) |
| (B10.A X A.BY)F$_1$ | a/b | (C57BL/10 X A.BY)F$_1$ | b/b | 6/39(15%) |
| Unirradiated controls | | | | |
| (C57BL/10 x A.BY)F$_1$ | b/b | | | 24/30(80%) |
| (B10.A X A.BY)F$_1$ | a/b | | | 4/20(20%) |

[1] Recipients received 900 Rads and then were reconstituted with 20 x 10$^6$ viable spleen and bone marrow cells. 2-3 months post-irradiation, all mice received 280 FFU B-tropic FV i.v. All mice were age and sex matched.
[2] Recovery was determined by resolution of palpable splenomegaly.

Table 2. H-2 Genotype of Nonleukemic Cells of the Spleen and Bone Marrow Determines the Incidence of Recovery

| Tolerized donor[1] | | Nonirradiated recipients[2] | | Recovered mice/total[3] |
|---|---|---|---|---|
| Strain | H-2 genotypes | Strain | H-2 genotype | |
| (C57BL/10 X A.BY)F1 | b/b | (B10.A X A.BY)F1 | a/b | 25/28(90%) |
| (B10.A x A/WySn)F1 | a/a | (B10.A X A.BY)F1 | a/b | 2/14(14%) |
| No cells transferred | | (B10.A X A.BY)F1 | a/b | 3/27(11%) |

[1]Donor mice were neonatally tolerized by injecting $20 \times 10^6$ viable spleen and bone marrow cells of (B10.A x A.BY)F1 into newborn (24 hr old) (C57BL/10 X A.BY)F1 or (B10.A X A/WySn)F1 mice. Tolerance was determined by viable, intact (B10.A X A.BY)F1 skin graft 40 days postgrafting.

[2]Recipient mice were given 280 FFU B-tropic FV i.v. and approximately 4-6 hr later received $40 \times 10^6$ viable spleen and bone marrow cells from tolerant donor mice.

[3]Recovery was determined by resolution of palpable splenomegaly.

on recovery.

We demonstrated the importance of the H-2 genotype of the nonleukemic cells of the spleen and bone marrow on recovery by mixing normal H-2$^{b/b}$ spleen and bone marrow cells with H-2$^{a/b}$ leukemia cells in vivo. To prevent a graft versus host reaction during this mixing experiment, we neonatally tolerized the H-2$^{b/b}$ donor mice to H-2$^{a/b}$. Tolerant H-2$^{b/b}$ nonleukemic spleen and bone marrow cells were given to FV inoculated H-2$^{a/b}$ mice receiving virus only (Table 2). When H-2$^{a/a}$ nonleukemic spleen and bone marrow cells, tolerized in the same manner, were given to FV inoculated H-2$^{a/b}$ mice, a low incidence of recovery was observed (Table 2). Because the donor H-2$^{b/b}$ and H-2$^{a/a}$ mice were neonatally tolerized to H-2$^{a/b}$, graft versus host disease was not observed in recipient mice. In other experimental systems in which donor mice were not tolerant to recipient H-2 alloantigens, regression of leukemia was accompanied by a severe graft versus host reaction (1). In our experiments, the H-2$^{a/b}$ recipient mice were not irradiated, and the majority of leukemia cells in all of these animals was of the H-2$^{a/b}$ genotype. The fact that H-2$^{a/b}$ leukemia cells were eliminated in mice which had received tolerized H-2$^{b/b}$ cells suggested that the H-2$^{b/b}$ cells (but not the H-2$^{a/a}$ cells) contained effector mechanisms capable of causing recovery from leukemia. Furthermore, these mechanisms were effective against leukemia cells of the low recovery genotype H-2$^{a/b}$ mice and in the splenic environment of H-2$^{a/b}$ mice.

The results of the cell transfers in Table 2 are compatible with an alternative interpretation. Leukemia cells of the H-2$^{b/b}$ high recovery genotype may be highly immunogenic. In our experiments, a small number of transferred H-2$^{b/b}$ cells could have been transformed by FV in the H-2-$^{a/b}$ recipients. These H-2$^{b/b}$ leukemia cells could have generated a strong immunological response resulting in recovery. We examined this possibility by presensitizing H-2-$^{a/b}$ mice with H-2$^{b/b}$ leukemia cells and then challenging these sensitized mice with FV. The presensitization of H-2-$^{a/b}$ with primary FV leukemic spleen cells of the H-2$^{b/b}$ genotype did not increase the incidence of recovery as compared to mice receiving virus only (Table 3). This result suggested that the immunogenicity of the FV leukemia cells was not influenced by their H-2 genotype, and thus supports our interpretation of the results in Table 2 that the nonleukemic cells of the spleen and bone marrow mediate the H-2 influence on recovery.

The mechanism of the H-2 influence on recovery from FV leukemia is unknown. Anti-FV antibody has been found in

Table 3. Presensitization with H-2b/b Leukemia Cells does not Increase the
Incidence of Recovery in H-2a/b Mice

| Donor | | Recipient | | Recovered |
| Strain | H-2 genotype | Strain | H-2 genotype | mice/total[3] |
|---|---|---|---|---|
| (C57BL/10 X A.BY)F₁ | b/b | (B10.A X A.BY)F₁ | a/b | 2/14(14%) |
| (C57BL/10 X A.BY)F₁ | b/b | (C57BL/10 X A.BY)F₁ | b/b | 13/14(93%) |
| No cells transferred | | (B10.A X A.BY)F₁ | a/b | 2/10(20%) |

[1] Donor FV leukemic spleen cells were obtained from mice 8 days after FV inoculation. Donor cells were treated with a monoclonal anti-Thy-1 antibody plus rabbit complement prior to transfer.
[2] Recipient mice received 40 x 10⁶ viable "T" lymphocyte depleted FV spleen cells. Approximately 4-6 hr later, all mice received 660 FFU B-tropic FV i.v.
[3] Recovery was determined by resolution of palpable splenomegaly.

both recovery and nonrecovery strains and appears to be
necessary, but not sufficient, for recovery (3). FV leukemia cells are susceptible to elimination by natural resistance mechanisms involved in rejection of hematopoetic
grafts (6).Furthermore, this resistance, possibly mediated
by natural killer (NK) cells, is controlled by genes in the
H-2D region (7). On the other hand, we do not believe that
this mechanism plays a major role in recovery from FV leukemia because the H-2D$^d$ genotype is associated with greater
NK activity then the H-2D$^b$ genotype (8), the inverse of
the genetic influence on the incidence of recovery observed
in our system. Also, in most systems in which NK cells or
natural resistance are seen, the inoculum of tumor or
hematopoetic cells is small (10), whereas in the FV system
recovery occurs even after massive leukemic splenomegaly
(2).

   Previous findings have suggested that FV-specific cytotoxic T lymphocytes (CTL) are necessary for recovery (4).
FV-specific CTL are demonstrable in recovered mice regardless of their H-2 genotype. By an appropriate virus inoculum, FV-specific CTL can be generated in both high and low
recovery H-2 genotypes, thus H-2 does not govern the absolute ability to generate FV-specific CTL (5). Currently we
believe that H-2 influences the kinetics of production of
CTL such that mice of the high recovery H-2$^{b/b}$ genotype
generate these CTL earlier than low recovery H-2$^{a/b}$ mice.
FV-specific CTL could have a greater influence on recovery
early in the disease when the leukemia cell burden is low.
Thus, the kinetics of the appearance of these CTL may have a
marked influence on the incidence of recovery observed.

## REFERENCES

1.  Bortin, M., Rim, A., Rose, W., and Saltzstein, E.
    Transplantation 18:280, 1974.
2.  Chesebro, B., Wehrly, K., and Stimpfling, J. J.Exp.-
    Med. 140:1457, 1974.
3.  Chesebro, B., and Wehrly, K. J.Exp.Med. 143:73, 1976.
4.  Chesebro, B., and Wehrly, K. J.Exp.Med. 143:85, 1976.
5.  Chesebro, B., and Wehrly, K. J.Immunol. 120:1081,
    1978.
6.  Cudkowicz, G., Rossi, G., Haddad, J., and Friend, C.
    J.Natl.Cancer Inst. 48:1972, 1972.
7.  Cudkowicz, G. Transplant.Proc. 7:155, 1975.
8.  Harmon, R., Clark, E., O'Toole, C., and Wicker, L.
    Immunogenetics 4:601, 1977.
9.  Lilly, F. J.Exp.Med. 127:465, 1968.

10. Petranyi, G., Kiessling, R., Povey, S., Lein, G., Herzenberg, L., and Wigzell, H.   Immunogenetics 3:15, 1976.

## DISCUSSION

Cudkowicz:   Friend virus-induced leukemic cells are extremely sensitive to natural killer cells.  Has Britt any experimental evidence that in his system NK cells might also play a role, rather than cytotoxic T cells?

Britt:   We really have no evidence for NK cells though I must admit that we have not searched exhaustively for them. In one experiment I cited, I had depleted the T lymphocytes with a monoclonal anti-Thy 1 serum.  Those cells were taken at a time when the mice were at the peak of their recovery, and I would assume that I left Thy-1 negative cells intact in those mice.  Those cells did not transfer recovery; based solely on that, I would not be sure that NK cells are important.

Cudkowicz:   I noticed that experiment, and I agree that in that cell transfer experiment NK cells were not implicated. But has Britt an experiment such as, for instance, thymectomizing neonatally the mice that he later infects with Friend virus, and then determining if they still recover.

Britt:   We have some data that neonatally thymectomized mice of the high recovery genotype have a low incidence of recovery as compared to normal.

Bennett:   Was Britt able to separate the cells which actually formed the leukemia, from the cells that would have formed an immune response?  I am a little confused by these experiments.

Britt:   I am not sure that I understood the thrust of Bennett's question entirely.  The neonatal tolerance experiment is complex.  What we did was to observe the effect twice and then proceed to explain the results.  Based on the experiment I presented here and other data, it does not appear that we were immunizing the mice with $H-2^{b/b}$ leukemic cells.  Also, the genotype of the leukemia cells does not seem to be important for its recognition and rejection.  Accordingly, we felt that we had eliminated two arms of the immune system and that the effect we got was from the transferred non-leukemic cells.

USE OF AN INFECTIOUS CENTER ASSAY TO STUDY $Fv-2^r$-MEDIATED
RESISTANCE OF MOUSE BONE MARROW CELLS TO FRIEND SPLEEN
FOCUS-FORMING VIRUS

Richard Steeves[1], Chalobon Yoosook[2]
and Frank Lilly[1]

[1]Department of Genetics
Albert Einstein College of Medicine
Bronx, N.Y. 10461
[2]Department of Microbiology
Faculty of Science
Mahidol University
Bangkok 4, Thailand

Since its identification a decade ago as a gene that
inhibits Friend virus [FV]-induced spleen focus formation
(5), the $Fv-2^r$ gene has been reported to inhibit other
parameters of FV infection, including: the replication of
spleen focus-forming virus [SFFV] (10), spleen colony formation by SFFV-infected leukemia cells (3), and the production of erythropoietin-independent, erythroid colony-forming
units (1,11). Even in "normal" mice that have not been infected exogenously with SFFV, the $Fv-2^r$ allele (as compared with $Fv-2^s$) has been associated with: resistance to N-
demethyl rifampicin effects on mouse spleen cells (7), reduced susceptibility to [3]H-thymidine suicide of erytroid
progenitor cells (12), reduced expression of endogenous,
SFFV-related, RNA sequences (6), lack of detectable SFFV-
specific cell surface antigen on normal hemopoietic cells
(8), and possible lethality during early development (2).

How can we reconcile this multiplicity of phenotypic
expression to the action of a single gene? Is the Fv-2 gene
really this pleiotropic? Perhaps there are two or more
closely linked genes on chromosome 9 that are responsible
for these various effects. Alternatively, the Fv-2 gene may
induce some fundamental change within the developing hemopoietic system that alters the state of normal erythroid
progenitor cells and thereby confers resistance to exogenous
SFFV infection as well.

To examine the latter possibility we used a target
cell assay (9), based on the capacity of Friend SFFV-infected cells to form infectious centers in the spleen, to study
the cellular basis of the resistance specified by the
$Fv-2^r$ gene. We were able to limit our examination to
Fv-2-mediated resistance without interference by other known
resistance genes from C57BL mice by using partially congenic

337

strains, DBA/2 ($Fv-2^S$) and D2.$Fv-2^r$ mice, which had been
bred in our laboratory (2). Thus, bone marrow cells from
DBA/2 and D2.$Fv-2^r$ mice were centrifuged, resuspended in
N-tropic FV to the concentration needed, and incubated at
37°C for 60 min. The infected cells were then washed twice
in Eagle's medium, diluted, and injected into (BALB/c X DBA-
/2)$F_1$ and (BALB/c X D2.$Fv-2^r$)$F_1$ recipients, respectively.
Nine days later their spleens were removed, fixed in Bouin's
fluid, and the colonies on the surfaces of the spleens were
counted. The results, expressed in infectious centers
(where one infectious center is the amount of cells required
to generate one colony, on the average, per recipient
spleen), are summarized in Table 1.

Table 1. Effect of Fv-2 Genotype and Hemopoietic Stress on
Availability of Target Cells to Generate Infectious Centers.

| Mouse strain | Hemopoietic stress (orbital bleeding) | Number of Infectious Centers/ml[*] ($\bar{x} \pm$ S.E.) |
|---|---|---|
| DBA/2 | No | $480 \pm 120$ |
| D2.$Fv-2^r$ | No | $350 \pm 80$ |
| DBA/2 | Yes | $1790 \pm 230$ |
| D2.$Fv-2^r$ | Yes | $370 \pm 60$ |

[*]$4 \times 10^7$ bone marrow cells were incubated with N-tropic FV
at a concentration of $4 \times 10^4$ FFU/ml, and after 60 min at
37°C they were washed, diluted and assayed for the number of
infectious centers in groups of 5 FV-1-resistant, histocompatible recipients.

Without any hemopoietic stress such as bleeding, the
bone marrow from D2.$Fv-2^r$ mice had a lower frequency of
potential target cells than DBA/2 bone marrow. (The difference here was consistent in several tests, even though not
statistically significant in any one test). However, if the
mice had been bled 2 and 3 days previously by taking 0.25 ml
from the retro-orbital sinus, the frequency of target cells
increased dramatically in the bone marrow of DBA/2 mice,
while there was no detectable effect of the bleeding on
D2.$Fv-2^r$ bone marrow. Therefore the Fv-2 gene controls

the availability of target cells for SFFV, and the $Fv-2^r$ allele prevented mice from responding "normally" (like $Fv-2^s$ mice) to a hemopoietic stimulus, even before the mice or their cells were ever exposed to SFFV.

In these in vitro infection experiments the time of incubation was only 60 min. Therefore, cells capable of forming infectious centers should be detectable just as rapidly after in vivo infection if a sufficient concentration of virus were inoculated. To compare the early events post-infection in mice differing at the Fv-2 locus, we bled DBA/2 and D2.FV-$2^r$ mice and infected them with a large dose ($10^5$ FFU) of FV. The concentration of infectious centers and the amount of virus (both SFFV and helper F-MuLV) recoverable from the spleens of the infected mice were assayed 1 hour and 2 days after infection.

As shown in Table 2, the Fv-2 gene had a profound effect upon the recovery of infectious centers, even as early as 1 hour post-infection. In contrast, there was no effect upon the recovery of either SFFV or F-MuLV, probably because we used a large input dose of virus and a short time until virus harvest.

Based on the similar amounts of virus recovered from DBA/2 and D2.Fv-$2^r$ mice by 1 hour after infection, it appears that SFFV and F-MuLV adsorbed to and infected the majority of their target cells at the same rate in both mouse strains. It can also be concluded that these viruses are able to multiply in a large population of cells other than the minor early population of infectious centers, because the genetic inhibition of the latter was not reflected in the virus titers. (In separate experiments in which smaller virus inocula and/or longer growth times were used, the Fv-$2^r$ gene did express itself in reduced viral yields).

To determine if the $Fv-2^r$ gene had any effect on later steps of the virus growth cycle or on the proliferative capacity of FV-infected cells, we tested for the capacity of infectious centers to generate secondary infectious centers and to release SFFV in irradiated, histocompatible recipients. The results (data not shown) indicate that the generation of secondary infectious centers per unit of primary infectious centers injected was 8-fold lower in mice injected with D2.Fv-$2^r$ bone marrow cells than in mice given DBA/2 bone marrow cells. However, there was only a 2-fold inhibition in the amount of SFFV recovered per infectious center. Therefore, it appears that the $Fv-2^r$ gene may inhibit the proliferation as well as the inital generation of infectious centers.

Suzuki and Axelrad (12) have recently shown that the Fv-2 locus controls the proportion of erythropoietic

Table 2. Recovery of Infectious Centers and Virus From the Spleens of Mice Shortly After Infection With a High Virus Dose[a]

| Mouse Strain | Time After Infection (hours) | Frequency of Infectious centers per $10^7$ cells ($x \pm$ SE) | Virus Titer ($\bar{x} \pm$ SE) | |
| --- | --- | --- | --- | --- |
| | | | SFFV (FFU/spleen)[c] | F-MuLV (PFU/spleen)[d] |
| DBA/2 | 1 | 159.5 $\pm$ 11.3 | 3.0 ($\pm$ 1.3) x 10 | 7.0 x $10^2$ |
| | 48 | 1128.0 $\pm$ 128.0 | 2.2 ($\pm$ 0.6) x $10^4$ | 3.1 x $10^5$ |
| D2.Fv-2[r] | 1 | 10.9 $\pm$ 2.7 | 2.3 ($\pm$ 1.7) x 10 | 5.0 x $10^2$ |
| | 48 | 53.5 $\pm$ 16.7 | 4.4 ($\pm$ 0.7) x $10^4$ | 3.8 x $10^5$ |

[a]Groups of bled DBA/2 and D2.Fv-2[r] mice were injected intravenously with $10^5$ FFU of N-tropic FV. After the times shown 3 mice were sacrificed, spleen cell suspensions were made, and these were assayed for IC, SFFV and F-MuLV.
[b]Measured in 7 CDF$_1$ mice.
[c]Measured in 6 DBA/2 mice.
[d]Measured in duplicate by XC assay.

progenitor cells (BFU-E) synthesizing DNA in normal mice. Meanwhile, Hankins et al. (4) have provided evidence which points to the same cell or a closely related one as the target cell for erythroid transformation by SFFV. In the present study we have brought these observations together by showing that the $Fv-2^r$ gene can control SFFV infection at a pre-infection stage, that is, at the level of the target cell, and that Fv-2 resistance is also manifested as early as 1 hour after infection through inhibition of the generation and proliferation of infectious centers, which may eventually lead to the inhibition of SFFV replication. Perhaps the many phenotypic expressions of the $Fv-2^r$ gene, like an umbelliferous plant, arise from one common genetic "stalk", but if this is so, then we still have many intriguing "branches" to explore.

## ACKNOWLEDGEMENT

This work was undertaken during the tenure of a Research Training Fellowship awarded (to C.Y.) by the International Agency for Research on Cancer. This research was supported by U.S. Public Health Service grant CA-19873 from the National Cancer Institute.

## REFERENCES

1. Axelrad, A.A., Suzuki, S., Van der Gaag, H., Clark, B.J., and McLeod, D.L. In ICN-UCLA Symposia on Molecular and Cellular Biology. D.W. Golde, M.J. Cline, D. Metcalf, and C.F. Fox (eds). New York: Academic Press, p69, 1978.
2. Blank, K.J., and Lilly, F. J.Natl. Cancer Inst. 59:-1335, 1977.
3. Blank, K.J., Steeves, R.A., and Lilly, F. J.Natl.-Cancer Inst. 57:925, 1976.
4. Hankins, W.D., Kost, T.A., Koury, M.J., and Krantz, S.B. Nature 276:506, 1978.
5. Lilly, F. J.Natl.Cancer Inst. 45:163, 1970.
6. Mak, T.W., Axelrad, A.A., and Bernstein, A. Proc.Natl-Acad.Sci.USA 76:5809, 1979.
7. Mitani, S., and Wakabayahi, K. Europ.J.Cancer 11:649, 1975.
8. Risser, R. J.Exp.Med. 149:1152, 1979.
9. Steinheider, G., and Steeves, R. Leuk.Res. 2:197, 1978.

10. Steeves, R.A., and Grundke-Iqbal, I.    J.Natl.Cancer
    Inst. 56:541, 1976.
11. Steeves, R.A., Lilly, F., Steinheider, G., and Blank,
    J.K.    In Differentiation of Normal and Neoplastic
    Hematopoietic Cells.   B. Clarkson, P.A. Marks, and
    J.E. Till (eds).    New York, Cold Spring Harbor
    Laboratory, p591, 1978.
12. Suzuki, S., and Axelrad, A.A.   Cell 19:225, 1980.


DISCUSSIONS


Chesebro:   I was wondering whether Steeves had looked at B6
or B10 $Fv-2^r$ mice and done the same infectious center
assay, putting the cells into other (B6 x DBA/2)$F_1$'s.

Steeves:   No we have not done that.  We have just kept to
the partially congenic mice because we wanted to really
limit ourselves to the analysis of the Fv-2 gene, and to
avoid having to worry about those other genes with which
Chesebro has been so fascinated (and we are too).  We hope
to have 16th back-cross mice available in the near future,
so that our mice truly will be fully congenic.

Wainberg: Does Steeves know whether the viral protein pro-
file are identical from each of the cell types he is testing?

Steeves:   That is an interesting thought, but we have not
really compared that.  I think it might be very interesting
to do it in virus fully adapted to cross the Fv-2 barrier.
We do have such virus, the BsB and the BB6, which can
effectively overcome the Fv-2 resistance;  perhaps not entirely, but at least it does not replicate as efficiently as
wild type virus.  It does not appear to recognize Fv-2 resistance and that particular virus might be interesting to
test. There is no evidence here that the virus is changed in
any way, but both kinds of studies might, nonetheless, be
done.

Cudkowicz:   Did I understand Steeves' message correctly,
that Fv-2, even though it is called Fv for Friend virus,
turns out to be a gene controlling some step in differentiation of erythroid cells?   I can appreciate that, merely
because Friend virus uses erythroid cells as targets, it
happens to affect leukemogenesis, but this should not be
allowed to obscure the message that its primary function is
something other than to control a host response or some

cellular response to the virus. At this meeting we have been faced with several such situations. Steeves may recall that earlier on O'Brien described mutants affecting macrophages, and then as a consequence affecting the resistance to infection with a particular microorganism. Are we here dealing with a similar situation?

Steeves: I think so. Cudkowicz is familiar, of course, with the "W" and "Steel" genes. We know that these affect the stem cells and secondarily the virus. The "Steel" genes and "W" genes were isolated first, whereas their resistance to Friend virus was discovered later on. In our case, we find a gene which seems to be unique to the C57BL family and was discovered on the basis of resistance to Friend virus. But I am not convinced that is its' only role. Suzuki and Axelrod demonstrated very nicely in a recent issue of Cell that this has a very clear-cut effect on the cycling of BFU-E. This is the real point of the present report, i.e., that this is very much the case.

Bang: The limitation of the growth of the infectious centers in the spleen raises the question as to what role different cells are playing there. Does Steeves have any idea whether lymphocytes play a role in this process?

Steeves: No, except that we have not observed substantial differences in nude mice (e.g., on the Balb/c background) that are infected with virus or injected with histocompatible cells. Also, there is no difference in antibody production; nor have we seen any difference in interferon production across differences at Fv-2. So we have not encountered any evidence so far for involvement of immunological phenomena or for interferon mediated phenomena at this genetic locus.

# GENETICALLY ACQUIRED RESISTANCE TO FATAL PICHINDE VIRUS INFECTION IN THE SYRIAN HAMSTER

Sydney R. Gee, Marcia A. Chan
David A. Clark and William E. Rawls

McMaster University
Hamilton, Ontario

Pichinde virus, a member of the arenavirus group, causes a lethal infection accompanied by high levels of viremia in the MHA strain of Syrian hamsters when inoculated intraperitoneally (IP), but not in the LSH or LVG strains (1). Survival and the ability to limit viremia were independent of virus dose over a range of 35 plaque-forming units (pfu) to $10^6$ pfu (data not presented), suggesting that resitance to the lethal infection was genetically acquired. Thus, individual $F_1$ and back-cross animals were injected with Pichinde virus and observed daily for survival (Table 1).

Table 1. Inheritance of Susceptibility to Fatal (IP) Pichinde Virus Infection in Syrian Hamsters

| | Number surviving/number tested[1] | | | | |
|---|---|---|---|---|---|
| | LVG | MHA | $F_1$ (LVG X MHA) | $F_1$ X LVG | $F_1$ X MHA |
| Experiment 1 | 15/15 | 2/15 | 32/40 | NT | NT |
| Experiment 2 | 5/6 | 2/6 | NT | 12/16 | 15/35 |
| Experiment 3 | 6/6 | 4/10 | 8/8 | 23/24 | 11/16 |
| Total | 26/27 | 8/31 | 40/48 | 35/40 | 26/51 |
| Percent Survival | 96.3 | 25.8 | 83.0 | 87.5 | 51.0 |

[1] Animals which had received an intraperitoneal (IP) injection of $2 \times 10^3$ pfu Pichinde virus were housed individually, and observed daily for survival.

Survival of $F_1$ (LVG X MHA) and $F_1$ X LVG progeny did not differ from that of the resistant LVG parent, (p>.10 by $x^2$ test), but was significantly different from the MHA parent (p<.001). Moreover, survival of $F_1$ X MHA progeny did not differ significantly from the values expected for a dominant characteristic controlled by a single gene or linked genes (p=0.9 by $x^2$ test).

When levels of viremia in these animals were determined 8 days after infection with Pichinde virus (Table 2), no

significant difference between levels of viremia in LVG and
$F_1$(LVG X MHA) hamsters was apparent, whereas levels of viremia in MHA hamsters were significantly greater than those
observed in either LVG or $F_1$(LVG X MHA) animals (p<.001).

Table 2.   Inheritance of Ability to Limit Viremia After IP
Pichinde Virus Infection

| Genetic Background | n | Phenotype | Mean Virus Titre $\pm$ SD[1] ($\log_{10}$ pfu/ml blood) |
|---|---|---|---|
| **Experiment 1** | | | |
| LVG | 9 | | 2.80$\pm$1.13 |
| MHA | 9 | | 6.52$\pm$0.64 |
| $F_1$(LVG X MHA) | 19 | 19 LVG[2] | 2.45$\pm$1.58 |
| $F_1$ X LVG | 21 | 17 LVG | 3.69$\pm$0.73 |
| | | 4 MHA | 5.94$\pm$0.26 |
| $F_1$ X MHA | 16 | 9 LVG | 3.83$\pm$0.82 |
| **Experiment 2** | | | |
| LVG | 5 | | 4.95$\pm$0.55 |
| MHA | 3 | | 7.74$\pm$0.42 |
| $F_1$ X LVG | 14 | 14 LVG | 3.71$\pm$1.24 |
| $F_1$ X MHA | 24 | 13 LVG | 3.78$\pm$1.46 |
| | | 11 MHA | 6.95$\pm$0.54 |

[1]Animals received an IP injection of $2\times10^3$ pfu Pichinde virus in Experiment 1, or $2\times10^5$ pfu in Experiment 2.  Individual animals were then bled by cardiac puncture 8 days after
infection.  Aliquots of blood were assayed for pfu on  monolayers of Vero cells.
[2]$F_1$ and back-cross progeny were classified as having an LVG
phenotype if their virus titers fell within 2SD of the mean
LVG titre.  All titres above this limit were said to manifest the MHA phenotype.

These results suggested that the ability to limit viremia
behaved as a dominant trait.  Among a total of 35 $F_1$ X LVG
back-cross progeny in Experiments 1 and 2, 31 (89%) had titres which resembled their LVG parent.  of 40 $F_1$ X MHA test-
cross animals, 22 (55%) had titres similar to their LVG parent, and 18 (45%) had titres comparable to the MHA strain.
These observations were consistent with the hypothesis that

a single dominant gene controls virus replication (.6<p<.7). Furthermore, no difference in survival or virus titre with respect to sex of the animal was observed. An analysis of coat colour in $F_1$ and back-cross progeny failed to reveal a linkage of genes controlling this trait to those genes responsible for survival and limiting viremia after Pichinde virus infection (data not shown).

Studies were then undertaken to determine the basis for the genetically acquired susceptibility of MHA hamsters to lethal Pichinde virus infection.    Death appeared to be a consequence of virus-induced necrosis within the reticuloendothelial system, suggesting that the basis for susceptibility or resistance resided in an ability to limit virus proliferation (5).  However, since peritoneal exudate cells and primary kidney cells from either strain supported virus replication equally well in vitro (1), attention was directed towards the role of the immune response in resistance to Pichinde virus infection.

The observation that cyclophosphamide abrogated resistance to Pichinde virus infection (1) suggested that immunity to the virus was an important component of resistance. Furthermore, resistance in LVG and LSH hamsters developed with age, in association with the maturation of the immune response.    Nevertheless, both resistant and susceptible hamster strains produced similar titres of antibodies against internal antigens of the virion and against antigens present on the infected cell (1).  Thus, immune recognition of virus antigens, assessed by the humoral response, was not deficient in the susceptible strain.

As a measure of cell-mediated immunity, the footpad swelling response to a primary inoculation of virus (8) was examined.    Both resistant hamster strains responded to a primary inoculation of Pichinde virus with swelling, as measured by calipers or a radioisotopic method (6).    A histological examination of the footpad revealed a cellular infiltrate consisting of lymphocytes and macrophages (data not shown).  In contrast, the susceptible MHA strain did not show the swelling response (Fig. 1).  This unresponsiveness appeared to be an inherited trait. The preliminary results, shown in Table 3, were consistent with the concept that a single (autosomal) dominant gene controlled the footpad swelling response to Pichinde virus (p<.001).

Despite the lack of reactivity, however, MHA hamsters survived the footpad inoculation of Pichinde virus, and limited virus replication to low levels (Table 4).  High titres of complement-fixing anti-viral antibodies were demonstrable, and the animals were protected against a normally lethal IP challenge of Pichinde virus. These

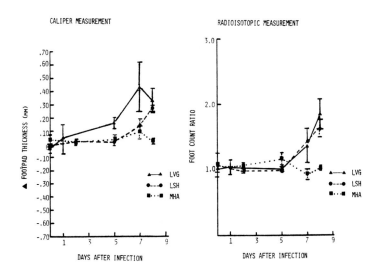

**Figure 1.** Animals were injected with $2\times10^3$ pfu Pichinde virus in the right rear footpad and with control cell supernate in the left rear footpad. One day before assay, each animal received an IP injection of $^{125}$I-labelled hamster serum albumin. On the next day, both hind feet were measured with spring loaded calipers. The feet were then amputated, and counted in a gamma counter. The results are expressed as the ratio: cpm-test foot/cpm-control foot.

parameters were independent of the dose of Pichinde virus injected into the footpad over a range of $10^3$-$10^6$ pfu (data not shown). These findings suggested that, when challenged by an appropriate route, the susceptible MHA strain of MHA strain of Syrian hamsters was capable of resisting Pichinde virus infection.

In further studies on cell-mediated immunity in hamsters undergoing Pichinde virus infection, natural killer (NK) cell mediated cytotoxicity against MAD hamster tumour cells was observed in the spleens of IP-injected animals (4).

Table 3. Genetics of the Footpad Swelling Response to Pichinde Virus in Syrian Hamsters

| Background | n | Phenotype | Mean Foot-Count Ratio $\pm$ SD[1] ($\frac{\text{test cpm}}{\text{control cpm}}$) |
|---|---|---|---|
| LSH | 20 | | 1.78$\pm$0.38 |
| MHA | 23 | | 1.20$\pm$0.15 |
| F$_1$ X LSH | 8 | 8 LSH[2] | 1.87$\pm$0.26 |
| | | 0 MHA | |
| F$_1$ X MHA | 26 | 13 LSH | 1.76$\pm$0.31 |
| | | 13 MHA | 1.18$\pm$0.10 |

[1] Animals received an inoculation of $2 \times 10^3$ pfu Pichinde virus in 25$\lambda$ in the right rear footpad, and 25$\lambda$ of supernate from uninfected cells in their left rear footpad on day 0. On day 7, $10^6$ cpm $^{125}$I-labelled hamster serum albumin was injected IP. Animals were sacrificed 8 days after infection, and the hind feet were amputated and counted in a gamma counter.

[2] Back-cross progeny were classified as having the LSH phenotype if their mean foot-count ratio fell equal to or above 1SD of the mean LSH ratio. Ratios equal to or below the range of 1SD of the mean MHA ratio were said to manifest the MHA phenotype.

Table 4. Effect of Footpad Route of Inoculation of the Pathogenesis of Pichinde Virus Infection in Syrian Hamsters

| Hamster Strain: Route of Injection:[1] | MHA | | LSH | |
|---|---|---|---|---|
| | IP | FP | IP | FP |
| Percent Survival | 25.8% | 100% | 96.3% | 100% |
| Mean Viremia, 8d after injection (log pfu/ml blood) | 6.52 | 3.90 | 2.80 | <2.70 |
| Mean antibody titre, 13d after infection (assayed by complement fixation) | 1:38 | 1:138 | 1:53 | 1:48 |
| Survival following secondary IP challenge | - | 100% | 100% | 100% |

[1] MHA and LSH hamsters were injected with $2 \times 10^3$ pfu Pichinde virus either by the intraperitoneal (IP) route or subcutaneously into the footpad (FP).

As shown in Table 5, levels of endogenous NK activity were significantly higher in the spleens of MHA hamsters than in the LSH strains (Students t test, p<.005). Moreover, Pichinde virus infection induced an augmented response in both strains (p<.005) but the magnitude of the augmented response in MHA hamsters was significantly greater than that observed in LSH hamsters (p<0.005). Furthermore, this pattern of response may be genetically controlled; induced NK activity in $F_1$(LSH X MHA) progeny was comparable to the level observed in LSH hamsters, and significantly lower than that observed in MHA hamsters (p<.0005).

Table 5. Levels of Splenic NK Activity in Control and Pichinde Virus-infected Syrian Hamsters

| | Mean % specific $^{51}$Cr release[1] | n | SD | SEM |
|---|---|---|---|---|
| Control LSH | 4.12 | 63 | 9.43 | 1.19 |
| Virus-infected LSH | 16.87 | 67 | 15.10 | 1.85 |
| Control MHA | 12.04 | 80 | 9.95 | 1.11 |
| Virus-infected MHA | 43.05 | 85 | 19.97 | 2.17 |
| Virus-infected $F_1$(LSH X MHA) | 17.75 | 83 | 15.94 | 1.75 |

[1] Data from 35 separate experiments in which spleen cells from control or Pichinde virus-infected MHA and LSH hamsters were assayed for cytotoxic activity against $^{51}$Cr-labelled MAD targets were analyzed. A mean % specific $^{51}$Cr release value was estimated for each group by summing the actual % release values at effector to target ratios of 100:1, 50:1 and 25:1 in all 35 experiments and dividing by the number (n) of values.

Analysis of infectious centres of Pichinde virus and cytotoxic activity in the spleen and popliteal lymph nodes of infected hamsters revealed that a population of infected target cells in the spleen of IP-infected MHA hamsters co-purified with a population of cells demonstrating NK activity. However, the comparable population of spleen cells in resistant LSH hamsters contained 10-fold fewer infectious centres (4). Similarly, in foot-pad inoculated hamsters, cytotoxic activity was found in a population of popliteal lymph nodes (PLN) cells and this population accounted for 100-fold more infected target cells in MHA hamsters compared to the same cytolytic fraction of LSH hamster PLN cells (Figure 2).

Velocity sedimentation of lymph node cells from foot-pad-inoculated hamsters

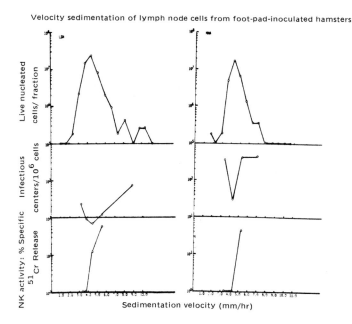

Sedimentation velocity (mm/hr)

Figure 2. Popliteal lymph node cells from 7-10 footpad-infected hamsters were layered on a gradient of BSA in a STA-PUT chamber. Cells were allowed to sediment for 3.5 hrs at 4°C under unit gravity. Fractions were collected and the cells were pelleted and counted. Sedimentation velocities were calculated for each fraction. Aliquots were then assayed for infectious centres of Pichinde virus, and for NK activity against [51]Cr-labelled MAD targets.

In conclusion, then, while Pichinde appears able to re-plicate in several cell populations, a key difference bet-ween susceptible and resistant hamsters is the presence of a population of cells in the susceptible MHA strain which con-tains at least 10-fold more infectious centres of Pichinde virus than the comparable LSH hamster population. While the co-purification of NK activity with this population of cells and the genetics of the response may be fortuitous associat-ions, the possibility that the MHA NK cell may actually be a target cell for Pichinde virus replication must be consider-ed. The lymphotropism of arenaviruses may be partly related to an ability to grow in NK cells. It has been noted that poly (ICLC) treatment, which is known to activate NK cells via interferon induction (3) increased the titres of viremia

in Rhesus monkeys inoculated with the arenavirus Machupo
(7). Thus, the genetically acquired susceptibility of MHA
hamsters to a lethal IP injection of Pichinde virus may depend on the genetically determined differences in the NK
cell population, such that the susceptible strain has a target cell for Pichinde virus replication that the resistant
strain lacks. Because hamster spleens appear to be a major
reservoir of NK cells (unpublished observations; 2), an intraperitoneal injection of Pichinde virus may lead to an
overwhelming proliferation of virus against which the host's
immune defenses are inadequate. In contrast, when virus is
inoculated by the footpad route, the relative paucity of
target cells in this location retards virus growth sufficiently to permit the host's defense mechanisms to clear the
relatively low virus load.

ACKNOWLEDGEMENT

Supported, in part, by a grant from the Eastburn Foundation and by the NCI of Canada.

REFERENCES

1.  Buchmeier, M.B., and Rawls, W.E. Infect.Immun. 16:413,
    1977.
2.  Datta, S.K., Gallagher, M.T., and Trentin, J.J.
    Int.J. Cancer 23:728, 1979.
3.  Djeu, J.Y., Heinbaugh, J.A., Holden, H.T., and
    Herberman, R.B. J.Immunol. 122:175, 1979.
4.  Gee, S.R., Clark, D.A., and Rawls, W.E. J.Immunol.
    123:2618, 1979.
5.  Murphy, F.A., Buchmeier, M.B., and Rawls, W.E.
    Lab.Invest. 37:502, 1977.
6.  Paranjpe, M.S., and Boone, C.W. J.Natl.Cancer Inst.
    48:563, 1972.
7.  Stephen, E.L., Scott, S.K., Eddy, G.A., and Levy, H.B.
    Texas Rep.Biol.Med. 35:449, 1977.
8.  Zinkernagel, R.M., Althage, A., and Jensen, F.C.
    J.Immunol. 119:1242, 1977.

# SUBACUTE SCLEROSING PANENCEPHALITIS IN INBRED HAMSTERS

R. Michael Massanari, Marcia L. Wilson
and Joel R. Leininger

University of Iowa
Iowa City, Iowa 52242

## INTRODUCTION

Hamster brain subacute sclerosing panencephalitis virus (HBS) produces a sporadic, inconstant encephalitis in random bred Syrian hamsters (3). Some animals are resistant to infection whereas others develop an acute fatal illness or a chronic persistent encephalitis. Byington and Johnson (3,4) reported that age and immune competence are important preconditions of the host which determine patterns of resistance and clinical manifestations of HBS encephalitis. Genetic constituents are also important determinants of host resistance to viral induced encephalopathies in several animal systems (6). Because the original studies of HBS encephalitis were conducted in random bred Syrian hamsters (3), the role of genetic factors in modifying host resistance to infection was not examined. This report summarizes preliminary experiments in which we examined the susceptibility of highly inbred hamster strains to the acute phase of HBS encephalitis. Our results indicate that the genotype is indeed an important determinant of host resistance to HBS infection.

## MATERIALS AND METHODS

Pregnant female and 4-week-old male $PD_4$ (A) and CB (B) inbred hamsters were purchased from Charles River Laboratory, Wilmington, MA. Four week-old male 87.20 (C), 15.16 (D), and $F_1d$ hybrid (CxD) hamster strains were purchased from Bioresearch Consultants, Cambridge, MA. Hamsters were housed in plastic cages at 22°C and fed and watered ad libitum.

HBS virus was kindly supplied by Drs. D.P. Byington and K.P. Johnson (San Francisco, CA). Adaptation to hamster central nervous sytem (CNS), preparation of the stock virus, and techniques for virus isolation have been described previously (2,5).

Dilutions of HBS virus were inoculated into the right cerebral hemisphere under light ether anesthesia. Hamsters from different strains were infected simultaneously with the

GENETIC CONTROL OF NATURAL RESISTANCE
TO INFECTION AND MALIGNANCY

same inoculum. Animals were observed daily for clinical
signs of encephalitis including ptyalism, myoclonic jerks,
seizures, paralysis, or death. In some experiments, hamsters were selected at random at predetermined intervals
following infection (PI), anesthetized with chloroform and
exsanguinated. CNS tissues were fixed in 10% neutral
buffered formalin and stained with hematoxylin eosin for
histology.

Hamster sera, stored at -20°C, were titrated for measles hemagglutination-inhibition (HI) antibodies using a
standard microtiter assay (7). Statistical methods used in
analysis of the data included chi square analysis, student's
test, and the Wilcoxon rank sum test.

RESULTS

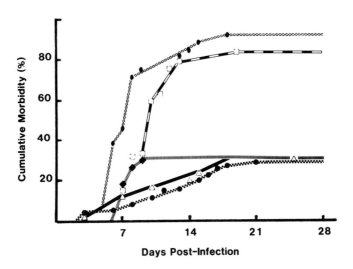

Figure 1. Cumulative morbidity following HBS infection.
Twenty to 40 hamsters from each strain were examined.
Strain A = ● , B = △ , C = □ , D = ◆ , E = ◖ .

Inbred hamster strains exhibited striking differences in patterns of resistance to the acute phase of HBS virus encephalitis. Figure 1 summarizes results from several experiments wherein 4-6 week-old inbred hamsters were infected with $10^{3.6}$ 50% tissue culture infective doses of HBS virus. In these experiments clinical signs of acute encephalitis (occurring before 28 days PI) were used as indicators of susceptibility to infection. Differences in resistance to HBS infection were most evident when the number of strain A hamsters with clinical encephalitis was compared with strain C ($x^2$ = 9.2, p <0.01). Clinical manifestations of encephalitis also differed between strains A and C, i.e. the incubation period for strain A was 6 days longer than strain C (t = 2.84, p <0.01) and the clinical course in the former was more protracted with fewer deaths. Whereas resistance to HBS infection in strain D was comparable to A and B, the $F_1d$ hybrid (CxD) behaved like the parental strain C.

Strain B hamsters, like their 4 week-old counterparts in strain A, were relatively resitant to HBS infection. Infection at 2 weeks of age, however, required a 10,000-fold reduction in the amount of HBS virus necessary to produce 50% mortality ($LD_{50}$), 2 logs less than the $LD_{50}$ for 2 week-old strain A hamsters. Thus, age as well as genotype were important determinants of host resistance to HBS encephalitis.

The histopathologic lesions in HBS-infected hamsters (4-6 week-old) were indistinguishable from strain to strain. Inflammation was present in the gray and white matter throughout the neuraxis. The most frequently observed lesions consisted of perivascular cuffing by mononuclear cells, including lymphocytes and plasma cells. Among animals with acute clinical disease, extensive areas of inflammation and necrosis were noted. These lesions were found predominantly in the gray matter and were characterized by mononuclear cell infiltration, gliosis and neuronophagia. Numerous eosinophilic nuclear and cytoplasmic inclusions, along with syncytial cells, were present in these foci (Figure 2). All histologic sections from animals sacrificed before day 7 PI, regardless of genotype, contained lesions of encephalitis (Table 1). Subsequent to this time (7-42 days PI), only 2/12 strain A hamsters exhibited histologic evidence of encephalitis whereas 3-50% of animals in other strains had CNS sections showing these inflammatory foci.

Despite evidence for oncoging inflammation, virus was rarely isolated (1/29) from hamster CNS tissue after day 14 PI. Of the CNS tissues examined before day 14 PI, 8/19 or approximately 40% of the tissues from the respective hamster strains contained low titers of HBS virus. In contrast to

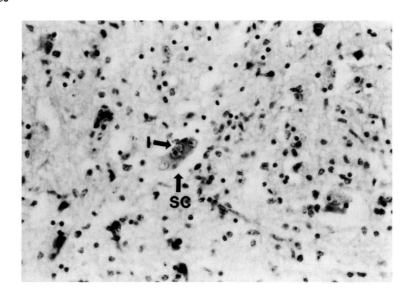

Figure 2.    Representative histologic lesion following
HBS   infection   which   demonstrates   gliosis,   necrosis,
syncitial cells (SC), and inclusions (I).

Table 1.  Histopathologic Evidence of HBS Encephalitis Among
          Hamsters (4-6 w/o) of Different Genotypes

| Hamster Strain | Days Post-Infection | | | | | Total |
|---|---|---|---|---|---|---|
| | 7 | 14 | 21 | 28 | > 28 | |
| A | 3/3* | 1/4 | 0/4 | 1/4 | 0/9 | 5/24 |
| B | 3/3 | 3/4 | 1/4 | 3/5 | 1/3 | 11/19 |
| C | 1/1 | 6/7 | | 1/2 | 1/3 | 9/13 |
| D | 1/1 | 0/1 | 0/1 | 1/2 | 0/4 | 2/9 |
| C x D | 5/5 | 4/4 | 2/2 | | 1/3 | 12/14 |
| Total | 13/13 | 14/20 | 3/11 | 6/13 | 3/22 | |

*Number postive/Number examined

other strains, no virus has been detected in strain A hamsters examined between days 7-10 PI.

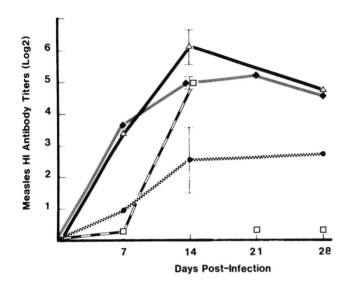

**Figure 3.**   Measles HI antibody responses following HBS infection.    Each  point  represents  a  geometric  mean  titer
($Log_2$)  and  bars  represent  standard  error  of  the  mean.
Strain A = ●, B = △, C = □, D = ◆, E = ❶.

The  variable  phenotypic  responses  to  HBS  encephalitis
among  hamsters  of  different  genotypes  were  also  reflected  in
the  humoral  immune  response  to  infection  (Figure 3).   Using
titrations  of  measles  HI  antibodies  as  a  measure  of  humoral
immunity,  differences  were  most  apparent  14  days  PI  when
titers  in  strain  B  exceeded  those  in  all  other  strains  tested  (p = 0.05).   Limited  sample  sizes  precluded  analysis  at
other  intervals  PI.

## DISCUSSION

The  clinical  consequences  of  HBS  infection  in  random
bred  Syrian  hamsters  are  highly  variable  (3).   The  susceptibility  to  infection  and  clinical  expression  of  the  disease
are  modified  by  the  age  and  immune  competence  of  the  host

(3,5). Infection of inbred weanling hamsters has demonstrated that the genetic background of the host is also an important determinant of host resistance to HBS encephalitis. Significant differences in patterns of resistance to infection, patterns of clinical disease and humoral immune responses were observed among the four hamster strains examined.

Histopathologic evidence of encephalitis in all CNS tissues examined before day 7 PI and increased susceptibility of 2 week-old hamsters to infection suggest that all hamsters, regardless of their genotype, possess the necessary milieu to support infection and replication of the HBS virus in CNS tissue. Based upon the early resolution of histologic lesions and absence of virus in strain A hamsters, spread of the virus is apparently curtailed early in infection among resistant strains (strain A), whereas it continues to replicate and spread in susceptible strains (strain C). These observations point to the probable role of the immune system in limiting the infection and suggest that genetic modulation of resistance to HBS infection may be mediated through immunological mechanisms. Differences in humoral immune responses among the hamster strains tested support his hypothesis; however, the disparity between the actual antibody titers and host resistance indicate that humoral immunity, alone, cannot explain the differences in resistance. Since cell mediated immunity is the principle mode of defense against paramyxovirus infections (1,5), genetic determinants may modulate resistance through the cellular arm of the immune system.

A comprehensive genetic analysis of resistance to HBS infection in hamsters is not possible from the information presently available. From observations in strains C, D, and $F_1{}^d$ hybrids (CxD), the trait for susceptibility to infection appears to be dominant. While preliminary results suggest that resistance may be modulated by a single gene, further backcross analyses are essential before drawing conclusions in this multifarious sytem.

ACKNOWLEDGEMENT


This study was supported by National Multiple Sclerosis Grant No. RG-1220-A-2.

The authors thank Mr. David Steiner for his technical assistance and Mrs. Linda Schauberger for her assistance in preparing the typescript.

REFERENCES

1.  Burnet, F.M.  Lancet ii:610, 1968.
2.  Byington D.P., Castro, A.E., and Burnstein, T.  Nature 225:554, 1970.
3.  Byington, D.P., and Johnson, K.P.  J.Infect.Dis. 126:18, 1972.
4.  Byington, D.P., and Johnson, K.P.  Lab.Invest. 32:91, 1975.
5.  Massanari, R.M., Paterson, P.Y., and Lipton, H.L. J.Infect.Dis. 139:297, 1979.
6.  Neighbour, P.A., Rager-Zisman, B., and Bloom, B.R. Infect.Immun. 21:764, 1978.
7.  Rosen, L.  Virology 13:139, 1961.

MAREK'S DISEASE IN CHICKENS: GENETIC RESISTANCE TO A VIRAL
NEOPLASTIC DISEASE. A REVIEW

Jan S. Gavora and J. Lloyd Spencer

Animal Research Institute
Research Branch
Agriculture Canada
Ottawa, Ontario K1A 0C6

Marek's disease (MD) is a lymphoproliferative disease
of chickens caused by a herpesvirus and the first neoplasm
for which an effective vaccine was developed. This communication will briefly review genetic aspects of MD resistance.

The highly cell-associated MD virus matures in the
feather follicle and is shed in the skin dander. Horizontal
transmission of infection is rapid and 2 to 3 weeks after it
is infected, the chicken begins to shed virus (10). In the
1960's the disease often killed 20 to 30% of a flock and was
responsible for high rates of condemnation of broiler
chickens at processing. The disease is characterized by
development of lymphoid tumors, consisting primarily of T
cells (9), in various tissues including nerves, muscle and
visceral organs. All chickens are susceptible to infection
with MD virus but the outcome of infection is influenced by
host factors such as genotype, age and sex, as well as by
the virulence of the virus.

The first progress in controlling MD was achieved by
breeding for genetic resistance. The commonly used procedure was selection of breeders based on the incidence of MD
in their progeny inoculated at 1 day of age with MD virus
and observed for 8-10 weeks. Using this procedure, Cole (3)
developed in only two generations of selection from a common
genetic base a resistant N line and a susceptible P line of
Leghorns with respective MD susceptibilities of 13 and 98%.
These procedures were costly, and when effective vaccines
against MD became available in the early 1970's, commercial
companies greatly reduced breeding for genetic resistance to
MD. However, protection from vaccination is not complete
and both genetic and vaccination-induced resistance are
necessary to maximize protection (17).

Effects of vaccination, genotype, age and sex on MD
resistance.
The first vaccine against MD was a live attenuated MD
virus (2). Other types of vaccine include low pathogenicity
field viruses (15), and a turkey herpesvirus (18). Vaccina-

tion dramatically reduced MD mortality and the benefit from the use of vaccines in the USA alone was estimated at $168 million annually (14).

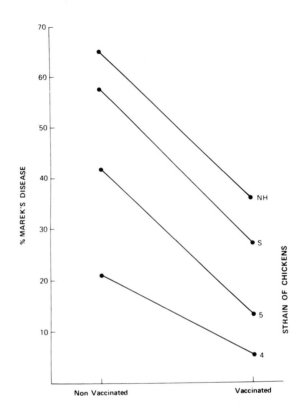

Figure 1.    Response of genotypes to vaccination against Marek's disease.  The Ottawa New Hampshire strain NH is naturally susceptible and Leghorn strains 4 and 5 are naturally relatively resistant to Marek's disease.  The Leghorn strain S was selected for Marek's disease susceptibility at Cornell University.  Females exposed to Marek's disease by contact at 3 weeks.   Based on lesions in birds that died or were killed at 133 days of age.

Figure 1 illustrates the genetic variation in MD resistance among strains of chickens and also shows that resistance to MD was highest in vaccinated chicks that had the highest degree of genetic resistance. The latent period before death tends to be longer in resistant birds. Chickens become more resistant to tumor development with increasing age at time of exposure. Sharma et al (16) suggested that age resistance is expressed through an ability of older birds to cause MD tumors to regress. Sex of chickens also plays a role in MD, with females being more susceptible (13).

## Mechanisms of genetic resistance to MD

The major histocompatibility complex (the B-system) of the chicken has been treated as a single genetic locus, although recent evidence suggests its greater complexity, perhaps similar to that of the HLA in humans and the H-2 in mice. The first suggestion of the involvement of the B-system in MD resistance was made by Hansen et al (8). Increased MD resistance of chickens carrying the $\underline{B}^{21}$ allele was later established by Longenecker et al (11) and Briles et al (1). As illustrated in Table 1, the association between the $\underline{B}^{21}$ haplotype and resistance to MD depends on the pairing of the $\underline{B}^{21}$ with other B-alleles and perhaps also on other resistance mechanisms.

Table 1. Incidence of Marek's disease in chickens of various histocompatibility genotypes (11).

| Population[a] | Histocompatibility genotype | Number of birds tested | Marek's disease (%) |
|---|---|---|---|
| 1 | $\underline{B}^{21}/\underline{B}^{21}$ | 23 | 8.7 |
|   | $\underline{B}^{2}/\underline{B}^{21}$ | 43 | 25.6 |
|   | $\underline{B}^{2}/\underline{B}^{2}$ | 29 | 44.8 |
| 2 | $\underline{B}^{21}/\underline{B}^{21}$ | 35 | 5.7 |
|   | $\underline{B}^{14}/\underline{B}^{21}$ | 40 | 10.0 |
|   | $\underline{B}^{14}/\underline{B}^{14}$ | 27 | 14.8 |
| 3 | $\underline{B}^{21}/\underline{B}^{21}$ | 65 | 0 |
|   | $\underline{B}^{2}/\underline{B}^{21}$ | 148 | .6 |
|   | $\underline{B}^{2}/\underline{B}^{2}$ | 67 | 19.4 |

[a]Populations 1 and 2 were exposed to Marek's disease virus by contact and killed at 109 days. Population 3 was injected with MD virus at 21 days and killed at 80 days. Based on lesions in birds that died or were killed at the termination of the experiments.

The discovery of the association of the $\underline{B}^{21}$ haplotype, detectable on red blood cells, with MD resistance represents a potential tool that can be used by the poultry industry for indirect selection for MD resistance. Several other genetic mechanisms possibly involved in MD resistance were suggested by various authors but none of them seem to have effects comparable in size to that of the major histocompatibility complex.

Improvement of genetic resistance to MD by selective breeding.

Based on the assumption of polygenic inheritance, estimates of heritability (proportion of additive genetic variation from total phenotypic variation) of MD resistance obtained by several authors ranged from .05 (12) to .61 (6). Rapid responses to selection for MD resistance or susceptibility (e.g.3) seem to support the higher heritability estimates. MD resistance shows a tendency to increase with earlier sexual maturity and higher egg production but to decrease with higher egg weight and more rapid body growth (6). Han and Smyth (7) suggested that factors increasing total body growth rate may also enhance neoplastic growth while factors causing a decrease in normal body rate of growth may also inhibit neoplastic development.

Simultaneous improvement of MD resistance and production traits by selection in meat-type chickens was reported by Friars et al (4) and preliminary data from an experiment in Ottawa (5) indicate that simultaneous improvement of MD resistance and egg production is also feasible. In the latter study, improvement of MD resistance was demonstrated in both vaccinated and non-vaccinated birds. Strain crosses were generally more resistant than pure strains and these heterotic effects were greater in non-vaccinated birds.

Although vaccines have dramatically reduced incidence of MD, it is still one of the most economically important poultry diseases. Breeding for genetic resistance, such as selection for specific histocompatibility genotypes, should be important in further reducing residual losses from MD in vaccinated flocks. More research on breeding for MD resistance and on MD resistance mechanisms is essential for economic reasons but may also contribute to the understanding of virus-induced malignancies in other species.

REFERENCES

1.    Briles W.E., Stone, H.A., and Cole, R.K.   Science 195:-
      193, 1977.

2.  Churchill, A.E., Payne, L.N., and Chubb, R.C.   Nature (London) 221:744, 1969.

3.  Cole, R.K.   Avian Dis. 12:9, 1968.

4.  Friars, G.W., Chambers, J.R., Kennedy, A., and Smith, A.D.   Avian Dis. 16:2, 1972.

5.  Gavora, J.S.   Proceedings, 28th National Breeders Roundtable, Memphis, Tennessee. p.33, 1979.

6.  Gavora, J.S., Grunder, A.A., Spencer, J.L., Gowe, R.S., Robertson, A., and Speckmann, G.W.   Poultry Sci. 53:889, 1974.

7.  Han, P.F.S., and Smyth, J.R.,Jr.   Poultry Sci. 51:975, 1972.

8.  Hansen, M.P., Van Zandt, J.N., and Law, G.R.J.   Poultry Sci. 56:1268, 1967.

9.  Hudson, L., and Payne, L.N.   Nature (New Biol.) 241:52, 1973.

10. Kenzy, S.G., and Biggs, P.M.   Vet Record. 19:565, 1967.

11. Longenecker, B.M., Pazderka, F., Gavora, J.S., Spencer, J.L., and Ruth, R.F.   Immunogenetics 3:401, 1976.

12. Lush, J.L., Lamoreaux, W.F., and Hazel, L.N.   Poultry Sci. 27:375, 1948.

13. Payne, L.N., Frazier, J.A., and Powel, P.C.   Int.Rev.-exp.Path. 16:59, 1976.

14. Purchase, H.G., and Schultz, E.F.,Jr.   World Poultry Sci.J. 34:198, 1978.

15. Rispens, H.H., Van Vloten, H., Masenbreck, N., Maas, H.J.L., and Schat, K.A.   Avian Dis. 16:108, 1972.

16. Sharma, J.M., witter, R.L., and Burmester, B.R.   Infect. and Immun. 8:715, 1973.

17. Spencer, J.L., Gavora, J.S., Grunder, A.A., Robertson, A., and Speckmann, G.W.   Avian Dis. 18:33, 1974.

18. Witter, R.L., Nazerian, K., Purchase, H.G., and Bungoyne, G.H.   Am.J.Vet.Res. 31:525, 1970.

# RELATIONSHIP BETWEEN TUMORGENICITY AND IMMUNOSUPPRESSION IN RESISTANT AND SUSCEPTIBLE STRAINS OF MICE INFECTED WITH FRIEND LEUKEMIA VIRUS

Steven Specter, Herman Friedman, and Walter S. Ceglowski*

Department of Medical Microbiology
University of South Florida
College of Medicine
Tampa, Florida
and
*Department of Microbiology and Immunology
Temple University
School of Medicine
Philadelphia, PA.

Genetic control of susceptibility to infection by Friend leukemia virus (FLV), a murine virus, is well established (6,9,12). Control of resistance has been demonstrated to be associated with both the major histocompatibility locus (H-2) and genes outside the H-2 locus (2,6,9,12). Resistance is closely associated with the $H-2^b$ genotype, while $H-2^d$ confers susceptibility. The heterozygote $H-2^{b/d}$ is susceptible, indicating the genetic dominance of this trait. Chesebro et al.(6) demonstrated that the responsible gene within H-2 maps close to the D end of the locus, and is related to recovery from Friend virus infection. This gene has thus been designated RFV-1.

Two genes not located within the H-2 complex have also been associated with susceptibility to FLV induced leukemogenesis (2,9). The gene designated Fv-1 regulates susceptibility to the lymphatic leukemia virus (LLV) component of the FLV complex, which acts as a helper virus for replication of the defective spleen focus forming virus (SFFV) component (5). Fv-1 has two alleles; $Fv-1^b$ which refers to the tendency to infect B-tropic (BALB/c) mice and $Fv-1^n$ which infect N-tropic (NIH Swiss) mice. The Fv-2 gene is believed to control susceptibility to SFFV, and alleles are referred to as $FV-2^s$ for susceptibility and $Fv-2^r$ for resistance (9).

While genetic control of leukemogenesis has been carefully studied and described in some detail, genetic factors controlling FLV induced immunosuppression have not; FLV, as well as many other oncogenic and non-oncogenic viruses, are well recognized as immunosuppressive agents (11). Ir gene(s) in the MHC have been postulated to genetically regulate susceptibility to immunodepression by FLV (9,10).

However, results from this laboratory suggest rather that susceptibility to immunosuppression is a direct result of genetic susceptibility to the leukemogenic process.

Genetically susceptible BALB/c mice ($H-2^d$, $Fv-1^b$, $Fv-2^s$) and resistant C57BL/6 mice ($H-2^b$, $Fv-1^b$, $Fv-2^r$) were used to assess the immunosuppressive effects of FLV. Immunoresponsiveness included: a) assessment of antibody responses to sheep erythrocytes in vivo (3,4) and in vitro, by the hemolytic antibody plaque forming cell (PFC) assay, and b) measurement of in vitro correlates of cell-mediated immunity assessed by macrophage migration inhibition (1) and lymphocyte mediated cytolysis (7) using allogenic tumor target cells. All assays for immune responsiveness included susceptible and resistant mice exposed to virus and unexposed controls.

Suppression of the primary antibody PFC responses for IgM were detectable when sheep red blood cell (SRBC) challenge occurred one day post infection of BALB/c mice. By 7 days post infection suppression approached 99% of control responses using $10^3$ $LD_{50}$. In resistant C57BL/6 mice suppression exceeded 90% by day 3 post-infection; however by day 7 responses had returned to normal.

Table 1.   Effect of FLV infection on immune responses of
           BALB/c and C57BL/6 mice.

| Immune Studies | BALB/c | C57BL/6 |
|---|---|---|
| Presence of virus in spleen | Chronic | Transient[a] |
| Leukemogenesis | Yes | No |
| In vivo 1° Ab response | Depressed | Transient depression |
| In vivo 2° Ab response | Depressed | Transient depression |
| In vitro 1° Ab response | Depressed | Depressed[b] |
| Macrophage Migration Inhibition | Depressed | Normal |
| Lymphocyte Mediated Cytolysis | Depressed | Transient depression |

[a]Splenic FLV infection is progressive in BALB/c mice and transient in C57BL/6 mice with no detectable virus by day 7.
[b]In vitro cultures show detectable FLV throughout 5 day culture period for both mouse strains.

Similar results were observed for both IgM and IgG PFC, when secondary responses were measured. When secondary SRBC challenge occurred 3 weeks after primary immunization both IgM and IgG responses were depressed by 90% or greater after 7 days in BALB/c mice and remained low until death of the animals at about 30 days. C57BL/6 mice demonstrated 90% depressed PFC response at 3 days post infection with recovery of normal IgM responses by day 7. IgG responsiveness recovered at a slower pace showing only 50% recovery by 7 days. Immune suppression appeared to be directly related to presence of FLV in the spleen since virus was detectable in BALB/c mice from 3 days post infection until death whereas in C57BL/6 mice virus was present by day 3 but was cleared from spleens before day 7.

In vitro antibody responses were depressed in both strains of mice when virus was added to normal spleen cells and sheep RBC and remained throughout the culture period as detected by immunofluorescence. Using a dose of $6 \times 10^3$ $LD_{50}$ PFC responses were only 40% of uninfected controls for both mouse strains. Thus the C57BL/6 mice were equally suppressed in vitro as long as virus was present. Studies in vitro using heat-killed virus or antibody neutralized FLV did not result in immunosuppression even in the highly susceptible BALB/c mice, indicating the need for active virus to induce suppression.

Migration inhibition (MI) studies were performed with BALB/c and C57BL/6 mice sensitized with killed mycobacteria and infected with FLV at various times before sensitization. Three weeks after sensitization splenocytes were removed and cells placed in capillary tubes. The tubes were then placed in Sykes-Moore chambers containing RPMI 1640 with or without 50μg PPD/ml. Areas of migration were measured 20 hours after culture initiation, and inhibition of migration of 20% or greater of control values was deemed to be significant. BALB/c mice infected for 3 days or longer showed reduced MI by 50-70%. C57BL/6 spleen cells from FLV infected mice never showed a decrease in MI versus uninfected controls, in sharp contrast to transient depression seen for other effects. Lymphocyte mediated cytolysis to allogeneic tumor target cells showed a progressive suppression of this activity in BALB/c mice. EL4 lymphoma cells were readily killed by immune BALB/c spleen cells with 50% cytotoxicity, occurring at an effector to target cell ratio of 20:1. With 5 day FLV infected BALB/c spleen cells cytotoxicity was only 10% at 20:1 ratios. Cytotoxicity of C57BL/6 spleen cells immune to P815 mastocytoma cells was not depressed at 5 days post infection, although at earlier times some depression was noted in the C57BL/6.

FLV infection and genetic control of immunologic impairment correlates directly with susceptibility to leukemo-

genesis and replication of virus. Resistance to leukemogenesis in C57BL/6 mice also resulted in a general resistance to immunosuppression by FLV. Migration inhibition was
not depressed in C57BL/6 mice and the other immune responses
that were measured showed only a transient immunosuppression
which could be directly correlated to the presence of virus.
In fact, when C57BL/6 spleen cells were infected, in vitro,
antibody formation was inhibited to the same degree as susceptible BALB/c mice. These C57BL/6 cultures did contain
detectable FLV. Such suppression again was associated with
presence of virus. Leukemogenesis in susceptible BALB/c
mice, which do not clear FLV, is closely associated with
chronic immunosuppression by the virus. Thus, in every instance where immune suppression was measured FLV was
present. Because of this it is not possible at this time to
ascertain if control of susceptibility to immunosuppression
is genetic or merely reflects viral presence resulting from
genetic susceptibility to leukemogenesis.

Lilly (8) has suggested that immune response genes,
which are located in the H-2 complex, control susceptibility
to effects of murine leukemia viruses. This close association of the genes controlling immune competence and susceptibility to murine leukemia virus is suggestive of genetic
control of immunosuppression by FLV, but remains to be
proven.

## REFERENCES

1.   Bloom, B., and Bennet, B.  Science 153:80, 1966.
2.   Ceglowski, W.S., Campbell, B.P., and Friedman, H.
     J.Immunol. 114:231, 1975.
3.   Ceglowski, W.S., and Friedman, H.  J.Immunol. 102:338,
     1969.
4.   Ceglowski, W.S., LaBadie, G.U., Mills, L., and
     Friedman, H.  In Virus Tumorigenesis and Immunogenesis.
     W.S. Ceglowski and H. Friedman, eds.  New York:
     Academic Press, p167, 1973.
5.   Cerny, J., Essex, M., Rich, M.A., and Hardy, W.D.Jr.
     Int.J.Cancer 5:351, 1975.
6.   Chesebro, B., Wehrly, K., and Stimfling, J.  J.Exp.Med.
     140:1457, 1974.
7.   Henney, C.S.  J.Immunol. 101:1558, 1977.
8.   Lilly, S.  Transp.Proc. 3:1239, 1971.
9.   Lilly, S., and Pincus, T.  Advances in Cancer Res. 17:-
     231, 1973.
10.  Mortensen, R.J., Ceglowski, W.S., and Friedman, H.
     J.Immun. 112:2077, 1974.

11.  Specter, S., and Friedman, H.   Pharm.Therap.A. $\underline{2}$:595, 1978.

12.  Tucker, H.S.G., Weens, J., Tsichlis, P., Schwartz, R.S. Khiroya, R., and Donnelly, J.  J.Immun. $\underline{118}$:1239, 1977.

# VIRAL IHIBITION OF LYMPHOCYTE MITOGENESIS: IMMUNOLOGICAL CHARACTERIZATION OF AN INHIBITORY FACTOR DERIVED FROM ADHERENT CELLS

Evelyne Israel[1] and Mark A. Wainberg[2]

Lady Davis Institute for Medical Research
Sir Mortimer B. Davis Jewish General Hospital
Montreal, Quebec, Canada
and
Department of Microbiology and Immunology
McGill University
Montreal, Quebec, Canada

Previous research from our laboratory and by others has shown that numerous viruses can non-specifically interfere with lymphocyte responses against mitogens (1) and allo-antigens (7). The effects obtained are independent of infection, and are seen using ultraviolet (UV) light-inactivated virus preparations, as well as lymphocyte-virus combinations for which the cells lack the receptors normally required for viral entry and penetration. We have postulated that membrane-membrane interactions involving the surfaces of both virus particles and cells account, in part at least, for these results (3). These findings, which suggest an important role for viruses in immune regulation, may help to explain the fact that patients with acute viral infection are often immunosuppressed.

This communication reports on our attempts to further elucidate the mechanism(s) of virus-mediated suppression of lymphocyte mitogenesis in vitro. In a previous paper, we showed that viruses can apparently induce macrophages to release a soluble activity with anti-mitotic properties (2). We now reiterate that this factor is made by an adherent cell, and show that it is active against cells of both syngeneic and allogeneic origin. Furthermore, the factor in question appears competent to directly activate an inhibitor cell population, which, if transferred to fresh syngeneic cultures, displays a dramatic anti-mitogenic effect.

## MATERIALS AND METHODS

Virus. The PrA and $B_{77}$ strains of avian retrovirus were propagated in cultures of chicken embryo fibroblast (CEF) cells as described (6), pelleted by centrifugation, and employed in lymphoid cell-incubation at concentrations beyond which further dilution abrogated any inhibitory effect (usually about 5-10 virus particules per cell (3).

<u>Lectin-driven mitogenesis assays.</u> These experiments were performed in RPMI medium using microtiter plates as described (3) with Concanavalin A (Con A, Difco) at a concentration of 4 µg/ml. Cultures (250,000 cells/well) were labelled for 16 hr with [3]H-thymidine (0.2 µCi/well) after 48 hr, and macromolecular material precipitated onto filter pads for scintillation counting. In some experiments, cultures contained not virus but dilutions (1:10 unless otherwise noted) of supernatant fluids derived from cells that had been co-incubated at 37°C with viruses for 24 hr. Such fluids were centrifuged for 15 min at 400 g to remove cellular debris and at 200,000 g for 3 hr to remove viral particles. Previous results have shown these supernatants to be free of both contaminating viral proteins and interferon activity (2).

**Table 1.** Ability of Different Cell Populations to Produce the Virus-Induced Inhibitory Factor

| Inhibitory factor induced by: | Cell population tested for factor production: | CPM following Con A stimulation | % Inhibition |
|---|---|---|---|
| - | - | 13,705 ± 1362 | - |
| RPMI | Whole spleen | 14,685 ± 543 | - |
| PrA | Whole spleen | 9,335 ± 1515 | 31.2 |
| RPMI | Sephadex G-10 filtered spleen | 22,240 ± 1756 | - |
| PrA | Sephadex G-10 filtered spleen | 16,727 ± 1361 | - |
| RPMI | Adherent spleen cells | 13,526 ± 706 | 1.3 |
| PrA | Adherent spleen cells | 6,075 ± 506 | 55.7 |
| RPMI | Whole thymus | 23,134 ± 2150 | - |
| PrA | Whole thymus | 15,333 ± 3693 | - |

## RESULTS

The data of Table 1 indicate that production of the virus-induced anti-mitogenic factor is apparently restricted to adherent cells. In this experiment, mouse B10.A spleen cells were filtered through a Sephadex G-10 column to remove macrophages and other adherent cells (5). The PrA strain of avian retrovirus was co-incubated for 24 hr with suspensions of each of unfiltered spleen cells, Sephadex G-10 filtered

spleen cells, whole thymus cells, or with macrophages from
B10.A spleen that have been allowed to adhere to 35 mm plastic petri dishes over 24 hr (about $10^6$ cells/plate). Virus-
free supernatant fluids were prepared as described and tested for ability to inhibit the proliferation of fresh spleen
cells in the presence of Con A.

Supernatant fluids obtained from non-virus-co-incubat-
ed, RPMI-containing cultures served as controls. Significant inhibition was obtained only with fluids derived from
virus pre-treated whole spleen cells or adherent cells. Removal of macrophages on Sephadex G-10 eliminated elaboration
of the inhibitory principle. Thymus cells, which contain
relatively few macrophages to begin with, were similarly unable to produce the inhibitory factor. These results also
indicate that control fluids derived from non-virus-treated
cultures are often stimulatory rather than inhibitory in
nature.

Having determined that the inhibitory factor was adherent cell-derived, we next sought to determine whether it
might only be active against syngeneic cells. Accordingly,
supernatant fluids, derived from co-incubation of mouse
B10.A splenic macrophages with the $B_{77}$ or PrA strains of
avian retrovirus, were diluted into splenic cultures of
B10.A, C3H, Balb/c or C57BL/6 origin. These various combinations include instances of significant overlap within
the major histocompatibility complex (MHC) with the B10.A
producer, as well as of complete disparity (C57BL/6). The
results (Table 2) indicate a lack of MHC restriction in
terms of the action of the inhibitory principle on target
cells.

Table 2. Effect of Mouse B10.A Macrophage-Derived
Inhibitory Factor on Con A-Driven Mitogenesis of Spleen
Cells of Different Mouse Strains

CPM when mouse strains tested were:

| Factor induced by: | B10.A | C3H | Balb/c | C57 Bl/6 |
|---|---|---|---|---|
| – | $10,744 \pm 884$ | $8990 \pm 172$ | $18,521 \pm 1292$ | $44,249 \pm 288$ |
| RPMI | $10,926 \pm 899$ | $6281 \pm 911$ | $32,534 \pm 1277$ | nt |
| $B_{77}$ | $2,331 \pm 396$ | $2600 \pm 10$ | $3,529 \pm 490$ | nt |
| PrA | $3,043 \pm 721$ | $5254 \pm 227$ | $5,331 \pm 736$ | $6,516 \pm 737$ |
| PrA | $5,549 \pm 793$ | $3743 \pm 157$ | $5,580 \pm 284$ | nt |

The fact that the inhibitory factor was adherent cell-derived prompted us to examine whether its effectiveness, when tested in vitro, might be dependent on the presence of an adherent cell population. Accordingly, Con A-driven mitogenesis assays were carried out using suspensions of each of whole spleen cells and Sephadex G-10 filtered spleen cells, to which a 1:25 dilution of mouse B10.A macrophage-derived inhibitory factor had been added. The results (Table 3) show that removal of adherent or accessory cells on Sephadex G-10 considerably diminished the basal level of mitogen responsiveness obtained. The residual responsiveness of Sephadex G-10 filtered cells appeared, however, to be relatively refractory to the effects of added inhibitory factor.

Table 3. Effect of Mouse B10.A Macrophage-Derived Inhibitory Factor on Con A-Driven Mitogenesis of Whole Spleen and Sephadex G-10 Filtered Spleen Cells.

|  | CPM when lymphocytes were derived from: | |
| --- | --- | --- |
| Factor induced by: | Whole spleen cells | Sephadex G-10 filtered spleen cells |
| - | 14,781 ± 1064 | 4,247 ± 380 |
| RPMI | 25,806 ± 5349 | 12,563 ± 770 |
| B$_{77}$ | 1,472 ± 305 | 2,862 ± 201 |
| PrA | 1,500 ± 441 | 3,529 ± 248 |

The above results cumulatively suggest the importance of adherent cells or macrophages in mediating the inhibition by virus particles of lectin-driven lymphocyte mitogenesis. In a further approach, different numbers of recovered plastic-adherent cells were added to whole spleen cells and the latter were then tested for responsiveness to Con A in the presence of virus. The results (Table 4) indicate that addition of syngeneic adherent cells apparently increased the extent of virus-mediated inhibition of lymphocyte stimulation otherwise seen.

Finally, we have previously shown (7) that addition of virus to splenic cultures can cause the appearance of a cell population with the ability to impede proliferative responsiveness of fresh lymphocyte suspensions to Con A. We endeavoured to determine whether the virus-induced, adherent-cell-derived inhibitory factor could directly activate such inhibitory cells. This was accomplished by preparing virus-free supernatant fluids from cultured macrophages that had

Table 4. Effect of Addition of Adherent Cells on
Virus-Mediated Inhibition of Con A-Driven Mitogenesis

| Expt | Mouse strain | Viral inhibitor | CPM when number of adherent cells added was: | | | |
|---|---|---|---|---|---|---|
| | | | 0 | $10^3$ | $5.10^3$ | $50.10^3$ |
| 1 | B10.A | – | 14,781 ± 1065 | 13,459 ± 1389 | 8,528 ± 448 | |
| | | $B_{77}$ | 2,212 ± 50 | 954 ± 85 | 809 ± 22 | |
| 2 | Balb/c | – | 73,218 ± 2409 | | | 11,097 ± 859 |
| | | PrA | 59,511 ± 5073 | | | 3,666 ± 488 |

been incubated for 24 hr in RPMI medium in either the presence or absence of avian retrovirus ($B_{77}$ or PrA strain).
Such fluids were then used at a 1:25 dilution in RPMI medium
to pre-treat $10^6$ whole spleen cells over 24 hr at 37°C.
These pre-incubated cells were then washed twice by centrifugation and added at various concenrations to fresh spleen
cells in the presence of Con A. The results

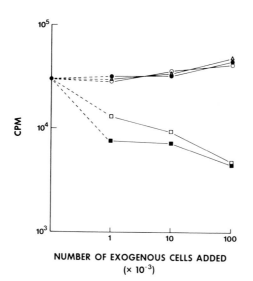

NUMBER OF EXOGENOUS CELLS ADDED
($\times 10^{-3}$)

Figure 1. Con A-driven mitogenesis of mouse B10.A spleen
cells in the presence of exogenously added syngeneic splenocytes. Addition of (O) newly-harvested cells; (●) RPMI pre-
incubated cells, (△) cells pre-incubated in normal macrophage supernatant, (□) (■) cells pre-incubated in supernatants derived from $B_{77}$- and PrA-treated macrophages, respectively.

(Figure 1) show that significant inhibition was attained only when culture fluids of virus co-incubated macrophages were used to pre-treat the spleen cells that were later added to fresh splenic cultures. Neither pre-treatment with normal macrophages fluids nor the pre-incubation period itself activated the inhibitory cells otherwise described.

## DISCUSSION

Our results are in accord with those of other investigators (4) who have also shown that adherent cells play a key role in mediating viral inhibition of lectin-driven mitogenesis. We show here that this role is notably accomplished through the elaboration of a factor with the ability to impede the proliferative responses of fresh spleen cells. We have found incidentally that this factor is produced to greater extent by spleen cells derived from B10.A than from Balb/c or C3H mice. The inhibitory principle derived from B10.A cells is equally active, however, against fresh spleen cells of any of Balb/c, C3H or B10.A origin. Therefore, synthesis of this factor but not its interaction with target tissue appears to be under genetic control. This factor may act through the activation of a cell population with direct inhibitory potential. Current efforts are aimed at the biochemical characterization of this substance, which, on the basis of preliminary results, is non-dialyzable and of molecular weight greater than 20,000. This task is made difficult by the instability of the inhibitory activity; the titre which initially may be as high as 1:3000 drops rapidly over a 2-month period even at -70°C.

On the other hand, it is hardly surprising that a potent immunosuppressive moiety, apparently induced as a consequence of exposure to virus, should be functionally unstable. We believe that these results may help to explain the transient immunosuppression that often accompanies acute viral infection in humans (8).

## ACKNOWLEDGEMENT

Supported by a grant to Mark A. Wainberg from the Medical Research Council of Canada.

[1]This research was performed by Evelyne Israel in partial fulfillment of the degree of Ph.D. in the Department of Microbiology and Immunology, McGill University.

[2]Chercheur-boursier of the Conseil de la Recherche en Santé du Québec.

## REFERENCES

1.  Hebebrand. L.C., Mathes, L.E., and Olsen, R.G.   Cancer Res. 37:4532, 1977.
2.  Israel, E., and Wainberg, M.A.   Immunology, 1980 (in press).
3.  Israel, E., Yu, M., and Wainberg, M.A.   Immunology 38:41, 1979.
4.  van Loon, A.M., van der Logt, J.ThM., and van der Veen, J.   Immunology 37:135, 1979.
5.  Ly, I.A., and Mishell, R.I.   J.Immunol.Meth. 5:239, 1974.
6.  Temin, H.M., and Rubin, H.   Virology 6:669, 1958.
7.  Wainberg, M.A., and Israel, E.   J.Immunol. 124:64, 1980.
8.  Willems, F.T.C., Melnick, J.L., and Rawls, W.E.   Proc.Soc.Exp.Biol.Med. 130:652, 1969.

# GENETIC CONTROL OF NATURAL RESISTANCE TO VIRAL INFECTIONS

## Chairman's Summary

D. Bernard Amos

Department of Microbiology and Immunology
Duke University Medical Center
Durham, North Carolina 27710

In summarizing their chapter on Innate and Acquired Immunity in "Topley and Wilson, Principles of Bacteriology and Immunology" the frustration of the authors Wilson and Miles at the complexities of the subject under consideration is evident from their conservative summary, "we have undoubted examples of heritable resistance to certain experimental infections; resistance which by breeding can be selected without exposure to the infection in question; and which in some cases has proved, in comparisons of resistant and susceptible strains to be associated with the high activity of certain tissue responses, including the immune response, that in other circumstances characterizes successful defence against microbial infection" (1). In principal, the whole basis of susceptibility or resistance to infection is genetic, yet we are attempting to understand through research extending back for relatively few years evolutionary processes that extend back to the creation of life. Because of the immense variety of organisms and the complexities of host defences there are few general cases; we are compelled to study individual processes affecting individual organisms with the hope of extending the studies to other infectious organisms, other routes of infection, and other hosts.

There have obviously been substantial gains in specific areas, although perhaps less than one would hope for. However there is a danger that in explaining these individual gains to scientists in other disciplines, failure to communicate effectively can lead to inadequate experimentation and fallacious conclusions. The literature is vast and few of us can be secure in our knowledge of our own field of specialization. The primary function of conferences such as this are to allow critical exchanges and to present specific relevant information. At this conference, as at others past and to come, attempts are made to relate infectious processes to genetic mechanisms, to immune responsiveness and to biophysical variability. To this observer, after reading the variety of papers included in this session, the attempt appears to have been more successful than most.

This summary attempts to highlight some of the contributions of the session on the Genetics of Viral Infection and will attempt to indicate where greater knowledge, or possibly greater care in interpretation may be required. The topic itself may have very urgent applications in the future. Little has been heard of regarding microbial tools in warfare in recent years, yet recombinant DNA technology could readily be applied to the generation of organisms of unprecedented virulence and completely novel antigenicity. While this possibility presently seems remote, prevention of pandemics through increased understanding of resistance mechanisms could be highly rewarding. The program also has the more prosaic, and hopefully more realistic, objective of advancing both basic and applied knowledge.

The general prerequisites of a successful viral infection are absence of pre-existing immunity, accessibility to a portal of entry and to suitable receptors as well as the appropriate conditions for binding, penetration and uncoating, the ability to replicate and finally to escape from the site of replication with freedom to re-infect. All of these processes involve genetic factors. Infection can, at least in theory, be arrested at any of these points although little attention is paid to some of them.

Receptors presumably subserve a normal physiologic function in the intact host and thus will differ from species to species, from tissue to tissue and will frequently be age and even sex dependent. The most dramatic example of the ability of a host to escape infection through lack of a receptor relates to the deletion of the gene for the red cell antigen Duffy (2). This genetic defect is common in African blacks and exceptionally rare in other populations. Duffy Null cells are essentially free from invasion by Plasmodium vivax since they lack the receptor for the malarial parasite. There seems to be little evidence regarding the genetics of expression of viral receptors. One approach would be to study individuals escaping infection when confronted with exposure to a new or variant organism such as occurs when an isolated arctic population encounters viruses transmitted to them from the crew of a supply ship. This would be a study in what has been called herd immunity, yet herd immunity has received little recent and systematic investigation, especially in human populations. Host variability within a herd is essential to survival of the species. We commonly think that the survival of the individuals in a herd exposed to a new infection is largely due to protection through prior exposure to cross-reactive environmental agents; one interesting exception, possibly worth

exploration, would be identification of individuals lacking
the receptor. These individuals, like those previously
immunized should escape infection. The epizootic which
followed the introduction of myxomatosis to the rabbits of
Australia killed over 99% of the rabbit population.
Obviously very few rabbits had the ability to respond in
time, or possibly some lacked the myxomatosis receptor. Unfortunately, absence of receptors might be largely restricted to receptors that were carbohydrates since individuals
lacking proteinaceous membrane components (Rh, HLA) tend to
have defective cells and to be at a selective disadvantage
while individuals with defective carbohydrate antigens
(Bombay) show no physical disability (3).

While genetically regulated generalized immunodeficiencies are important and frequent causes of increased susceptibility to viruses, this topic is not discussed in this
session since it is extensively described in many texts and
monographs. Instead, one very dynamic and incompletely exposed area of acquired immunosuppression does form the bases
for contributions to this section; these are immunosuppression secondary to viral infection. This topic urgently
needs extensive investigation. The paper by Kirchner et
al. relates virally related immunodepression to decreased
interferon production and impaired NK activity. The genetic
control of interferon production is itself a topic of
interest. In this session it is most formally developed by
Haller et al. who present evidence for a gene $\underline{Mx}$ for interferon regulation, but the regulation of interferon is also
discussed or implied in several other papers. Gee et al.
suggest that NK is inhibited in virus infections because
activated NK effectors are susceptible to the virus; this
has previously been shown by Bloom and his colleagues (4)
for latent infection of T lymphocytes. The infected cells
die when stimulated and prophylactic immunostimulation, e.g.
for the virus-related tropical pemphigus, may be hazardous.
While the role of NK $\underline{in\ vivo}$ is still disputed, especially
in tumor surveillance, genetic control of NK is invoked by
Britt and Chesebro in an interesting manner in their experiments on the reconstitution of Friend virus infected mice
with cells of a resistant genotype. Specter and Friedman
studying other immunological parameters also show genetically determined immunosuppression by Friend virus.

The Friend erythroleukemia model has long served Lilly
and his colleagues as a model for highly detailed studies of
the genetics of viral resistance or susceptibility. At
least 4 genes are implicated. One of the most interesting
is $\underline{Fv-2}$. The paper from Dr. Lilly's laboratory included in
this monograph (Steeves et al.) shows an exquisite sensitiv-

ity to the difficulties of the problem. The $Fv-2^r$ gene exhibits a complex variety of phenotypic effects. While $Fv-2$ may turn out to be part of a genetic complex, pleiotropy of gene expression may be a very important and little investigated phenomenon in disease susceptibility or resistance.

It is encouraging to see that further genetic studies are being pursued in hamsters by Massanari et al. and in chickens by Gavora and Spencer. To this observer, the type of genetic investigation that uses second and higher generation crosses of resistant and susceptible strains or individuals even in the absence of fully inbred and highly characterized strains needs continuing exploitation.

Genetic studies should always have redundancy built into their experimental design. This was pointed out many years ago by the great geneticist Sewall Wright. Under certain conditions polydactylia appeared to be inherited as a single mendelian trait (5). In fact, polydactylia is polygenic. If crosses involving different lines are set up, this complexity becomes apparent. In preliminary linkage studies of the gene $G_{IX}$ (controlling the virion 69-71 glycoprotein), loose linkage to $H-2^b$ appeared probable (6). When a different $H-2^b$ parental line was used the linkage disappeared (7). Thus it is always advisable to cross check a genetic conclusion by setting up a different cross. A valid observation should give (approximately) the same result.

It is fashionable, but inadequate to pinpoint the location of the genetic regulator at an exact point within a genetic system, such as H-2 without adequate segregation and other supporting genetic data. Because two mice have the same H-2 serotype there is no assurance that they have identical haplotypes. There is, unfortunately, a widespread misconception dating back over 20 years that congenic mice are essentially co-isogenic. Indeed two members of an H-2 congenic pair may easily differ by a segment of the 17th chromosome as extensive as 13 centimorgans in length (8). The foreign segment often includes the Qa-Tl segment of the 17th chromosome (9). This region, which includes many functionally active genes, should probably be included as part of the H-2 complex (10). In this context it is interesting that Bancroft et al. while finding some general correlation between NK and H-2 type, point out that one mouse strain B10.BR ($H-2^k$) exhibits only slight NK augmentation after infection although it is basically highly resistant and wisely conclude that other factors are important. These investigators used a variety of mouse strains and congenics. In another study, Chalmer attempts to map resistance to cytomegalovirus in congenics on BALB, C3H, and B10 backgrounds to the K-I-A subregion. However she has encountered numerous complications which she attributes to genes at or outside the D region. Realising the difficulties involved in studies relying on congenics, she also employed a series of hybrids between conventional strains to further document regulation; unfortunately segregating crosses have not been analysed in the study this far. Congenic mice must obviously be used with great caution and the widely held view that immune response genes are primarily dominant in expression is gradually being discarded. For example Dorf and his colleagues have shown that not only can Ir genes be recessive but that complementation even by genes within the H-2 complex can be encountered (11). Besides ignoring Qa and other regions of the 17th chromosome remote from the D and K region, most investigators studying immunity in mice also ignore the Mls genes although it has been found by Fitch and his colleagues that Mls can provide help for T cell reactivity (12). Early studies on the immune response gene Ir1 to the synthetic peptide (T,G)-A-L suggested that all $H-2^k$, (except AKR) all $H-2^d$, all $H-2^b$ haplotypes (13) were identical. More recent studies are casting doubt on this. Either the haplotype of two strains typing identically for H-2 is not really identical, or other genes, not on the 17th chromosome may be included by translocation or recombination during the formation of congeneic line.

H-2 congenics and H-2 mutants are undoubtedly of the greatest importance but there are other genetic models that should be exploited more extensively. One of these are the recombinant inbred lines as developed by Bailey (14) and also by Taylor (15) in which many separate sublines derived from one original cross between mice of two inbred strains differing at many loci have been characterized for an extensive library of marker genes. Mice of these lines are available from the Jackson Laboratory and can be used for initial screening exactly as congenics are used now.

By establishing which of the lines are high and which are low responders (or which are resistant and which susceptible) it is possible to determine which of many genes appear to influence the outcome. The next step would be to select high responder lines and low responder lines and to test $F_1$ hybrids and backcross or $F_2$ segregants. Because of the rich variety of recombinant inbred lines it is possible to confirm (or refute) the data by setting up other series of crosses between the recombinant inbreds. The Biozzi high and low responder lines are also becoming increasingly well characterized (16).

In this session many different facets of the genetic
control of immunity have been presented. These studies describe several different classes of virus and different
hosts. In attempting an integration and interpretation of
genetic mechanisms it must be stressed that there is no
single pattern of resistance just as there is no single
portal of entry. Anti-viral antibodies and T cell mediated
immunity are of known importance in the prevention and
control of such disease entities as measles, cytomegalovirus
and poliomyelitis. Antibody dependent cell mediated cytotoxicity (ADCC) may be an important host response mechanism
but little information is available regarding ADCC. Lymphokines such as the interleukons, the various interferons,
prostaglandin and what might be thought of as immunological
agents of broad specificity such as NK, NC and macrophage
mediated lysis of virally infected or virally altered cells,
as well as phagocytosis by macrophages and interference by
noninfectious particles all have relevance to different
facets of viral immunity. Obviously while many of these
topics have not been covered by the papers or by this overview, there is rapid progress in this fascinating interface
between genetics, immunology and infectious disease.

## REFERENCES

1.   Wilson, G.S., and Miles, A.A. (Editors) In Topley and
     Wilson's Principles of Bacteriology and Immunology.
     Arnold 6th Edition, 1975.
2.   Miller, L.H., Mason, D.J., Clyde, D.F., and McGinnis,
     M.H. New Eng.J.Med. 295:302, 1976.
3.   Bhende, Y.M., Despande, C.K., Bhatia, H.M. Lancet
     1:903, 1952.
4.   Bloom, B.R., Senik, A., Stoner, G., Ju, G., Nowakowski,
     M., Kano, S., and Jimenez, L. Cold Spring Harbor
     Symp. Quant.Biol. 41:73: 1977.
5.   Wright, S. Genetics 19:537, 1934.
6.   Stockert, E., Old, L.J., and Boyse, E.A. J.Exp.Med.
     133:1334, 1971.
7.   Stockert, E., Boyse, E.A., Sato, H., and Itakura, K.
     Proc.Natl.Acad.Sci.U.S.A. 73:2077, 1976.
8.   Flaherty, L. Immunogenetics 2:325, 1975.
9.   Klein, J., Flaherty, L., VandenBerg, J.J., and
     Schreffler, D.C. Immunogenetics 6:489, 1978.
10.  Klein, J. Science 203:516, 1979.
11.  Dorf, M., and Benacerraf, B. Proc.Natl.Acad.Sci.U.S.A.
     72:3671, 1975.
12.  Glasebrook, A.L., and Fitch, F.W. J.Exp.Med. 151:876,
     1980.

13. McDevitt, H.O., and Herzenberg, L.A.   Ann.Review of Genetics 2: 237, 1968.
14. Bailey, D.W.  Transplantation 11:325, 1971.
15. Taylor, B.A.   In Origins of Inbred Mice.   H.C. Morse III (ed).  Academic Press,p 423, 1978.
16. Mouton, D., Heumann, A.M., Bouthillier, Y., Mevel, J.C., and Biozzi, G.  Immunogenetics 8:475, 1979.

# GENETIC CONTROL OF IN VITRO NK REACTIVITY AND ITS RELATIONSHIP TO IN VIVO TUMOR RESISTANCE

Rolf Kiessling, Klas Karre and Gunnar Klein
Department of Tumor Biology
Karolinska Institutet
S-104 01 Stockholm 60
Sweden

## INTRODUCTION

The NK system of the mouse is now widely being recognized as one of the most important host defence mechanisms against tumor growth. Most, if not all, of the basic understanding of the in vivo role of NK cells stems from the use of mouse experimental systems. Much of this understanding has been obtained by the analysis of the genetic control of NK activity. Here it has been possible to use the early finding that NK cells seem to be under genetic control in order to analyze the tumor resistance to NK sensitive tumors in vivo. We will in this chapter briefly review the work carried out in our group on the genetic control of mouse NK activity and the evidence that this activity is responsible for tumor resistance in vivo. Some more recent data relating to this field will also be discussed.

## STRAIN DISTRIBUTION OF NK REACTIVITY

The basis of the genetic analysis in the NK system was the finding that mouse strains could be grouped according to their levels of in vitro cytolytic NK activity (8,9). This observation has later led to a more extensive genetic analysis aimed at understanding the mode of inheritance of the genes conferring high NK reactivity, as well as mapping their position within the mouse genome. The initial classification of mouse strains was performed with the highly NK-sensitive tumor YAC-1, but subsequently several other less NK-sensitive tumors were used as well. In Table 1, we summarize the NK reactivity of 15 different mouse strains, as tested on the YAC-1 target. The same classification, however, also applies to most other NK targets tested (for discussion on this point see Table 1).

The least reactive group includes the A strain, the A congenic resistant strains A.CA, A.SW and A.BY, as well as the AKR, the 129/J and the SWR/J strains. Highest reactivity is invariably seen using effector cells from the CBA or the C3H strains. The C57BL,C57Leaden and the DBA/2 strains should be classified as an intermediate group.

Table 1.  Grouping of mouse strains according to their
          levels of NK reactivity.

| High reactive strains | | |
|---|---|---|
| CBA/J | C3H/J | C3H/St |

Intermediately reactive strains

| C57BL/6 | C57BL/10 | C57Leaden DBA/2 |
|---|---|---|

Low reactive strains

| A/Sn  A/J | AKR  129/J | SWR/J  A.BY  A.CA  A.SW |
|---|---|---|

## NK REACTIVITY IN F1 CROSSES

When the low reactive A strain was crossed with various
other strains, and cells from these F1 hybrids tested
against the semisyngeneic YAC lymphoma of A origin for NK
activity, reactivity resembled the high reactive parent
(17). Thus, in these crosses, high reactivity was found to
be dominant. In subsequent studies using other F1 crosses
we found evidence of an inheritance pattern which is not a
simple dominance of high reactivity, but rather suggests a
genetic "complementation". Thus, in the C57BL x DBA/2 F1
hybrid, NK reactivity exceeded that observed with either
parental strain (29). A similar complementation phenomenon
in the NK system was also found when comparing the NK activity of certain CR strains with that of the background and
the H-2 donor strains (13).

## NK REACTIVITY IN BACKCROSSES BETWEEN HIGH REACTIVE F1 HYBRIDS AND LOW REACTIVE PARENTAL STRAINS

In trying to map the number and the position of the NK
regulating genes we have analyzed the offspring from various
backcrosses between high reactive F1 hybrid crosses back to
low reactive parental strains. Having in mind the importance of H-2 linked factors in virus induced leukemogenesis
and in the hybrid resistance phenomenon against transplantable tumors (16,23), it is natural that considerable interest in this analysis has been focused on the possible involvement of H-2 linked genes controlling levels of NK
activity.

The following backcrosses have been analyzed:

(A x C57BL) x A (18), (A x C57Leaden) X A (18), and (DBA/2 x
C57BL) x C57BL (29). The conclusions to be drawn from these
experiments are as follows: a) Several different genes
seem to be active in regulating high NK reactivity (18).
This was concluded by studying the distribution of reactivities in the offspring from the (A x C57BL) x A backcross
which distributed widely in between the high reactive F1
hybrid and the low reactive parental and argued against
models of one or two gene control. b) At least one of
these genes seems to map on chromosome 17. Thus, a clear
H-2 linkage was seen in all three backcrosses mentioned
above, indicated by the significantly higher reactivity
among H-2 heterozygotes as compared to H-2 homozygous littermates. No clear linkage was seen in the (A x BL) x A
backcross with 10 other genetic markers (18). Since an H-2
linkage was seen both in the (A x BL) x A (H-2$^{a/b}$ more
reactive than H-2$^{a/a}$) and the (DBA x BL) x BL (H-2$^{d/b}$
more reactive than H-2$^{b/b}$) backcrosses, it must be
concluded that evidence exists from these studies both for
an H-2$^b$ and an H-2$^d$ linked gene. The existance of
H-2$^d$ linked reactivity genes has also been borne through
in the CR analysis studies reviewed below.

## NK REACTIVITY IN CONGENIC RESISTANT (CR) AND H-2 RECOMBINANT MICE

In accordance with the observed H-2 linkage in the
backcross analysis, evidence for H-2 linkage of NK activity
has also been obtained by using CR or H-2 recombinant mouse
strains. Originally, Harmon et al. (7) using CR or H-2 recombinant mice on B10.A background showed that heterozy-
gosity within or near the D-end of the H-2 complex was sufficient to give high NK reactivity against the C57BL lymphoma EL-4. In confirmation of their data, also our group has
found evidence for the H-2$^d$ linked reactivity gene maps in
the D-end of the H-2 complex. First, in F1 crosses between
H-2 recombinant mice and C57BL strains, mice heterozygotes
in the D-end were found more NK active than the H-2 homozygote ones (29). This is examplified by the experiment shown
in Fig. 1, where (B10.A x C57BL) (H-2D$^d$/H-2D$^b$) mice are
more NK reactive than the H-2 homozygote (B10.A(2R) x C57BL)
(H-2D$^b$/H-2D$^b$) animals when tested against three different tumor targets.

In a more extensive study we have recently further investigated the importance of H-2D linked factors by testing
eleven B10 congenic or B10.A recombinant mice for NK activity (14). In this study the H-2D$^d$ strains B10.A, B10.T-
(6R), B10.S(7R), B10.HTT and B10.D2 were all more reactive

than B10, B10.S, B10.G, B10.A(2R) and B10.BR, that do not
carry the d allele at the H-2D locus.  While this confirms
the H-2D$^d$ association of a reactivity gene, an exception
was found in the B10.A(5R) strain that was low reactive in
spite of the fact that it carries H-2D$^d$.  Altogether, however, these data support the notion that the H-2$^d$ linked
gene maps are within or in close promimity to the D-end of
the H-2 complex.

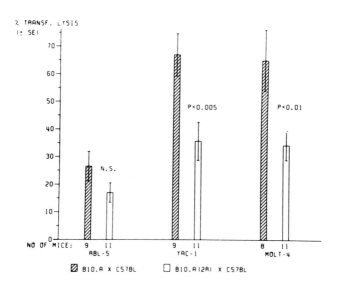

## Figure 1.

As regards the H-2$^b$ linked factor(s), which were revealed by the (A x C57BL) x BL backcross results mentioned
above, the mapping of this gene on chromosome 17 is not yet
clear.    Indications  from  the  A.BY  and  the  AKR-H-2$^b$  CR
strains, carrying the H-2$^b$ haplotype, argue for the idea
that this factor is located at some distance from the H-2
complex on chromosome 17, since none of these two strains
displayed significantly higher reactivities than did their
NK low reactive background strains (17,29).    Alternatively,
the H-2$^b$ linked reactivity gene is not fully expressed unless it receives some type of complementary help from other,
non-H-2 linked gene(s) present in the C57BL and C57Leaden
genomes but absent from strains with an A or AKR background.
For the purpose of this discussion, this hypothetical contribution is tentatiely designated as "background reactivity" (BR) gene(s).    At present it is not possible to exclude
any of these alternatives.

Furthermore, the exceptionally high reactivity of the B10.D2 strain seen in this study is reminiscent of the "complementation" effect we previously described in the B6 x DBA/F1 hybrid, with the hybrid showing a consistently higher NK-lysis than either one of the two parental strains. This result would suggest that complementation has occurred between the $H-2^d$ linked reactivity gene of DBA/2 and the "background" genome of the B10 strain.

## IS THERE A UNIQUE GENETIC PATTERN OF NK ACTIVITY DEPENDING ON THE TARGET CELL GENOTYPE?

NK cells can lyse a broad range of syngeneic, allogeneic and xenogeneic tumor targets (for review see 12). Since mouse strains can be divided into high- and low-reactive strains, one important question is to what extent the target cell genotype influences the genetic "pattern" of high- and low-reactivity of the effector strain. In other words, is it possible to detect a unique genetic pattern of high-versus low-reactive strains on targets depending on their genotypes? This question would be important to resolve when discussing the NK system in relation to the resistance to bone marrow grafts ("hybrid resistance"), where it has been postulated that the rejection is directed against Hh-1 determined antigens expressed on bone marrow grafts of certain genotypes only (3).

Previous results from our group using a variety of mouse and human lymphoma targets demonstrated a similar strain distribution and H-2 linkage regardless of the tumor genotype (29), but results from others have pointed to a unique genetic regulation of NK cells at the "target cell level" (30). To pursue the analysis of this question, we have in a recent genetic study used primary thymocytes and peritoneal macrophages as NK targets. The advantage of using normal tissue as targets for this type of analysis would be to avoid the "individuality" that each tumor line possesses, apart from their genetically determined cell surface antigens.

Figure 2 shows the results from this study in which LCMV-induced NK effector cells from 4 different mouse strains (C3H/St, Balb/c, SWR/J and A/J) were tested against thymocytes (Fig. 2A) or peritoneal (Fig. 2B) cell targets from the same mouse strains. The YAC-1 tumor line was included in these experiments as well. The important point to be made from these experiments is that the same genetic pattern of high or low reactive strains was seen regardless of the genotype of the target cell (thymocyte) donor. Thus, the C3H/St strain invariably showed highest activity against

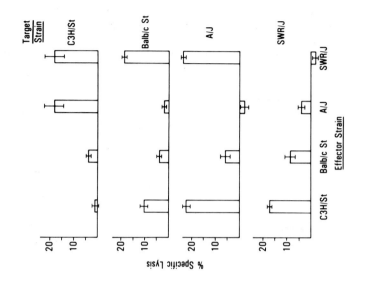

**Figure 2A:**

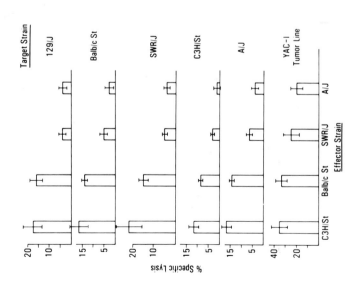

**Figure 2B.**

thymocytes of all genotypes, closely followed by the BALB/c
strain. The SWR/J and the A/J strains were both considerably less reactive against all five target genotypes. The
same genetic pattern was also seen against the YAC-1 lymphoma target (Fig. 2A).

In sharp contrast to the thymocyte-YAC-1 assay, an entirely different genetic regulation seems to be active in
the lysis of adherent peritoneal cells. Here, a unique pattern of reactivity is seen for each effector cell genotype,
dependent on the strain origin of the target cell (Fig. 2B).
In line with previous findings (28) syngeneic combinations
of effector-target cells yielded little, if any, reactivity
while various allogeneic combinations showed considerable
levels of activities. Taken together, these two NK systems
can clearly be distinguished by differences in their genetic
pattern of lysis. One crucial question is whether the same
effector cells which are active against thymocytes and YAC-1
cells, are active against PC cells. Cell fractionation experiments and experiments with the mouse mutants nude (normal or enriched in NK) and beige (deficient in NK) clearly
indicate that the effector cells active in the thymocyte as
well as in the PC system are natural killer cells. There
is, however, evidence that various "subtypes" of NK-like
cells may exist (1,24,30). It is therefore possible that
also in regards to lysing normal cells we may be demonstrating various subpopulations of NK cells.

## EVIDENCE THAT NK CELLS ARE INVOLVED IN REJECTION OF TUMOR TRANSPLANTS

Several lines of evidence from murine experimental systems now strongly suggest that NK cells are involved in rejection of tumor cells. These are briefly listed in Table
2. For a more extensive discussion on this point the reader
is referred to a recent review (12). It is notable, however, that the knowledge of the in vitro genetics of the NK
system has been more important in analyzing the in vivo role
these cells play in rejecting tumor transplants. Thus, the
first evidence came from comparing levels of in vitro NK
reactivity with those of in vivo tumor resistance to small
tumor inocula in semisyngeneic mice, where a high correlation was found between the in vitro activity and in vivo
resistance (10). In this first study, only the MLV-induced
lymphoma YAC was used, but it was subsequently extended to
involve a large number of different tumor-host combinations,
aiming at understanding the role of NK cells in the "hybrid
resistance phenomenon" against tumors. The results from
these studies are discussed in another chapter in this

volume. These studies support the idea that NK cells probably are one of the most important factors active in the
hybrid resistance against lymphomas, but further studies
would seem necessary to evaluate the role of T-cells as well
as other T-cell independent host resistance factors. The
knowledge of NK genetics was also used in another experimental in vivo model, where we demonstrated that high tumor
resistance in vivo can be transferred to low resistant genotypes by bone-marrow or fetal liver from NK high reactive
animals (6). These "NK chimeric" mice also served to prove
that NK cells are derived from the bone-marrow (6).

Table 2.  Evidence that NK cells are involved in genetically
          controlled in vivo rejection of tumor grafts.

|   |   | Reference |
|---|---|---|
| 1. | High correlation between in vitro NK reactivity and in vivo tumor resistance in various semisyngeneic F1 crosses. | 10 22 29 7 |
| 2. | NK activity and in vivo tumor resistance influenced by H-2 linked factors in backcross analysis and in CR-resistant mice. | 18 29 7 |
| 3. | High NK reactivity and in vivo tumor re-sistance in T-cell deficient mice to certain tumors. | 11 26 |
| 4. | Similar age-dependency of NK activity and tumor resistance. | 22 6 |
| 5. | High tumor resistance in vivo can be transferred to low resistant genotypes by bone-marrow from NK high reactive animals. | 5 6 |
| 6. | NK-sensitive tumors are more easily re-jected than NK insensitive ones. | 26 20 |
| 7. | The mouse mutant beige with a selective defect in NK reactivity is less resistant to tumor growth and to metastasis. | 15 25 |
| 8. | Short-term rejection of $^{125}$IUdR labeled tumor cells in vivo correlates with NK-activity. | 19 20 15 |

When trying to evaluate the role of NK cells in "immune surveillance" against syngeneic tumors, it could be criticized that the semisyngeneic F1 model involves H-2 miss-match between tumor graft and host. A better model for the analysis of anti-tumor effector mechanisms in the intact syngeneic host was recently discovered by the use of the beige mutation on the C57BL mouse strain background (21). The recessive beige gene ($bg^J$) which affects melanosome and granulocyte lysosome functions, also causes a profound depression of NK-activity whereas other anti-tumor effector mechanisms mediated by T-cells and macrophages remain relatively intact (31). Although beige mice have some NK activity, particularly after boosting of reactivity with potent interferon inducers such as LCMV virus (27), the beige model offers an unique possibility to test the effect of low NK activity on an otherwise NK high reactive genotype.

In the first part of this study we tested the benzpyrene-induced EL-4 and the Rad-LV-induced P52-127-166 leukemias of C57BL/6 origin, both previously shown to be highly resisted by certain C57BL-F1 hybrids that have high NK-activity in vitro (7,29). Here, low dose inocula of the in vivo maintained ascite lines of the two leukemias behaved similarly. Subcutaneous inoculation in a transplantation test yielded higher tumor take incidence in bg/bg mice (o--o) than in heterozygous littermates (x—x), as shown in Fig.3. In addition to the increased incidence of takes in mutant mice, the progressively growing tumors appeared with a shorter latency than in controls. Since this short period before tumor appearance in the bg/bg mice indicated that the defect in natural resistance of these animals involved early events after tumor inoculation, we also used a test system whereby the short-term survival of intravenously injected [125]IUDR-labelled leukemia cells is monitored (2,19). This test has been proposed as a most appropriate in vivo assay for NK-cells, since it has been shown to reflect a rapid non-immune rejection mechanism sharing many characteristics with NK activity. the heterozygous control mice elminated P-52-127-166 ascites cells more efficiently than beige mice, measured either as total, pulmonary or splenic radioactivity retained 18 hrs after i.v. injection (Fig. 4: beige mice 0, control X), although differences were detectable already after 4 hrs in the spleen (data not shown). The results suggest that bg/bg mice may lack an important mechanism for rapidly eliminating tumor cells e.g. as blood-borne metastases in the lungs and spleen. In line with these findings, Talmadge et al. (25) recently found that the B16 malignant melanoma had an increased metastatic capability in bg compared to control mice.

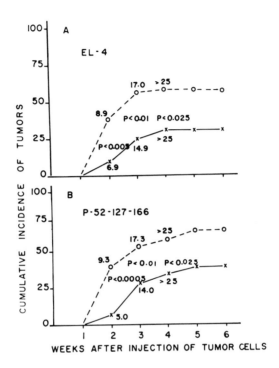

WEEKS AFTER INJECTION OF TUMOR CELLS

Figure 3.

Our findings in in vivo tests correlate well with the
in vitro measured splenic NK-activity against both tumors
tested.  In vitro cultured EL-4 or P-52-127-166 cells had a
low, but significant, sensitivity to ±/bg spleen cell cytotoxicity (5-10% specific lysis) whereas bg/bg spleen consistently gave values below 3% specific lysis.  An augmentation
of the low NK-levels against EL-4 and P-52-127-166 occurred
in mice receiving the low tumor cell dose used in the transplantation tests.  The NK activities of ±/bg as well as bg/
bg mice were increased, although relative differences between the groups were maintained.  In both tumor inoculated
and control groups bg/bg mice gave values corresponding to a
9-fold dilution of ±/bg splenocytes in terms of lytic units.
It is important to keep in mind that such augmented NK-activity, induced during the transplantation tests, may account

for <u>in</u> <u>vivo</u> resistance against tumor cells which show very
low susceptibility to <u>in</u> <u>vitro</u> lysis by NK-cells from normal
mice.

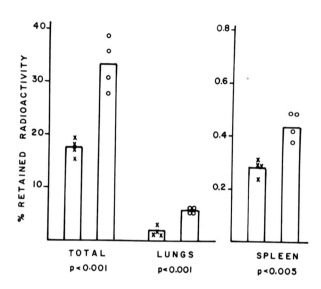

Figure 4.

Several different phenotypic manifestations of the
beige mutation may be partly responsible for the low natural
resistance against transplanted tumors in <u>bg/bg</u> mice observed here. However, our results from the two <u>in</u> <u>vivo</u> test
systems suggest that early events are of major importance
for the final outcome of tumor growth, which would argue
against adaptive mechanisms requiring proliferative expan-
sion of specific clones, as in a cytotoxic T-cell response.
Furthermore, the more efficient <u>in</u> <u>vivo</u> elimination of
leukemia cells in ±/bg mice was paralleled by a greater cell
mediated cytotoxicity <u>in</u> <u>vitro</u> against the same tumors which
was independent of adherent cells, arguing against the involvement of macrophages and monocytes.

Finally, <u>bg/bg</u> mice have previously been shown to generate highly efficient T killer cells <u>in</u> <u>vivo</u> after injection
of P815 tumor cells and anti-tumor effects mediated by
macrophages were also normal (31). Thus, our results
strongly suggest that NK-cells play a major role in the
cell-mediated <u>in</u> <u>vivo</u> resistance against transplanted tumors
observed in syngeneic phenotypically normal (±/bg) mice.
This has important implications for the evaluation of NK-
cell influences on primary tumor formation and growth in the

normal autochthonous host. If the high NK-cell activity of nude mice is the explanation for their low or "normal" incidence of tumors and their ability to resist growth of certain murine as well as human transplanted tumors, it is clear that a double mutant combining the beige and the nude defects would be a useful tool for future research. Such a defect is not lethal, and we have recently been able to produce double mutant mice by a series of crosses and intercrosses between C57BL/6 bg/bg and C57BL/6 ±/nu mice. These C56BL/6 bg/bg nu/nu mice are presently being characterized immunologically.

In conclusion, the experimental model provided by the beige mutation has given strong additional support to the notion that NK-cells may play a role in anti-tumor surveillance in vivo. It is interesting to note that humans bearing the same or similar Chediak-Higashi gene have an even greater impairment (500-fold) in NK function (32 this volume) and a corresponding increase in the incidence of a spontaneous lymphoproliferative disorder which is thought to be malignant (4).

## ACKNOWLEDGEMENTS

This investigation was supported by Grant No. IROI CA 14054-C7. awarded by the National Cancer Institute, DHEW, and by grants from the Swedish Cancer Society.

## REFERENCES

1. Burton, R. "Natural cell mediated immunity against tumors". R. Herberman (ed.). Academic Press, New York, (in press).
2. Carlsson, G.A., and Wegman, T.G. J.Immunol. **118**:2130, 1977.
3. Cudkowicz, G., and Bennett, M. J.Exp.Med. **134**:1513, 1971.
4. Dent, P.B., Fish, L.A., White, J.F., and Good, R.A. Lab.Invest. **15**:1634, 1966.
5. Haller, O., Hansson, M., Kiessling, R., and Wigzell, H. Nature **270**:609, 1977.
6. Haller, O., Kiessling, R., Orn, A., and Wigzell, H. J. Exp. Med. **145**:1411, 1977.
7. Harmon, R.C., Clarke, E., O'Toole, C., and Wicker, L. Immunogenetics **4**:601, 1977.
8. Herberman, R.B., Nunn, M.E., and Lavrin, D.H. Int.J.-Cancer **16**:216, 1975.

9. Kiessling, R., Klein, E., and Wigzell, H. Eur.J.-Immunol. 5:112, 1975.

10. Kiessling, R., Petranyi, G., Klein, G., and Wigzell, H. Int.J.Cancer 15:933, 1975.

11. Kiessling, R., Petranyi, G., Klein, G., and Wigzell, H. Int.J.Cancer 17:1, 1976.

12. Kiessling, R., and Wigzell, H. Immunol.Rev. 44:165, 1979.

13. Klein, G., Karre, K., Klein, G., and Kiessling, R. J.Immunogenetics, 1980 (in press).

14. Kumar, V., Bennett, M., and Eckner, R.J. J.Exp.Med. 139:1093, 1974.

15. Karre, K., Klein, G., Kiessling, R., Klein, G., and Roder, J. Nature (in press).

16. Lilly, F., and Pincus, T. Adv.Cancer Res. 17:231, 1973.

17. Petranyi, G., Kiessling, R., and Klein, G. Immuno-genetics 2:53, 1975.

18. Petranyi, G., Kiessling, R., Povey, S., Klein, G., Herzenberg, L., and Wigzell, H. Immunogenetics 3:15, 1976.

19. Riccardi, C., Pucetti, P., Santoni, A., and Herberman, R.B. (submitted for publication).

20. Riesenfeld, I., Orn, A., Gidlund, M., Axelberg, I., Alm, G., and Wigzell H. Int.J.Cancer (in press).

21. Roder, J.C., and Duwe, A.K. Nature 278:451, 1978.

22. Sendo, F., Aoki, T., Boyse, E.A., and Buofo, C.K. J.Natl.Cancer Inst. 55:603, 1975.

23. Snell, G.D. Transpl.Proc. 8:147, 1976.

24. Stutman, O., Paige, C.J., and Feo Figarella E. J.Immunol. 121:1819, 1978.

25. Talmadge, J., Meyers, K., Prieur, D., and Starkey, J. Nature (in press).

26. Warner, N.L., Woodruff, M.F., and Burton, R.C. Int.J.-Cancer 20:146, 1977.

27. Welsh, R., and Kiessling, R. Scand.J.Immunol (in press).

28. Welsh, R.M., Zinkernagel, R.M., and Hallenbeck, L.A. J.Immunol. 122:475, 1979.

29. Klein, G., Klein, G., Karre, K., and Kiessling, R. Immunogenetic 7:391, 1978.

30. Kumar, V., Luevano, E., and Bennet, M. J.Exp.Med. 150:531, 1979.

31. Roder, J.C., Lohmann-Matthes, M.L., Domzig, W., and Wigzell, H. J.Immunol. 123:2174, 1979.

32. Haliotis, T., and Roder, J.C. (this volume).

DISCUSSION

Kaplan: Kiessling observed that in the killing of peritoneal cell targets by NK cells, cytotoxicity for syngeneic cells is less than for allogeneic cells. Could he give the reasons for this?

Kiessling: That is the case in the peritoneal cell assay. The basis for this difference is not at all known. This could involve some kind of interaction between the Ia antigens of macrophages and NK cells but, for now, that is pure speculation.

Kaplan: One might raise the possibility that, if what is perceived on these target cells are different types of antigens such as histocompatibility antigens, then Kiessling might find autochthonous cold-target inhibition, were he to use autologous targets.

Kiessling: Yes, I agree; that would be very interesting to do with the peritoneal cells.

Roder: My query is one I generally put to interferon experts, but I never get a very clear answer. Perhaps Kiessling could tell us whether the NK-enhancing effects of interferon are species specific? In the experiment where xenogeneic targets were not well protected by mouse interferon, did added human interferon prove to be protective?

Kiessling: We don't have much information. That experiment should be done.

Haller: As Kiessling pointed out, it is well known from the work by Gresser that interferon enhances expression of H-2 structures on cells. I wonder whether he knowns if the decrease in NK sensitivity is due to interferon decreasing the amount of NK sensitive structures on the target cell surface.

Kiessling: As it appears from assays of competitive inhibition, it is clearly evident that NK sensitive targets also have a lower binding capacity, and that they compete less well after interferon treatment. That would argue more for a change of NK target structure than for sensitivity to lysis. These cells are also clearly more sensitive to lysis by cytotoxic T cells, probably because here too the expression of allo-antigens is increased in those targets.

Dupuy:   Would Kiessling comment on the regulation of NK cells and the possible effect of suppressor cells.

Kiessling:   This question is best put off until Roder's presentation as he will be dealing with issues pertaining to regulation of NK activity.

Winn:   Kiessling promised to come back to the matter of complementation in DBA/2XB6 hybrids.  Would he do so now?

Kiessling:   In congenic resistant mouse strains we see the same complementation if we look at a B10.D2 congenic resistant strain, which is more reactive than both the B10 background strain and the DBA H-2 donor strain.  That similarity will be then in that situation.

Winn:   But what if one crosses B10.D2 with B10?

Kiessling:   We haven't done that.  The fact is that we haven't formally proven true complementation.

Winn:   Is the increase in H-2 on thymocytes referable to the cortical or the medullary thymocytes?

Kiessling:   I think that what happens in vivo is that if one treats the thymocytes with interferon these cells are then driven towards differentiation to a more mature state.  So precursors would be mature medullary thymocytes, increased by this treatment.  As has been pointed out, this inverse relationship between H-2 and NK sensitivity can also be seen in other situations such as, for example, with lymphomas. Upon transplantation of lymphomas, the H-2 display generally decreases but NK activity grows, and vice-versa.

Lopez:   Does Kiessling know whether the antigens on thymocytes dilute out the activity against YAC cells?

Kiessling:   They do.  There appears to be a sharing of antigenic specificity because there is a criss-cross competition situation between thymocytes and YAC cells.

Bennett:   Would Kiessling comment on the observation that NK cells are absent in germ-free animals, with the possibility therefore that the H-2 restriction of NK cell activity is the result of response to pathogens?

Kiessling:   I believe it is clearly possible that H-2 linkage could be indirect, as Bennett implies, possibly due to sub-clinical infections with viruses or bacterial pathogens, which are capable of continuously stimulating NK activity. This is possibly regulated by some <u>H-2</u> linked resistance factor. The literature provides conflicting data on this point. For instance, Herberman and ourselves find quite a degree of reactivity in stereospecific infection in germ-free mice, whereas Clark has found that most of these mice are devoid of reactivity but can regain reactivity when transferred to a "conventional" environment. I would say that this issue is not yet resolved.

# DIFFERENT GENES REGULATE TUMOR CELL RECOGNITION AND CYTOLYSIS BY NK CELLS IN THE MOUSE

John C. Roder

Department of Microbiology and Immunology
Queen's University
Kingston, Ontario K7L 3N6, Canada

## INTRODUCTION

Two of the most important questions in the biological sciences today concern the "switches" which control eukaryotic gene expression and the membrane receptors which function as the cell's sense organs, signalling the state of the surrounding environment. The model under investigation involves a cell-mediated, cytolytic system in which various defined cell populations (effector cells) are capable of binding and destroying appropriate cells of another type (Targets) in a unidirectional interaction. The effector cell is thought to recognize various surface molecules on the target by means of complementary receptors. When these receptors interact with the target molecules of appropriate specificity a signal is delivered to the effector cell which triggers the translation, activation, or delivery of proteins involved in a lethal killing event. Since the lytic cycle is complex and multi-factorial it was necessary to devise a system for visualizing early stages of target-effector interaction.

## 1. Target Cell Recognition

The removal of adherent cells on nylon wool columns leaves a population of non-adherent lymphocytes which bind selectively to various target cells as previously shown (7). As shown in Table 1 these target binding cells (TBC) were a reliable estimate of the frequency of natural killer (NK) cells. The level of TBC and the level of lysis in a population were closely correlated in kinetics experiments and under varying biological conditions of age, organ site, phenotype and reactivity on a panel of target cells. Inhibition of TBC formation with EDTA inhibited subsequent lysis of the target cell, thereby indicating that the binding event was a necessary prerequisite for lysis. In more direct experiments, cell populations enriched or depleted in TBC by velocity sedimenttion showed a corresponding increase or decrease in the ability to lyse YAC targets and the majority of single TBC isolated in droplets or monodispersed

in agar killed the target to which they were attached (8).
These results suggest that the majority of TBC detected
(80%) are indeed NK cells.

Table 1.  Evidence that TBC are Killer Cells

| Experiment | Covariance Between % Lysis and % TBC |
|---|---|
| Strain Survey (n=9) | r=0.94, p<.001 |
| Target Survey (n=14) | r=0.90, p<.001 |
| Organ Distribution (n=5) | r=0.98, p<.01 |
| Age Development (n=6) | Parallel |
| H-2 Linkage in Backcross (n=20) | p<.005 |
| Dominant in Low X high, F1 (n=6) | p<.001 |
| Kinetics (n=30) | r=0.86, p<.001 |
| Inhibition with EDTA | Yes |
| Enrich or deplete TBC | Yes |
| Isolated conjugates | Yes |

NK frequency = 0.6-2.4% of total lymphocytes in spleen, per
ipheral blood and lymph node.  The data in this table are
summarized from Roder et al. (7,8).

Trypsinization of the effector (or treatment with
papain and pronase) abolished target cell binding and cytolysis.  Both functions regenerated in a parallel time course
in the absence of cycloheximide which is compatible with the
suggestion that binding occurs prior to lysis and is mediated by a protein-like cell surface recognition structure.
Prolonged (3 hr) treatment with puromycin and cycloheximide
alone also prevented TBC formation, possibly by blocking the
synthesis of recogniton receptors.  Theserecognition structures are at least partially specific since preincubation of
effectors with solubilized target cell antigens inhibited
subsequent binding to the intact target in a specific manner
as demonstrated in cross inhibition assays (5,10).

2.  H-2 Linked Control of Targetr Cell Recognition

As shown in Table 2 the F1 progeny of high responder
strains mated with low responder strains exhibited the cytolytic and target binding characteristics of the high reactive parent.  In contrast a hybrid between two low responders
(A/Sn and A.SW) maintained low levels of lysis and target
cell binding.  A backcross between C57BL/6 and C57BL/6 x
DBA/2 F1 mice revealed that the level of responsiveness in
TBC activity was at least partially controlled by genes
linked to the H-2 complex.  Hence spleen cells from hetero-

Table 2. Genetic Control of TBC

| STRAIN | % LYSIS | % TBC |
|---|---|---|
| CBA | 50 | 20 |
| A/Sn | 21 | 6 |
| CBA x A/Sn $F_1$ | 40 | 20 |
| C57B1/6 | 38 | 12 |
| C57B1/6 x A/Sn $F_1$ | 52 | 20 |
| A.SW | 13 | 7 |
| A.SW x A/Sn | 12 | 5 |
| DBA/2$^d$ | - | 17 |
| C57B1/6$^b$ | - | 12 |
| C57B1/6$^b$ x DBA/2$^d$ $F_1$ | - | 19 |
| (C57B1/6 x DBA/2) $F_1$ x<br>   C57B1/6 - H-2$^{d/b}$ | - | 22 |
| (C57B1/6 x DBA/2 $F_1$ x<br>   C57B1/6 - H-2$^{b/b}$ | - | 12 (p<.005) |

Spleens were pooled from 6 age-matched mice per group and passed over nylon wool columns. Lymphocytes were assayed for frequency of target-binding cells (TBC) and lysis of $^{51}$Cr labelled YAC cells at a 50/1 E/T ratio. Twenty offspring were tested individually in the backcross experiment and differed significantly at the p<.005 level. The data in this table is summarized from Roder and Kiessling (7). Standard deviations were always <10% of the mean values shown.


zygous backcross progeny which were typed as H-2$^{d/b}$ and tested individually had greater numbers of TBC than homozygous H-2$^{b/b}$ progeny. A similar H-2 linkage of cytolysis has been shown in the same backcross (1,2,3). These results suggest that the initial stage of target-effector interaction is regulated by dominant genes some or all of which may be linked to the H-2 region of chromosome 17. These genes would appear to control the size of the NK population expressing the putative recognition receptor. Whether these genes directly code for the recognition receptor or regulate some other aspect of cell differentiation cannot be ascertained at present.

3. Non H-2 Linked Genes Controlling the Cytolytic Mechanism

Since target cell recognition was only the first step in a complex series of events leading to target cell lysis we began a search for mutations which might affect discrete steps in the lytic pathway subsequent to target effector binding.

Table 3. NK Function in Beige Mice

| Genotype | % Lysis | % TBC |
|----------|---------|-------|
| C57Bl/6-+/+ | 50 | 20 |
| C57Bl/6-+/bg | 51 | 20 |
| C57Bl/6-bg/bg | 10 | 21 |

Nylon wool column passed cells from pools of 4 mice were assayed for frequency of TBC or % lysis of $^{51}$Cr labelled YAC cells at a 50/1 E:T ratio in a 4 hr cytolytic assay.

As shown in Table 3 the recessive beige mutation (bg) in C57BL/6 mice led to a marked impairment of NK cell mediated lysis. The heterozygous littermate controls (+/bg) responded as well as the wild type (+/+). With the exception of antibody dependent cell-mediated cytotoxicity (ADCC) against tumor cells, all other forms of cell-mediated immune function in homozygous beige mice were normal as summarized in Table 4, thereby indicating that the NK defect may be selective. Since beige mice had a normal frequency of TBC (Table 3) it is inferred that the NK defect may lie within the lytic machinery of the cell rather than at the level of population size or recognition receptors. A similar defect has recently been discovered in the human analog of the beige mutation, in the form of the Chediak-Higashi syndrome (Haliotis and Roder, this volume).

## 4.  Conclusions

Table 4.    Immune Function in Beige Mice

| FUNCTION | BG/BG | +/BG |
|---|---|---|
| - NK cytolysis (All ages, organs, targets enrichments, B.M. transfers) | Low | High |
| - NK - TBC | High | High |
| - ADCC vs. Tumor Cells | Low | High |
| - ADCC vs. CRBC | High | High |
| - CTL - MLC | High | High |
| - in vivo alloimmune | High | High |
| - Lectin induced | High | High |
| - Skin graft | High | High |
| - T cell - mitogens | High | High |
| - B cell - mitogens | High | High |
| - IG production | High | High |
| - ACT. MPH. cytolysis (BM) | High | High |
| - ACT. MPH. cytolysis (PEC) | High | High |
| - PRO-MPH cytolysis - spontaneous | High | High |
| - ADCC | High | High |
| - NK Interferon boost | Low | High |
| - Lysosomal Enzymes | Low | High |

The data supporting this summary can be found in Roder et al. (4,6,9,).

A picture of the NK cytolytic mechanism is emerging in which various genes control and regulate discrete steps in the lytic cycle.  H-2 linked genes on chromosome 17 control the initial stage of target effector recognition either through the regulation of population size and/or the

putative recognition receptor itself. Target-effector contact is postulated to trigger a series of events which lead
to the activation of the actual lytic moiety. These intervening steps are susceptible to the action of genes regulating the production of or response to interferon. Finally
the terminal stages of the cycle close to the lethal hit are
regulated by the beige gene in the mouse on chromosome 13
and the CH gene in the human. The beige mouse provides a
valuable model for investigation of the genes controlling
various steps in the cytolytic pathway and is also being
used to validate the role of NK cells in immune surveillance
against tumor development.

## REFERENCES

1.  Harmon, R.C., Clark, E., O'Toole, C., and Wicker, L.
    Immunogenetics 4:601, 1977.
2.  Klein, O., Klein, G., Kiessling, R., and Karre, K.
    Immunogenetics 6:651, 1978.
3.  Petranyi, G., Kiessling, R., Povey, S., Klein, G.,
    Herzenberg, L., and Wigzell, H. Immunogenetics 3:15,
    1976.
4.  Roder, J.C. J.Immunol. 123:2168, 1979.
5.  Roder, J.C., Ahrlund-Richter, L., and Jondal, M.
    J.Exp.Med. 150:471, 1979.
6.  Roder, J.C., and Duwe, A. Nature 278:451, 1979.
7.  Roder, J.C., and Kiessling, R. Scand.J.Immunol. 8:135,
    1978.
8.  Roder, J.C., Kiessling, R., Biberfeld, P., and
    Andersson, B. J.Immunol. 121:2509, 1978.
9.  Roder, J.C., Lohmann-Matthes, M.L., Domzig, W., and
    Wigzell, H. J. Immunol. 123:2174, 1979.
10. Roder, J.C., Rosen, A., Fenyo, E.M., and Troy, F.
    Proc.Natl Acad.Sci USA. 76:1405, 1979.

## DISCUSSION

Cudkowicz: Roder has shown us several correlations between
NK activity and a number of target binding cells. Has he
done an experiment with anti-NK antisera? There are now
several available which, under certain conditions, are fairly selective for NK cells. If he treats such cells with
antisera and complement, would the number of conjugates be
reduced or would they disappear all together?

Roder: Yes, if one treats with such antisera, one can reduce the capacity to form conjugates by over 50% (actually
70% in several experiments). Furthermore, in a more direct
kind of study where we stain conjugates with a fluorescent
technique, we show that the majority of conjugates do light
up when one stains them with antisera to other markers reported to be on NK cells. One we haven't yet looked at is
the NK 1.1 alloantigen.

Winn: Would Roder identify this particular antisera? We
know that anti-Ly5 isn't very helpful because that antigen
is present on many other cells.

Roder: The antiserum I employed is made against ganglioside
GM-1 from which sialic acid has been cleaved. In all killing assays with complement, it removes NK activity without
any effect on cytolytic T-cells or mitogen responsiveness.

Winn: What happens to viability with trypan blue exclusion
if one adds antibody and complement to these spleen cell
suspensions?

Roder: The antiserum kills 10-20% of spleen cells.

Winn: So that represents a degree of killing quite a bit
more than the NK cells themselves which I recall Roder saying was about 0.6 to 2.4%.

Roder: That's true. Probably the antiserum is acting on a
subpopulation of T cells as well, possibly immature T cells.

Cudkowicz: About the Chediak-Higashi cells, could Roder
tell us something about the correction of their defect or
restoring their activity with cyclic GMP.

Roder: Some experiments were recently carried out by Paul
Katz at NIH. He could significantly increase the response
with interferon in vitro, possibly 10-fold, but this is
still 100-fold less than the controls in terms of lytic
units. So this is nowhere near a complete restoration, but
Paul Katz did then subject these cells to a brief preincubation with cyclic GMP, or 8-bromo-cyclic GMP, or dibutero-
cyclic GMP. He found that a 30 minute preincubation and
wash of effectors yielded complete restoration. So it is a
very dramatic reversal. This observation is just now being
followed up.

Gold: Could you comment: In beige mice with the NK defect

or loss of cell, what is the overall incidence of spontaneous cancer, or the efficacy of tumor induction chemically
or oncogenically with viruses?

Roder:  Such tests are now in progress but we have no hard
data yet.  As far as spontaneous incidence of neoplasia,
this has not been followed long enough, but up to 6 months
there has been no marked increase, although we are finding
some spontaneous tumors comping up.  I know of good data
with experimental tumors (B16 melanoma) that show in beige
mice much greater metastases and greater tumor takes.

# HETEROGENEITY OF NATURAL KILLER CELLS: A SEROLOGICAL STUDY WITH SPECIFIC ANTI-NK ALLOANTISERA

Robert C. Burton[1], Scott P. Bartlett
and Henry J. Winn

From the Transplantation Unit
General Surgical Services
and the Department of Surgery
Harvard Medical School
at the
Massachusetts General Hospital
Boston, Massachusetts 02114

## INTRODUCTION

The range of neoplastic and normal cells which is susceptible to natural killing, and the associated variations
in the conditions under which maximal levels of in vitro
lysis are observed have led to the suggestion that a heterogeneity of natural killer (NK) cells might exist (7,8). The
recent discovery of alloantisera with specific activity directed against the NK cells in fresh spleen cell preparations which lyse lymphoma targets ($NK_L$ cells), has provided a powerful tool with which to further analyze the effectors of natural killing (1,6). We describe herein the definition of the NK-1 system of $NK_L$ cell alloantigens, and
the use of anti-NK 1.2 serum, and other serological reagents, in an examination of the relationships between $NK_L$
cells, NK cells which lyse non-lymphoma targets ($NK_S$
cells), culture induced NK cells ($NK_C$ cells) and cytotoxic
T cells (Tc).

## METHODS

The inbred mice used in these studies were purchased
from Jackson Laboratories, Bar Harbor, Maine, and the backcross F1 and F2 mice were bred in our laboratory. Together
with the tumor cell lines employed they have been described
in detail elsewhere (2,3,4), as have the techniques used to
prepare spleen cell suspensions containing $NK_L$ and $NK_S$
cells (3) induce Tc and $NK_C$ in vitro (2,4), treat cells
with antibody and complement (4,9) and assay NK cells and Tc
by $^{51}Cr$ release from tumor targets (1,3). The serological
reagents: CBA anti-CE (anti-NK-1.1), CE anti-CBA (anti-NK-
1.2) C3H anti-ST (anti-NK-2.2), C3H anti-CBA (anti-LyM-1.2),
AKR anti-CBA (anti-Thy-1.2), B6AF1 anti-B10.D2 (anti-$K^d$)
and rabbit anti-mouse serum (RAMS) were prepared by hyper-

immunizing recipients with spleen and lymph node cells as
described elsewhere (4,9).  Monoclonal anti-Thy- 1.2 IgM
antibody (MC anti-Thy 1.2) was purchased from New England
Nuclear, Boston, MA.  (C3HxBALB/c)F1 anti-CE (anti-NK-1.1)
and (CExNZB)F1 anti-CBA (anti-NK-1.2) sera were kindly supplied by Dr. G. Koo and Dr. N.L. Warner respectively.

RESULTS

A.  The NK1 system of alloantigens

The CE anti-CBA serum was tested on fresh spleen cells
from individual mice of two backcross types (CExCBA)F1 x CE
and (CExC57BL/6)F1xCE.  The results (4; Burton and Winn, MS
submitted for publication) indicated that the anti-NK activity of this serum was directed at the product of a single
segregating locus which was expressed on a minor subpopulation of spleen cells which lysed YAC in vitro ($NK_L$ cells).
The C3H anti-ST serum was tested in a similar fashion
against spleen cells from (C3HxST)F1 x C3H backcross mice,
with results which lead to the same conclusion as the above.
Since C3H is a high and CE a low NK reactive strain, the
backcross mice positive for the NK alloantigen and negative
in the trypan blue test (9) have been backcrossed to C3H in
order to develop an NK congenic line on this background.  To
date, this line has reached the fourth backcross, and when
spleen cells from these mice were tested with C3H anti-ST
serum and C they were negative in the trypan blue test and
positive for removal of NK activity.
A backcross analysis of the (C3HxBALB/c)F1 anti-CE serum has shown that it too detects an NK specific alloantigen
which appears to be determined by a single gene (Dr. G. Koo,
personal communication).  The relationships between the NK
alloantigens detected by the various alloantisera have been
examined by comparing the strain distribution of the alloantigens detected by the various sera (Table 1), and also by
testing the spleen cells from individual (CBA x CE)F2 mice
simultaneously with all three of the above sera.  This analysis (Burton and Winn, submitted for publication) indicates
that there are a minimum of 4 alleles at the NK-1 locus and
that the C3H anti-ST serum detects an NK specific alloantigen which is not part of the NK-1 system.

B.  Heterogeneity of NK cells

A panel of tumor cell lines was tested for lysis by
fresh BALB/c spleen cells and levels of specific lysis >5%
were detected for all but two (EMT-6 and P-815) in 4-16 hour

Table 1. Strain distribution of NK alloantigens

| Antiserum | CBA C3H | C57BL/6 ST | NZB Ma/My | BALB/c DBA/2 | DBA/1 |
|---|---|---|---|---|---|
| anti-NK-1.1 | | | | | |
| CBA anti-CE | − | + | + | − | − |
| (BALB/c x C3H) anti-CE | − | + | + | − | − |
| anti-NK-1.2 | | | | | |
| CE anti-CBA | + | + | − | + | − |
| (NZB x CE)Fl anti-CBA | + | + | − | + | − |
| anti-NK-2.2 | | | | | |
| C3H anti ST | − | + | + | + | + |

*Mouse Strains* header spans CBA C3H, C57BL/6 ST, NZB Ma/My, BALB/c DBA/2, DBA/1

assays. Fresh spleen cells that had been treated with anti--NK-1.2 + C were then tested against 5 of these "lysable" tumors in a 16 hour assay, and it was found that NK activity against the 3 lymphoid tumors had been abolished, while NK activity against the two non-lymphoid tumors remained unchanged; thereby defining the $NK_L$ and $NK_S$ subclasses of NK cells in fresh spleen. The existence of these 2 subclasses had been suggested by Stutman et al. (8) and the results briefly described herein (Table 2), and reported in detail elsewhere, definitively etablish their existence (4).

Table 2. Susceptibility of various tumors to NK cell mediated lysis

| Tumor | Type | Susceptibility to Lysis | | |
|---|---|---|---|---|
| | | $NK_L$ | $NK_S$ | $NK_C$ |
| YAC | T-lymphoma | + | − | + |
| Cl.18 | plasmacytoma | + | − | + |
| PU-5 | macrophage tumor | + | − | n.t. |
| P-815 | mast cell tumor | − | − | + |
| FLD-3[a] | myeloid leukemia | − | + | + |
| WEH1-164 | fibrosarcoma | − | + | + |
| EMT-6 | carcinoma | − | − | + |

[a]Data from collaborative experiments with Dr. V. Kumar and Dr. M. Bennett.

Tumors were tested as targets in 6-16 hour assays using BALB/c spleen cells that had been cultured for 6 days as effectors. Levels of specific lysis >20% were observed in 6 hours for all targets, and EMT-6 and WEHI-164 were the most susceptible targets (Table 2). This finding in itself distinguishes this cultured cytotoxic effector cell ($NK_C$) activity from that of $NK_L$ and $NK_S$ cells.

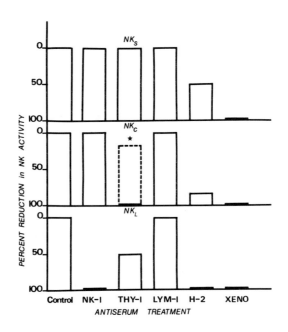

Figure 1.   Serological reactivity of NK cells.

A summary of the serological analysis of NK cells which lyse WEH1-164 and YAC appears in Figure 1. As can be seen, $NK_L$ cell activity is readily distinguished from $NK_S$ and $NK_C$ cell activity by virtue of its total sensitivity to anti-NK-1.2 + C treatment. Experiments with C57BL/6/-bg/bg (beige) mice, which have a near absolute defect in $NK_L$ cell activity against YAC have further confirmed the existence of $NK_L$ and $NK_S$ cell types, because $NK_S$ activity is normal in these mice (4). None of the NK cell subclasses expressed the B cell LyM-1 alloantigen (9).

The relationship between $NK_S$ and culture induced cytotoxic effector cells is complicated by what appears to be a heterogeneity of effectors induced by in vitro culture of lymphoid cells (2,4).

Table 3. A comparison of alloreactive Tc and culture induced Tc and $NK_C$

| BALB/c effector cells | Treatment | Percent Specific Lysis | | |
|---|---|---|---|---|
| | | YAC | | |
| BALB/c anti CBA | C | 53 + 3 | | |
| | anti-Thy-1.2 + C | 10 + 1 | | |
| | MC anti-Thy-1.2 + C | 5 + 1 | | |
| | | | P-815 | WEH1-164 |
| Cultured spleen | C | 30 | 29 | 49 |
| (means of 2-8 Expts) | anti-NK-1.2 + C | 31 | 31 | 32 |
| | anti-Thy-1.2 + C | 19 | 27 | 45 |
| | MC anti-Thy-1.2+C | 7 | 0 | 20 |
| | anti-LyM-1.2 + C | 22 | 24 | 44 |
| | anti-H-2$K^d$ + C | 5 | 0 | 15 |
| | RAMS + C | 0 | 0 | 5 |

A summary of the serological analysis of culture induced effectors is shown in Table 3, where it can be seen that at least 2 cytotoxic effector cell types appear to develop in cultures of spleen cells by themselves. Anti-Thy 1.2 serum treatment sharply distinguishes alloreactive Tc induced in vitro, and tumor specific Tc induced in vitro (4,5) from both of these culture induced effectors. However, treatment of cultured spleen cells with MC-anti-Thy 1.2 indicates that some at least of the culture induced effectors (those mediating all of the lysis of P-815, much of the lysis of YAC, and some of the lysis of WEHI-164) express Thy 1.2 (represented by a * in Figure 1). Therefore these cells are probably Tc with a low density of Thy 1.2 expression. This finding distinguishes these "spontaneous" Tc both from the remaining cultures induced effector cells, now designated $NK_C$, and also from $NK_S$ cells. The target preference and sensitivity to anti-$K^d$ treatment of these culture induced Tc and $NK_C$ further serve to distinguish them from $NK_S$ cells.

The relationship between $NK_L$ or $NK_S$ cells and $NK_C$ cells has been examined by culturing BALB/c spleen cells treated with anti-NK-1.2 or anti-H-$2K^d$ serum + C and untreated C57BL/6-bg/bg spleen cells for 6 days, and then testing them on YAC and WEHI-164. The results (4 and unpublished observations) indicate that $NK_L$ cells play no part in either $NK_C$ or spontaneous $T_C$ generation, and that $NK_S$ cells are probably the "precursors" of $NK_C$ cells but not of the spontaneous Tc.

## ACKNOWLEDGEMENT

This study was supported by Grants CA-17800 and CA-20044 awarded by the National Cancer Institute, Bethesda, Maryland and by Grants AM-07055 and HL-18646 from the National Institutes of Health, Bethesda, Maryland.

The authors acknowledge the excellent technical assistance of Mrs. J. Fortin and Mrs. K. Stenger.

[1] Robert C. Burton is a National Health and Medical Research Council of Australia Fellow in Applied Health Sciences.

## REFERENCES

1. Burton, R., Thompson, J., and Warner, N.L. J.Immun.Meth. 8:133, 1975.
2. Burton, R.C., Chism, S.E., and Warner, N.L. J.Immunol. 119:1329, 1977.
3. Burton, R.C., Grail, D., and Warner, N.L. Br.J.Cancer 37:806, 1978.
4. Burton, R. In Natural Cell Mediated Immunity to Tumors. R.B. Herberman (ed.). New York, Academic Press, 1980 (in press).
5. Burton, R.C., and Plate, J.M.D. Cell. Immunol., 1980 (in press).
6. Cantor, H., Hasai, M., Shen, F.W., Leclerc, J.C., and Glimcher, L. Imm.Rev. 44:3, 1979.
7. Paige, C.J., Figarella, E.F., Cuttito, M.J., Cahan, A., and Stutman, O. J.Immunol. 121:1827, 1978.
8. Stutman, O., Paige, C.J., and Figarella, E.F. J.Immunol. 121:1819, 1978.
9. Tonkonogy, S.L., and Winn, H.J. J.Immunol. 116:835, 1976.

# THE CHEDIAK-HIGASHI GENE IN HUMANS CONTROLS NK FUNCTION

Tina Haliotis and John C. Roder

Department of Microbiology and Immunology
Queen's University
Kingston, Ontario, Canada K7L 3N6

The immunodeficiency disorders have been instrumental in elucidating the development and interaction of the various B and T lymphoid components in the immune system of man. Natural killer (NK) cells represent one recently described but ill-defined subpopulation of lymphocytes which is thought to play an important role in surveillance against tumor development (9). Mice homozygous for the beige gene were found to have a selective deficiency in NK function (17; Roder this volume) and were more susceptible to transplantation of syngeneic tumors as predicted (8; Kiessling, this volume). We have recently reported that patients carrying the analogous, autosomal recessive Chediak-Higashi (CH) gene have a profound defect in their ability to spontaneously lyse various tumor cells in vitro by either antibody-dependent or independent mechanisms (6,10,19). Since other cell-mediated cytolytic functions were relatively normal, these results suggest that the beige or Chediak-Higashi gene in both man and mouse controls NK function.

The Chediak-Higashi syndrome in man is a rare, genetically determined disease manifested clinically by abnormal leukocyte granulation, defective pigmentation and an increased susceptibility to infections (22). Humoral immunity and delayed type hypersensitivity are normal (13) and children usually die of pyogenic infection, presumably resulting from a host defense abnormality related to defective granules in their polymorphonuclear (PMN) leukocytes (21,22). Survivors generally succumb to a lymphoproliferative disorder which may be malignant (4).

To investigate NK function, peripheral blood was separated by standard Ficoll-Hypaque gradient centrifugation and the mononuclear cell band was selectively depleted of most (90%) monocytes by adherence to microexudates of detached kidney cell monolayers. As shown in Table 1 lymphocytes from both CH patients were profoundly depressed in their ability to lyse K562 target cells, a human cell line of myeloid leukemia origin which is the most sensitive NK target described in the human. Data pooled from this and several repeat experiments revealed $85\pm12$ lytic units [LU/$10^6$ (n=6)] for age and sex matched normals and <0.1 LU/$10^6$ (n=2)

**419**

for the CH patients when LU were calculated at 20% lysis.
Thelow response in the CH patients was not altered by prolonged incubation time (up to 24 hr) and was evident in
tests of 6 different NK sensitive target cell lines including MOLT-4, Alab, CEM, MDA and human fetal fibroblasts (6).
The NK defect persisted during a 7 day incubation in vitro
with or without stimulator cells (10). As shown in Table 1,

Table 1. Defective NK and ADCC Activity in Lymphocytes from
CH Patients

| Donors | % Lysis* | | % TBC[++] |
|---|---|---|---|
| | NK | ADCC | |
| Normals | $60 \pm 5(66)$ | $70 \pm 3(200)$ | $24 \pm 4$ |
| CH patients | $7 \pm 1(<0.1)$ | $15 \pm 2 (2)$ | $25 \pm 2$ |

*Mean % lysis at 50/1 E:T ratio in a 4 hr $^{51}$Cr release assay
with lytic units/10$^6$ shown in brackets as calculated at a
20% level of lysis. The NK target was K562 and the ADCC
target was Chang pre-coated with rabbit anti-Chang antibody. Lysis of non-antibody coated Chang was 12% and 2% for
normals and CH respectively at a 50/1 E/T ratio.
++Nylon wool passed PBL were mixed with a 10 fold excess of
K562 cells and the % of target binding cells (TBC) was
enumerated (16).

lysis of Chang cells, precoated with an optimum dose of
rabbit anti-Chang antibody was also severely depressed. The
degree of cytolytic depression was similar against antibody-
coated Daudi targets, a human lymphoblastoid cell line and
lysis of antibody-coated RBL-5, a murine tumor, was also
markedly impaired although less so than the response against
human tumors (unpublished observation) (6). The failure of
CH lymphocytes to efficiently lyse human tumor cells was not
due to a generalized block in ADCC mechanism. Hence mononuclear effector cells and polymorphonuclear leukocytes
(PMN) from CH patients lysed antibody-coated human

erythrocytes (RBC) in a normal fashion (Table 2). When combined with the cell fractionation studies (19) these results
suggest that the defect in ADCC and NK in CH patients is
confined to a subpopulation of FcR+, non-adherent lymphocytes selectively blocked in their ability to lyse tumor
cell targets.

The selectivity of the antibody-independent NK cell defect is shown in Table 2. Lymphocytes were blocked in their
ability to spontaneously lyse tumor cell targets whereas
spontaneous cytolysis of tumor cells by monocytes was normal
(line 5). Surprisingly, cytostasis by neutrophils from CH
patients against K562 cells was also normal (line 8), as was
lectin generated killing by this cell type (line 7). Since
lysosomal enzymes and degranulation are abnormal in CH patients (reviewed in 22;21) these results suggest that lysosomal granules are not involved in PMN cytostasis or cytolysis against these target cell lines. The population of T
killer cells, as measured by lectin dependent cytolysis was
normal in one patient (Le) but low in the other (La, line
6). Therefore a definitive statement on the status of cytolytic T cells in these patients awaits a larger study. However, T cell mediated immunity in general was previously
shown to be normal in these and other patients as judged by
skin testing and proliferative responses to T dependent
mitogens (5).

Further experiments suggested that the CH defect may
lie within the lytic pathway rather than at the level of
population size. Nonadherent lymphocytes from CH patients
were completely normal in their ability to bind and lyse
K562 (Table 1). MOLT-4 was also bound whereas P815, an NK
insensitive target, was not bound to lysed by CH or normal
donors (6). Most of the TBC detected in this system have
been shown to represent NK cells in the mouse (15) and in
the human TBC can be specifically inhibited by pre-incubation of effector cells with solubilized glycoproteins from NK
sensitive targets (16). Therefore if the relative number of
TBC in a heterogeneous human lymphocyte population is a reliable estimate of the frequency of NK cells, as in the
mouse, then these results sugest that NK cells are present
in CH patients but do not function.

Suppressor cells in the NK system appear primarily to
be adherent, macrophage-like cells (reviewed in 3). Suppressor cells did not appear to be responsible for the low
NK response of CH patients since removal of FcR cells or
cells adherent to Sephadex G-10, nylon wool or microexudates
did not restore the low NK response in CH patients (6). In
addition no suppression of cytolysis was seen in mixtures of
CH and normal lymphocytes, even at the highest ratios tested

Table 2. Other Immune Functions in CH Patients

| Effector Function | Target | Normals | CH Patients |
|---|---|---|---|
| **A). This Study** | | | |
| 1. NK (lymphocyte) | tumor cells | + | - |
| 2. ADCC (lymphocyte) | tumor cells | + | - |
| 3. ADCC (mononuclear) | erythrocytes | + | + |
| 4. ADCC (neutrophil) | erythrocytes | + | + |
| 5. Spontaneous (monocyte) | tumor cells | + | + |
| 6. Lectin induced (lymphocytes) | tumor cells | + | +/- |
| 7. Lectin induced (neutrophils) | tumor cells | + | + |
| 8. Spontaneous cytostasis (neutrophils) | tumor cells | + | + |
| 9. Proliferation (PHA, ConA, PWM) | | + | + |
| **B). Previous Studies** | | | |
| 10. Serum Ig and complement | | + | + |
| 11. Antibody response to S. typhosa endotoxin and common vaccines | | + | + |
| 12. Delayed type hypersensitivity to mumps, Candida, DNCB and SKSD | | + | + |
| 13. Proliferative response to mitogens (PHA, ConA, PWM) | | + | + |

The summary of A (this study) is taken from data in Ref. 6,10, and 19. Previous studies (B) on the same patients have been gathered from data summarized by Blume and Wolff (1).

+, indicates a normal response whereas - indicates a severely impaired response.

(2/1).

In summary we have described the first immunodeficiency disorder in humans with an apparently selective deficit in effector functions mediated by NK cells and cells involved in ADCC. Other studies of the more familiar immunodeficiencies, involving impairments of both B and T cells, failed to reveal significant defects in NK function (14) except in the case of severe combined immunodeficiency (11). Impairments of ADCC are more widespread (reviewed in Pross et al. 14) and in one study of X-linked agammaglobulinemia ADCC was defective whereas NK activity was normal (11). In view of the complexity involved it is not surprising that different genes would control unique steps in an otherwise common cytolytic pathway in a single cell, possibly mediating both ADCC and NK activity.

The precise location of the defective gene product in the cytolytic pathway is not known but may involve an impairment of cGMP mediated triggering of NK cells since (i) cGMP causes a small but significant enhancement of NK activity in mice whereas cAMP decreases the level of cytolysis (18), (ii) cGMP or inducers thereof have been shown to improve other defects in CH patients such as abnormal granule morphology (12) and chemotaxis (2), and (iii) interferon, which boosts NK activity in CH patients (19) is known to cause a transient increase in cGMP levels in lymphoid cells (20) and finally in the most direct experiments a short preincubation of CH lymphocytes with cGMP restored the NK response to within normal levels (Katz, Roder, Fauci and Herberman, unpublished observations).

It is intriguing to note that CH patients surviving early infections almost invariably succumb to a lymphoproliferative disorder which is thought to be malignant (4). Eighty-five percent of the 53 cases on record had clearly entered the lymphoma-like stage (1). Closer scrutiny of this phenomenon may provide the first direct evidence that NK cells in the human are involved in surveillance against spontaneous tumor development.

## REFERENCES

1.  Blume, R.S., and Wolff, S.M. Medicine 51:247, 1972.
2.  Boxer, L.A., Watanabe, A., Rister, M., Besch, H., Allen, J., and Bachner, R. N.Eng.J.Med. 295:1041, 1979.
3.  Cudkowicz, G., and Hochman, P.S. Immunol.Rev. 44:13, 1979.
4.  Dent, P.B., Fish, L.A., White, J.F., and Good, R.A. Lab.Invest. 15:1634, 1966.

5.   Gallin, J.I., Elin, R.J., Hubert, R.T., Fauci, A.S.,
     Kaliner, M.A., and Wolff, S.M.  Blood 53:226, 1969.
6.   Haliotis, T., Roder, J., Klein, M., Ortaldo, J., Fauci,
     A.S., and Herberman, R.B.  J.Exp.Med. 151:000, 1980.
7.   Herberman, R.B., Djeu, J.Y., Kay, H.D., Ortaldo, J.R.,
     Riccardi, C., Bonnard, G.D., Holden, H.T., Fagnani, R.,
     Santoni, A., and Puccetti, P.   Immunol.Rev. 44:43,
     1979.
8.   Karre, K., Kiessling, R., Klein, G., and Roder, J.
     Nature, 1980 (in press).
9.   Kiessling, R., and Wigzell, H.   Immunol.Rev. 44:165,
     1979.
10.  Klein, M., Roder, J., Haliotis, T., Korec, S., Jett,
     J.R., Herberman, R.B., Katz, P., and Fauci, A.S.
     J.Exp.Med. 151:000, 1980.
11.  Koren, H., Amos, B., and Buckley, R.   J.Immunol.
     120:796, 1978.
12.  Oliver, J., and Zurier, R.B.   J.Clin.Invest. 57:1239,
     1976.
13.  Page, A.R., Berendes, H., Warner, J., and Good, R.A.
     Blood 20:330, 1962.
14.  Pross, H., Gupta, S., Good, R.A., and Baines, M.G.
     Cell.Immunol. 43:160, 1979.
15.  Roder, J.C., Kiessling, R., Biberfeld, P., and
     Andersson, B.  J.Immunol. 121:2509, 1978.
16.  Roder, J.C., Ahrlund-Richter, L., and Jondal, M.
     J.Exp.Med. 150:471, 1979.
17.  Roder, J.C., and Duwe, A.K.   Nature (Lond) 278:451,
     1979.
18.  Roder, J.C., and Klein, M.  J.Immunol. 123:2785, 1979.
19.  Roder, J.C., Haliotis, T., Klein, M., Korec, S., Jett,
     J.R., Ortaldo, J., Herberman, R.B., Katz, P., and
     Fauci, A.S.  Nature, 1980 (in press).
20.  Tovey, M.G., Rochette-Egly, C., and Custagna, M.
     Proc.Natl.Acad.Sci. USA. 76:3890, 1979.
21.  Vassalli, J.D., Cranelli-Piperno, A., Griscelli, C.,
     and Reich, E.  J.Exp.Med. 147:1285, 1978.
22.  Windhorst, D.B., and Padgett, G.  J. Invest. Dermatol.
     60:529, 1973.

# ANALYSIS OF THE GENETIC CONTROL OF NATURAL KILLER CELL ACTIVITY MAY REQUIRE STUDIES OF GENETICS WITH SEGREGATING ALLELES AMONG LITTERMATES

R. Michael Williams and Roger Melvold

Section of Medical Oncology
Department of Medicine and Microbiology-Immunology
and the Cancer Center
Northwestern University
Chicago, Illinois

## INTRODUCTION

Numerous immunological phenomena including natural killer cell activity (NKCA) appear to depend on the major histocompatibility complex (MHC) (1,3,4). Some original demonstrations of MHC effects resulted from studies of appropriately MHC typed backcross populations while many other studies have utilized MHC congenics which differ only by the many genes which are included in the MHC.

As part of a general program to define MHC dependent phenomena more precisely, our laboratory has embarked on a systematic program to evaluate H-2 dependent immune responses in mice with mutant H-2 alleles. Because most H-2 mutants probably differ from the wild type by a single gene, the mechanism underlying immunological differences observed between two such partner strains may be potentially deciphered at the molecular level. However, it is essential to rule out possible confounding environmental effects. Since siblings offer the most rigorous control for such effects, any truly H-2 linked phenomenon should be maintained among appropriately typed segregating backcross populations. We observed a significant differences in natural killer cell activity between C57BL/6Kh (B6) and B6.C-H-2$^{bml}$ mice, but the H-2 dependence of this observation was not substantiated in typed backcross populations.

## MATERIALS AND METHODS

All mice were bred, splenectomized, and skin grafted in the closed colony of H.I. Kohn at the Shields Warren Radiation Laboratory, Harvard Medical School. To avoid possible effects of skin grafting on NKCA, littermate animals were splenectomized for NKCA determination at 8 weeks of age. Then the genotype of each mouse was subsequently determined by skin grafting. This approach also meant that the indivi-

dual H-2 genotypes were not known until long after the NKCA
values were determined. NKCA was determined utilizing YAC-1
cells as targets by a method previously described in detail
(5). In brief, several splenocyte to target ratios are
tested and the data are fitted to the anticipated straight
line of log % 4hr corrected $^{51}$Cr-release vs log splenocyte
to target ratio. The correlation coefficient $r$ is calculated as that splenocyte to target ratio which gives 25% corrected $^{51}$Cr-release (L.U.$_{25}$ ratio). A killer unit (K.U.) is
defined as 6250 divided by the LU$_{25}$ ratio.

    Since the sensitivity of different preparations of
$^{51}$Cr-labelled YAC-1 preparations may differ, comparisons
among experimental groups are strictly valid only when individuals from each are tested on the same target preparation. Unfortunately, it is nearly impossible to study large
numbers of age matched and H-2 typed individuals in a single
experiment. The data in Figures 1 and 2 were obtained in a
single experiment. The data presented in Figure 3 represent
results obtained in three separate experiments and individuals from each are identified by separate symbols.


                              RESULTS


    Groups of littermate animals chosen from among the
following different mutant genotype strains were compared to
wild type C57BL/6Kh for NKCA: B6.C-H-2$^{bm1}$, B6.H-2$^{bm5}$,
B6.H-2$^{bm8}$, and B6.C-H-2$^{bm9}$. BALB/cKh was also compared
to BALB/c-H-2$^{dm2}$. The only significant difference from
wild type observed was apparently diminished NKCA among B6.-
C-H-2$^{bm1}$ mice (Figs. 1 and 2).

    The data in Figure 1 show the mean % corrected $^{51}$Cr re-
lease for groups of B6 and B6.C-H-2$^{bm1}$ mice. Table 1
contains the data calculated from the curve of % corrected
$^{51}$Cr-release vs splenocyte/target ratio for each individual
spleen cell preparation. The transformation of these data
to killer unit values for individual animals is shown in
Figure 2. By any reasonable type of analysis the wild type
H-2$^b$ mice appeared to have superior NKCA. The calculated
ratio for 25% $^{51}$Cr-release was lower (38 ± 10 vs 146 ± 30)
and thus the NKCA in killer units was higher (194 ± 38 vs 53
± 10). While there was no difference in missions of cells
per spleen (95 ± 5 vs 110 ± 6), the H-2$^b$ mice had more
lytic units per spleen (120 ± 25 vs 36 ± 5). Thus, we conducted the appropriate backcross experiments to verify expected H-2K$^b$ linkage of NKCA.

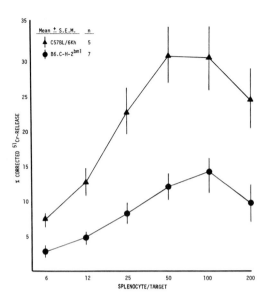

Figure 1. Natural Killer Cell Activity in C57BL/6 (H-2$^b$) and B6.C-H-2$^{bm1}$.

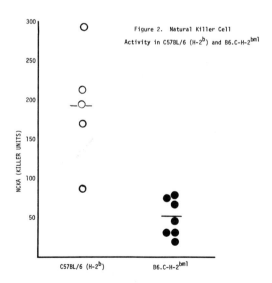

Figure 2. Natural Killer Cell Activity in C57BL/6 (H-2$^b$) and B.6C-H-2$^{bm1}$.

Table 1. Calculated Parameters for NKCA for Individual C57BL/6Kh and B6.C-H-$2^{bm1}$ mice.

| C57BL/6Kh | $r^2$ | L.U.$_{25}$ ratio[3] | Killer[4] Units | Cells/ Spleen ($\times 10^{-6}$) | L.U.$_{25}$/Spleen[5] |
|---|---|---|---|---|---|
| 1 | .983 | 21.1 | 297 | 93 | 177 |
| 2 | .987 | 70.2 | 89 | 83 | 47 |
| 3 | .987 | 32.0 | 195 | 106 | 132 |
| 4 | .996 | 28.8 | 217 | 107 | 149 |
| 5 | .995 | 36.3 | 172 | 87 | 96 |

| B6.C-H-$2^{bm1}$ | | | | | |
|---|---|---|---|---|---|
| 1 | .950 | 89.7 | 70 | 97 | 43 |
| 2 | .998 | 186.2 | 34 | 125 | 27 |
| 3 | .986 | 76.8 | 81 | 108 | 56 |
| 4 | .998 | 80.0 | 78 | 87 | 44 |
| 5 | .993 | 181.4 | 34 | 120 | 27 |
| 6 | .998 | 128.5 | 49 | 111 | 35 |
| 7 | .995 | 278.3 | 22 | 125 | 18 |

[1] In this particular experiment the total cpm for 25,000 $^{51}$Cr-labelled YAC-1 cells was 8000 and spontaneous release was 9% in 4 hours.
[2] Correlation coefficient for log % $^{51}$Cr-release vs splenocyte/target ratio based on splenocyte/target <100.
[3] Calculated splenocyte/target ratio which would produce 25% corrected $^{51}$Cr-release.
[4] 6250 ÷ L.U.$_{25}$ ratio.
[5] Lytic units per spleen.

The NK (killer units) of individual mice from both possible backcross populations is shown in Figure 3. The values span a range (21-718) which is greater than that for either parental strain. F1 hybrids were not tested since the genotype H-$2^b$/H-$2^{bm1}$ is reproduced in both back-crosses.

Clearly, there was no difference in mean NKCA among any of the genotypes. Except for a single extraordinarily high value of 718 KU obtained from one H-$2^{b/b}$ animal (this single value was excluded in calculations of mean NKCA), the means for each genotype (denoted by the horizontal lines in Figure 3) are nearly identical.

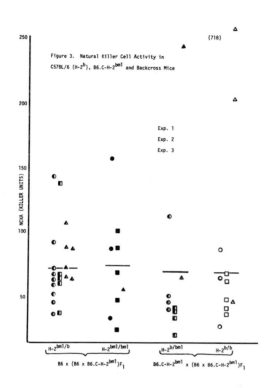

Figure 3. Natural Killer Cell Activity in
C57BL/6 (H-2$^b$), B6.C-H-2$^{bm1}$ and Backcross Mice

**Figure 3.** Natural Killer Cell Activity in C57BL/6(H-2$^b$), B6.C-H-2$^{bm1}$ and Backcross Mice.

## DISCUSSION

The recent flurry of investigations concerning natural killer cell activity have characterized the cells involved in some detail but little concrete information has developed to further our understanding of the purported H-2 influence. Thus, the apparent findings of a difference in NKCA between two strains which differ only by a mutation at the H-2K$^b$ gene seemed to offer some potential for giving more precise information. The fact that this difference did not persist among typed segregating littermates justifies a speculation that many apparently genetic differences observed between non-littermate strains, including congenics, could be artifacts. Indeed, even if NKCA depends on exposure to specific pathogens as recently suggested (2) the variations seen in this work appear to be independent of H-2 phenotype and thus are apparently not genetically controlled. Whether any aspect of NKCA depends directly on the MHC is an open question. Also, experiments comparing $H-2^{b/b}$ vs $H-2^{bml/bml}$ littermates of an F2 generation would be required to address the remote possibility that homozygosity is required to detect true single gene H-2 effects on NKCA.

REFERENCES

1.  Clark, E.A., and Harmon, R.C.  Adv.Cancer Res. 31:227, 1980.

2.  Clark, E.A., Russell, P.H., Egghart, M., and Horton, M.A.  Int. J.Cancer 24:688, 1979.

3.  Petranyi, G., Kiessling, R., and Klein, G. Immunogenetics 2:53, 1975.

4.  Petranyi, G., Kiessling, R., Povey, S., Klein, G., Herzenberg, L., and Wigzell, H.  Immunogenetics 3:15, 1976.

5.  Williams, R.M.  In Immune Mechanisms and Disease. D.B. Amos, R.S. Schwartz, and B.W. Janicki (eds).  New York: Academic Press, p163, 1979.

GENETIC RESISTANCE TO TUMORS:   ROLES OF MARROW-DEPENDENT AND
-INDEPENDENT CELLS

Michael Bennett, Vinay Kumar, Elinor Levy and Pamela Rodday
Departments of Pathology and Microbiology
Boston University School of Medicine
Boston, Massachusetts 02118

The immunogenetics of resistance to grafts of normal hemopoietic cells involves the recognition Hybrid or Hemopoietic histocompatibility (Hh) antigens (1,9) by radioresistant effector cells (10,11). The Hh antigens are inherited as recessive traits, and this is the basis of "hybrid resistance" to hemopoietic cell grafts.   Hybrid resistance was discovered by transplanting marrow cells into irradiated mice but was extended in studies of neoplastic hemopoietic cell grafts in unirradiated mice (8). The precise nature of the effector cells responsible for hybrid resistance has not been determined.   The weakening of hybrid resistance by administration of silica particles suggested that they were macrophages (31) even though stimulation of macrophages by heat-killed Corynebacterium parvum organisms abrogated hybrid resistance and resistance to H-2 allogeneic marrow resistance to marrow grafts by mice treated with the bone-seeking isotope, $^{89}$Sr, suggested that the effector cells were marrow-dependent (M) cells (2).   The discovery of "natural killer" (NK) cells (19,21)and the observation that $^{89}$Sr treatment depresses NK cell function (17) led to the conclusion by some that NK cells must be the effectors of resistance to grafts of normal and neoplastic hemopoietic cells.   The simultaneous observations that Hh antigens were responsible for recognition of EL-4 lymphoma cells in vivo and that natural killer cells for EL-4 tumor cells recognized Hh (6,18) must have cemented this concept in the minds of many interested in hybrid resistance.

However, there are controversies and uncertainties regarding the nature of the effector cells responsible for genetic resistance to tumor cells.   There are two major reasons for this.   Firstly, it is becoming increasingly clear that natural killer cells themselves are heterogeneous (vide infra).   Secondly, treatment of mice with $^{89}$Sr not only suppresses NK effector function but also increases the numbers/functions of suppressor cells and their precursors in the body (23,29,33).   Such findings have led some to doubt the existence of M cells and to postulate that all of the immunological defects of mice treated with $^{89}$Sr can be explained by the presence of suppressor cells (12).   We describe here a review and up-date of our work in this field.

GENETIC CONTROL OF NATURAL RESISTANCE
TO INFECTION AND MALIGNANCY

There is certainly not enough information available about effector cells and suppressor cells for one to draw final conclusions about these controversial points.

## BIOLOGICAL EFFECTS OF ADMINISTRATION OF LARGE DOSE OF $^{89}$Sr (100 µCi) TO MICE

$^{89}$Sr is a long-lived beta ray emitting isotope which is very energetic but does not penetrate its effects much more than 1 mm; it is a calcium antagonist or competitor and is incorporated into many tissues initially. However, it is considered a bone-seeking isotope because it remains in bone tissue for long periods of time. In the mouse, the marrow tissue is chronically irradiated and becomes hypoplastic, i.e., the marrow cavity contains primarily mature RBC and granulocytes.

The spleen takes over all of the stem cell functions of the body (2,16). Histologically, the white pulp is preserved and contains germinal centers in follicles (B cell areas) and well-populated periarteriolar lymphatic sheaths (T cell areas). The red pulp of the spleen is expanded by intense myelopoiesis, i.e., erythropoiesis, granulocytopoiesis and megakaryocytes. There are numerous phagocytic cells in the spleen. Lymph nodes contain follicles and inter-follicular lymphocytes. There is a mast cell infiltration of the thymus, lymph nodes and spleen (3). Normally, mast cells are restricted to the connective tissue surrounding these organs. Multiple small collections of maturing granulocytes can often be detected in the thymus and lymph nodes. Similar collections of granulocytes can be seen in mice which have been irradiated and repopulated with marrow cells. The effect of the mast cells or granulocytes ectopically located in lymphoid tissue has not been determined.

Mice treated with $^{89}$Sr are able to reject skin allografts rapidly and are able to generate normal numbers of antibody-forming cells in response to T-dependent antigens. The mice were quite sensitive to the immunosuppressive effects of low doses of total-body irradiation, however (16). Spleen cells of $^{89}$Sr-treated mice can respond to SRBC antigens upon adoptive transfer to irradiated mice (2), but pre-culturing the cells eliminates that capacity (33).

The genetic resistance of (C3H X C57BL)F1 mice, following irradiation, to grafts of incompatible parental-strain C57BL or allogeneic DBA/2 marrow cells is lost (2). Similarly, the genetic resistance of NZB or (NZB X C57BL)F1 mice, following iradiation, to grafts of allogeneic C3H graft-versus-host cells is weakened, although to a lesser extent (3). The genetic resistance of (C57BL/6 X DBA/2)F1 unirradiated mice to grafts of parental-strain EL-4 lymphoma cells is lost (32).

The genetic resistance of (C57BL/6 X DBA/2)F1 mice to early stages of infection with the facultative intracellular bacterium, Listeria monocytogenes, is impaired (4). There was no increase in susceptibility to infection with the extracellular bacterium, Yersinia pestis, a finding consistent with the concept that granulocytic function is intact. The genetic resistance to infection with Herpes Simples Virus-1 is also lost; the mice trated with $^{89}$Sr die of encephalomyelitis with minimal histological changes in the spinal cord or brain (30).

There is a loss of the genetically determined ability of NK cells to lyse YAC-1 and RL 1 lymphoma cells (17,27). The numbers of "target-binding cells" in the spleen are normal but the cells do not kill YAC-1 target cells even after the administration of interferon inducers or preparations containing types I or II interferon (28). Antibody-dependent cellular cytotoxicity, or "killer" (K) cell function is depressed if the appropriate target cell and antibody preparation are studied (Table 1). K cell function was normal if chicken RBC were the target cells (3).

Table 1.   Effect of $^{89}$Sr on NK(YAC-1) activity and on K(EL-4) activity of spleen cells.

| Treatment of B6D2F1 mice | Assay | Mean % Specific Cytotoxicity at E:T ratios of: | | | |
|---|---|---|---|---|---|
| | | 50:1 | 25:1 | 12.5:1 | Student's t test |
| Vehicle | NK(YAC-1) | 54.1 | 35.8 | 21.5 | |
| $^{89}$Sr[a] | NK(YAC-1) | 9.7 | 11.4 | 10.4 | p<0.01 |
| Vehicle | K(EL-4)[b] | 13.7 | 10.4 | 6.9 | p<0.01 |
| $^{89}$Sr | K(EL-4) | -3.3 | 2.7 | 1.9 | |

[a]  100 µCi i.p. twice at a monthly interval; assay done 4 weeks later.

[b]  1:1000 A anti-B6(H-2b) serum; 6-hour incubation for both assays.

There is a loss of the genetic resistance of C57BL/6 mice to the erythroleukemic (Fv-2$^{rr}$) and immunosuppressive (Fv-3$^{rr}$) effects of Friend virus complex (22,23,24,25,26).

Certain strains of Friend virus induces a leukemia which spontaneously regresses (35);  pretreatment of mice with $^{89}$Sr prevents the regression of the leukemia (15).

Long-term administration of $^{89}$Sr to (NZB X NZW)F1 mice lessens the severity of autoimmune disease associated with glomerulonephritis (40). Life span was not increased due to a high incidence of sarcomas in the treated mice. It was reasoned that T suppressor cell function would increase in these mice after $^{89}$Sr treatment so as to weaken autoimmune reactions.

Treatment of C57BL/6 mice with $^{89}$Sr results in the inhibition of cell-mediated lympholysis (CML) responses to the syngeneic tumor, EL-4 (14). Similar treatment of (C57BL/6 X DBA/2)F1 mice results in a poor CML response of their spleen cells to parental-strain C57BL/6 cells, i.e., hybrid resistance by T cells in vitro (12,29). CML responses to H-2 allogeneic spleen cells is either normal or only moderately suppressed.

Suppressor cells appear in the splen which are capable of inhibiting antibody formation in vitro and, following a 24-hour incubation, can inhibit antibody formation in vivo (33). This suppressor cell abnormality is transferable to lethally irradiated recipient mice by spleen cells of mice treated with $^{89}$Sr (29). This suppressor cell can be generated in athymic nude mice by $^{89}$Sr treatment, indicating that it is not a T cell (33). Following the 24-hour incubation, we have observed that spleen cells of these mice can inhibit responses to mitogens but cannot inhibit lysis of YAC-1 target cells by NK effectors from normal mice.

## IS MARROW A CENTRAL LYMPHOID ORGAN?

In support of the concept that marrow is the central lymphoid organ for NK ells capable of lysing YAC-1 tumor cells and for effector cells capable of mediating rejection of bone marrow allografts were the findings that long-term administration of estradiol to mice resulted in osteopetrosis with the loss of marrow tissue and loss of those effector functions (38,39). Congenital osteopetrosis (mi/mi) was associated with loss of NK cell function, also.

We have implanted single tibias into mice previously injected with $^{89}$Sr in an attempt to restore the marrow microenvironment. Five or six weeks after bone implantation, the spleens were removed and the portion of the spleen with the implant was dissected away. The remainder of the spleen was assessed for NK (YAC-1) cell function. As a percentage of age-control cytotoxicity values at a 50:1 effector: target cell ratio, the implants improved NK activity from 18 $\pm$ 5.4 to 48 $\pm$ 6.0 (p <0.01). NK cell function was still significantly less than control values, indicating a partial restoration of function. We are now assessing a variety of functions after similar bone implants in mice treated with [89]Sr.

Let us examine the alternative proposal that marrow is not a central lymphoid organ and that the presence of suppressor cells can explain the immune abnormalities of [89]Sr- or estradiol- treated mice. It is certainly true that the spleens of such mice do take over the functions of bone marrow with respect to myelopoiesis and yet retain lymphoid cell function. We have detected suppressor cells in normal bone marrow of mice (7) that share very similar properties to those in spleens of mice treated with [89]Sr (Table 2). The only difference we detected was the result of cell transfer to irradiated mice. Spleens of mice repopulated with marrow cells do not contain the suppressor cells whereas spleens of mice grafted with spleen cells of [89]Sr-treated mice do contain suppressor cells with similar properties (29). In that study, some of the defects observed in mice treated with [89]Sr were not detected in mice repopulated with spleen cells. For example the recipient mice were perfectly able to reject incompatible marrow cells after irradiation (29).

If NK cells are not M cells, what are they? It was logical to suggest that NK cells were pre-T cells (20) since their activity could be partially suppressed by anti-Thy-1.2 serum plus complement. Moreover, nude mice have high NK cell function. However, if one defines pre-T cells as those cells capable of repopulating the thymus of irradiated mice, NK cells do not appear to be pre-T cells. Marrow cells were stimulated with thymopoietin and later treated with anti-Thy-1.2 serum plus complement. The marrow cells (B6D2F1) were used to repopulate irradiated BALB/c mice in order to be able to distinguish between donor and host cells later. This procedure prevented repopulation of the thymus by approximately 65% but did not inhibit the generation of NK cells 4 to 8 weeks after cell transfer. One might even argue that pre-T cells (or some pre-T cells) are themselves marrow-dependent from a study by Stutman (41). He observed that adult, but not fetal yolk sac, stem cells could repopulate the thymus of recipient mice treated with [89]Sr.

## HETEROGENEITY OF NATURAL KILLER CELLS

The first indication that NK cells may be heterogeneous was presented by Stutman (42). Cells cytotoxic for Meth A sarcoma cells were present in spleens of neonatal mice,

Table 2. A Comparison of Non-T Suppressor Cells Found in Normal Bone Marrow and the Spleen of 89Sr Treated Mice.

| Characteristic | Bone Marrow Cell | 89Sr Suppressor Cell |
|---|---|---|
| T-independent antibody synthesis in vitro | Suppressed | Suppressed |
| T-dependent antibody synthesis in vitro | Suppressed | Suppressed |
| Induction of suppressor for mitogenic response by preculturing | + | + |
| Induction of suppressor for in vivo antibody response by preculturing | + | + |
| Reversal of suppression by mitomycin C pretreatment | | |
| a) AB synthesis in vitro | + | + |
| b) Mitogen | - | - |
| Radiation sensitivity (1000R in vitro) | | |
| a) Antibody synthesis in vitro | + | + |
| b) Antibody synthesis in vivo | - | - |
| c) Mitogen | - | - |
| Cell size | Large cell | Large cell |
| Adherent to Sephadex G-10 | + | + |
| Present in nude mice | + | + |
| Suppressor function transferred to lethally irradiated recipient spleen | - | + |

whereas NK cells cytotoxic for YAC-1 lymphoma cells do not mature until three weeks of age (19,21). The NK cells capable of lysing EL-4 target cells are also functional in neonatal mice (27) and differ from NK(YAC-1) cells in that they are functional in spleens of mice treated with $^{89}$Sr. The immunogenetics of the NK(EL-4) and NK(YAC-1) also differ. The NK(EL-4) appears to recognize Hh-1$^{\underline{b}}$ antigens (6,18) and Ir-like genes which regulate in vivo responses to C57BL-(Hh-1$^{\underline{b}}$) marrow grafts are reflected in this assay (27). The "promonocyte" natural killer cell differs from the "conventional" NK cell in that the beige (bg) mutation results in no loss of promonocyte NK lysis of YAC-1 cells whereas the bg mutation results in the loss of the conventional NK lysis of the same target cells (36,37).

In an attempt originally designed to study the mechanism of Fv-2 gene function, we developed an NK assay using Friend virus-transformed cells grown in vitro, FLD-3 cells. FLD-3 cells are BALB/c origin (13) and release large amounts of Friend virus complex. Whereas YAC-1 cells are lysed within 4 hours, FLD-3 and EL-4 cells are not lysed well until 18-24 hours. Lysis of all three targets is stimulated by pretreatment of mice with interferon inducers, is suppressed by pretreatment with cyclophosphamide, and is mildly suppressed (if at all) by pretreatment with silica particles. $^{89}$Sr-treatment inhibits NK(YAC-1) cells strongly, but inhibits NK(EL-4) and NK(FLD-3) only a fraction of the times tested. Infant mice and bg/bg (C57BL background) mice have normal NK activity against FLD-3 but not against YAC-1 cells. NK(FLD-3) cells can be distinguished from the NK-(YAC-1) and NK(EL-4) cells by their functional loss from spleens of mice 3 days after exposure to 800 R of total-body irradiation (Table 3). All strains of mice tested have good NK(FLD-3) cell function.

Table 3. Effect of pre-iradiation on NK cell functions

| Target cells | Mean % Specific Cytotoxicity* | | | |
|---|---|---|---|---|
| | 800 R on Day 0 | | 800 R -3 days | |
| YAC-1 | 57.6 | 33.8 | 70.3 | 63.8 |
| EL-4 | 17.5 | 9.3 | 27.0 | 19.0 |
| FLD-3 | 20.2 | 20.9 | 6.2 | 1.0 |
| E:T | 50:1 | 25:1 | 50:1 | 25:1 |

*B6D2F1 splenic effector cells; 18-hour incubation.

DO K CELLS MEDIATE GENETIC RESISTANCE AGAINST NORMAL AND
LEUKEMIC HEMOPOIETIC CELLS IN VIVO

    Rabbit anti-mouse brain (RAMB) serum treatment of mouse
bone marrow cells in vitro inhibits stem cell functions in
vivo by a complement-independent mechanism (5,43).  Due to
the close association between NK(YAC-1) cells and K cells
for tumor target cells (34 and Table 1), we decided to test
the hypothesis that K cells mediate the suppression of stem
cells pretreated with RAMB serum.  Marrow cells were incubated with RAMB serum (1:50 dilution) and complement (1:10
dilution of guinea pig serum), were washed, and inocula of 2
x $10^6$ nucleated cells were infused into irradiated (800 R)
mice.  Some of the mice had been treated 1 day earlier with
2.5 mg silica particles i.v. to suppress "marrow allograft
reactivity".  Silica particles "revived" the marrow stem
cells, as determined by measuring the uptake of 5-iodo-2'-
deoxyuridine-$^{125}$I(IUdR) in spleens 5 days after cell transfer (Table 4).  Cells treated with only complement grew
slightly better than cells treated with RAMB serum and infused into mice treated with silica (data not shown).  Another method of inhibiting the rejection of incompatible
marrow cells, i.e., 500 R 10 days prior to 800 R and cell
transfer, also allowed growth of syngeneic marrow cells pretreated with RAMB serum.

    Table 4.  Effect of silica pretreatment on the growth of
marrow cells treated with rabbit anti-mouse brain (RAMB)
serum in irradiated mice.

| Donor strain | Host strain | Geometric mean (95% C.L.) splenic IUdR uptake (%) | | Treat-ment |
| --- | --- | --- | --- | --- |
| | | Vehicle | Silica | |
| B6D2F1 | B6D2F1 | 0.12(0.09-0.18) | 0.48(0.36-0.62)* | |
| C3H | B6D2F1 | 0.22(0.15-0.32) | 0.69(0.44-1.11)* | |
| WB | WB | 0.16(0.10-0.51) | 0.92(0.63-1.35)* | |

* p<0.001, silica v. vehicle.  Marrow cells were treated
with RAMB serum as described in the test.  Isotope assay
performed 5 days after cell transfer.

The growth of inocula of $10^6$ FLD-3 tumor cells in spleens of irradiated syngeneic BALB/c mice was also suppressed by pretreatment with RAMB plus complement, as measured by splenic IUdR uptake (%) 5 days after cell transfer. Treatment of prospective recipient mice with silica particles allowed the cells to grow very well (10-fold effect). Thus K cells, under certain conditions, may inhibit the growth of normal and neoplastic hemopoietic progenitor cells. Presumably, silica treatment inhibits the function of those K cells.

FLD-3 cells were resisted by irradiated mice of a number of strains, some of which were H-2$^d$. These included B10.D2, DBA/2, (BALB/c X B10.D2)F1 (all H-2$^d$) and B6D2F1, WB and C3H strain mice. We decided to test the possibility that NK(FLD-3) and silica-sensitive effector cells both functioned in vivo against FLD-3 cells. Prospective recipient B6D2F1 mice were irradiated (8000 R) 3 days prior to infusion of FLD-3 cells, injected with 2.5 mg silica 1 day before irradiation and cell transfer, irradiated 3 days, and injected with silica 1 day, before challenge with FLD-3; or were irradiated 1 day before they were challenged with inocula of $10^6$ FLD-3 cells. The geometric mean IUdR uptake (%) values 5 days after cell transfer were 0.04 (controls), 0.14 (800 R -3 days), 0.33 (silica -1 day) and 2.89 (800 R -3 days, silica -1 day). This degree of synergism is consistent with the possibility mentioned. Alternatively, both treatments may have adversely affected a common cell type.

## CONCLUSIONS

We conclude that effector cells capable of mediating genetic resistance against tumor cells, particularly leukemia and lymphoma cells, are heterogeneous. NK cells may be conveniently classified by the antigens which they express, by the antigens on tumor cells which they kill, and by the effects of a variety of immunoregulatory treatments on their function. Only future experiments can determine if marrow really is a central lymphoid organ and if all of the immunological deficits of [89]Sr- or estradiol- treated mice can be explained by the presence of suppressor cells. It is not impossible that NK(YAC-1) cells are functionally absent in spleens of mice treated with [89]Sr, and at the same time, the spleens contain cells capable of suppressing NK(YAC-1) function. The difficulty some workers have in detecting suppressor cells in spleens of mice treated with [89]Sr or estradiol may be due to the presence of suppressor cells in spleens of normal mice. Thus NK cell function may be the net result of NK cells v. NK suppressor cells in lymphoid

cell suspensions. Spleens of mice treated with estradiol or
[89]Sr would have a high ratio of suppressor cells to NK
cells. It is conceivable that "pre-M" or "pre-NK" cells
accumulate in the spleens, retain the ability to bind to
target cells and suppress NK function by preventing contact
between tumor cells and competent NK effector cells.

## ACKNOWLEDGEMENTS

We thank Dr. Robert Burton for use of his antisera and
helpful discussion concerning the K cell assay (Table 1).
This work was supported by Grants CA-15369, CA-21401, CA-
25039 and HL 24201 from the National Institutes of Health.
This is publication number 007 from the Hubert H. Humphrey
Cancer Research Center of Boston University.

## REFERENCES

1.   Bennett, M.   Transplantation 14:289, 1972.
2.   Bennett, M.   J.Immunol. 110:510, 1973.
3.   Bennett, M., Baker, E.E., Eastcott, J.W., Kumar, V.,
     and Yonkosky, D.   J. Reticul.Soc. 20:71, 1976.
4.   Bennett, M., and Baker, E.E.   Cell. Immunol. 33:203,
     1977.
5.   Berridge, M.V., and Okech, N.   J.Immunol. 124:732,
     1980.
6.   Clark, E.A., Harmon, R.C., and Wicker, L.S.   J.Immunol.
     119:648, 1977.
7.   Corvese, J.S., Levy, E.M., Bennett, M., and Cooperbanc,
     S.R.   Cell.Immunol. 49:293, 1980.
8.   Cudkowicz, G.   "The proliferation and spread of neo-
     plastic cells". XXI Annual M.D. Anderson Symposium on
     Fundamental Cancer Research.   Baltimore: Williams and
     Wilkins Co. p661, 1968.
9.   Cudkowicz, G., and Stimpfling, J.H.   Immunology 7:291,
     1964.
10.  Cudkowicz, G., and Bennett, M.   J.Exp.Med. 134:83,
     1971.
11.  Cudkowicz, G., and Bennett, M.   J.Exp.Med. 134:1513,
     1971.
12.  Cudkowicz, G., and Hochman, P.S.   Immunol.Rev. 44:13,
     1979.
13.  Dube, S.K., Pragnell, I.B., Kluge, N., Gaedicke, G.,
     Steinheider, G., and Ostertag, W.   Proc.Natl.Acad.Sci.-
     USA 72:1863, 1975.
14.  Fitzgerald, P.A., and Bennett, M.   Immunol.Prospect,

1980 (in press).

15. Furmanski, P., Dietz, M., Fouchey, S., Hall L., Clymer, R., and Rich, M.A. J.Natl.Cancer Inst. 63:449, 1979.

16. Gurney, C.W., Klassen, L., Birks, J., and Allen, E. Exp.Hematol. 22:27, 1972.

17. Haller, O., and Wigzell, H. J.Immunol. 118:503, 1977.

18. Harmon, R.C., Clark, E.A. O'Toole, C., and Wicker, L.S. Immunogenetics 4:601, 1977.

19. Herberman, R.B., Nunn, M.E., and Lavrin, D.H. Int.J.-Cancer 16:216, 1975.

20. Herberman, R.B., and Holden, H.T. Adv.Cancer Res. 27:305, 1979.

21. Kiessling, R., Klein, E., Pross, H., and Wigzell, H. Eur.J.Immunol. 5:117, 1975.

22. Kumar, V., Bennett, M., and Eckner, R.J. J.Exp.Med. 139:1093, 1974.

23. Kumar, V., and Bennett, M. J.Exp.Med. 143:713, 1976.

24. Kumar, V., Caruso, T., and Bennett, M. J.Exp.Med. 143:728, 1976.

25. Kumar, V., Goldschmidt, L., Eastcott, J.W., and Bennett, M. J.Exp.Med. 147:442, 1978.

26. Kumar, V., Resnick, P., Eastcott, J.W., and Bennett, M. J.Natl.Cancer Inst. 61:1117, 1978.

27. Kumar, V., Luevano, E., and Bennett, M. J.Exp.Med. 150:531, 1979.

28. Kumar, V., Ben-Ezra, J., Bennett, M., and Sonnenfeld, G. J.Immunol. 123:1832, 1979.

29. Levy, E.M., Bennett, M., Kumar, V., Fitzgerald, P.A., and Cooperband, S.R. J.Immunol. 124:611, 1980.

30. Lopez, C., Ryshke, R., and Bennett, M. Infect.Immun., 1980 (in press).

31. Lotzova, E., and Cudkowicz, G. J.Immunol. 113:798, 1974.

32. Luevano, E., Kumar, V., and Bennett, M. 1980 (submitted).

33. Merluzzi, V.J., Levy, E.M., Kumar, V., Bennett, M., and Cooperband, S.R. J.Immunol. 121:505, 1979.

34. Ojo, E., and Wigzell, H. Scand.J.Immunol. 7:297, 1978.

35. Rich, M.A., Clymer, R., and Karl, S. J.Natl.Cancer Inst. 42:571, 1969.

36. Roder, J.C. J.Immunol. 123:2168, 1979.

37. Roder, J.C., Lohmann-Matthews M-L, Domzig, W., and Wigzell, H. J.Immunol. 123:2174, 1979.

38. Seaman, W.E., Blackman, M.A., Gindhart, T.D., Roubinian, J.R., Loeb, J.M., and Talal, N. J.Immunol. 121:2193, 1978.

39. Seaman, W.E., Gindhart, T.D., Greenspan, J.S., Blackman, M.A., and Talal, N. J.Immunol. 122:2541,

1979.

40. Seaman, W.E., Blackman, M.A., Greenspan, J.S., and Talal, N. J.Immunol. 124:812, 1980.

41. Stutman, O. Ann. Immunol.(Inst.Pasteur) 127C:943, 1976.

42. Stutman, O., Paige, C.J., and FeoFigarella, E. J.Immunol. 121:1819, 1978.

43. van den Engh, G.J., and Platenberg, M. Exp.Hematol. 6:627, 1978.

## DISCUSSIONS

Kiessling: Bennett seems to be making a distinction, at the genetic level, between the EL4 and the YAC system, implying the EL4 system is more similar to the hybrid bone marrow system while the YAC system is not. Could he elaborate on this point?

Bennett: Yes, the most dramatic differences are seen in vivo with DBA/2, CBA, C3H and Balb/c. They do not reject C57BL bone marrow cells very well. They are considered either low responders or intermediate responders; and yet they lyse YAC cells quite well, at an intermediate or high level. Spleen cells from these animals are not very effective in lysing EL4 where they are effective in lysing YAC. Now the B6 animal itself lyses the YAC at an intermediate level, while against EL4, it is quite inactive. This is a situation where there is no killing of syngeneic targets.

Kiessling: We could see this $H-2^d$-linked resitance factor in vitro against a wide panel of different targets, some of which are totally unrelated to the C57BL background, so that would support an argument that, in our hands, regulation does not control the specific recognition of a certain target structure but, more likely, the overall reactivity.

Bennett: That is correct.

Steeves: Bennett mentioned that [89]Sr interfered with the normal resistance of C57BL mice to Friend virus, specifying the Fv-2 gene. Would he not also include abrogation of resistance mediated by Fv-3 on the basis of results?

Bennett: Yes, I mentioned that Fv-3 gene is the gene regulating the resistance or susceptibility to the immunosuppressive effects of Friend virus and this too is abrogated by treatment with $^{89}$Sr via a T-suppressor cell.

Ralph: In agreement with others, we found that injection of BCG i.p. yields a suppressor cell in the spleen for YAC NK activity that is effective in a 6 hour assay. This involves stimulation of NK in the peritoneal cavity but depressed activity in splenic cells. In our case the NK cell was theta negative and non-adherent. Has Bennett done any such studies on the suppressor he mentioned?

Bennett: The suppressor is to the EL4 target. It is adherent in Sephadex G-10 columns. That is about all I can contribute to what Ralph has detailed.

Karre: Did Bennett use a 4 hour chromium release assay for the YAC targets?

Bennett: Usually we did, but after $^{89}$Sr treatment it did not matter if incubation was as short as 4 hours or as long as 18 hours. They were suppressed all the time.

Karre: So the differences are not dependent upon the macrophages.

# H-2 DEPENDENT AND INDEPENDENT NATURAL RESISTANCE TO LEUKAEMIA TRANSPLANTATION IN IRRADIATED AND NONIRRADIATED MICE

George A. Carlson[1] and Grant Campbell

Department of Immunology
University of Alberta
Edmonton, Alberta, Canada T6G 2H7

By several criteria, spontaneous cell-mediated cytotoxicity or natural killer (NK) activity appears to be the _in vitro_ counterpart of nonadaptive or natural resistance against transplantation of normal or malignant cells of the haemopoietic system (10). For example, both _in vitro_ NK activity and _in vivo_ resistance are independent of normal thymic function, but can be abrogated by treatment with anti-macrophage agents or $^{89}$Sr. However, the first observed manifestation of nonadaptive resistance to tumor transplantation in mammals, the hybrid effect (15), was shown to be dependent on H-2 nonidentity between the host and the graft at the major histocompatibility complex (MHC). Subsequently, resistance to bone marrow or tumour transplantation in irradiated (3) and nonirradiated (1) mice was also shown to be most strongly expressed against H-2 nonidentical cells. In contrast, with few exceptions, _in vitro_ NK activity is independent of H-2 nonidentity between the effector and target cells (eg. 12).

Using the technique of Hofer et al. (8) to directly monitor the death and metastatic distribution of $^{131}$I-IdUrd prelabelled tumour cells _in vivo_, we have previously demonstrated that rejection occurs in all strains of mice tested which are H-2 nonidentical with the tumour cells at either the K or D end of the MHC (1). In irradiated C57BL mice, non-H-2 genes provide radioresistant rejection capability and H-2D (Hh-1) nonidentity between the tumour and the host is a prerequisite for resistance (2). This H-2 dependent natural resistance in both irradiated and nonirradiated mice is antibody and T-cell independent, but is susceptible to pretreatment with either silica or $^{89}$Sr. Mechanistically and genetically, Hh-dependent resistance by irradiated mice appears to be a subset of a more general H-2 dependent nonadaptive rejection mechanism. Although NK activity is functionally similar with H-2 dependent resistance, the strain distribution of high NK as opposed to low NK activity is different than that for radioresistant and radiosusceptible rejection _in vivo_, and most investigators find no evidence

GENETIC CONTROL OF NATURAL RESISTANCE
TO INFECTION AND MALIGNANCY

that H-2 serves as the "target antigen" in natural killing (12,14). This apparent discrepancy between the genetic control of in vitro NK activity and the H-2 dependence of natural resistance in vivo has been a subject of our investigations. In this report, we describe evidence indicating that an H-2 independent resistance, with genetic control similar to that observed with in vitro NK activity, can also be quantitated in vivo.

As reported previously (2), treatment with silica or $^{89}$Sr, which abrogate H-2 dependent resistance, also increases the number of injected leukaemia cells which survive in the spleens and lungs of H-2 identical recipients. For example, CD2F$_1$ (H-2$^{d/d}$ - (BALB/c x DBA/2)F$_1$) mice treated with $^{89}$Sr as described by Bennett (16) were injected with $10^6$ $^{131}$IdUrd prelabelled L1210 cells (H-2$^{d/d}$) and the amount of remaining radioactivity in the spleens and lungs 2 days later was compared with that in untreated mice. The $^{89}$Sr treatment increased the survival of the leukaemia cells in the spleens of the H-2 identical mice, as indicated by the per cent of the remaining radioactivity, from $3.9 \pm 0.7$ ($\pm$S.D.)% to $8.8 \pm 1.3$% and in the lungs from $2.3 \pm 0.4$% to $5.3 \pm 1$%. Similar results were obtained with silica treated H-2 identical animals. Results such as these suggested that there may be an H-2 independent resistance operating concurrently with H-2 dependent resistance.

Table 1. Potentiation of Natural Resistance to Leukaemia Transplantation by Treatment with Poly I:C

| | | Percent (±S.D.) of Remaining $^{131}$I-L1210 on day 0.9 in | | |
|---|---|---|---|---|
| Mice | Treatment | Spleen | Liver | Lung |
| DBA/2 | saline | 7.1 ± 1.8 | 77.9 ± 6.5 | 10.0 ± 2.0 |
| DBA/2 | poly I:C | 3.9 ± 0.5 | 76.7 ± 5.5 | 6.5 ± 1.3 |
| C3D2F$_1$ | saline | 3.3 ± 0.8 | 84.0 ±12 | 6.2 ± 2.3 |
| C3D2F$_1$ | poly I:C | 0.7 ± 0.3 | 81.1 ± 6.0 | 2.7 ± 0.9 |

All differences in spleens and lungs between poly I:C treated and control mice are significant to at least the P< 0.01 level as is the hybrid resistance (C3D2F$_1$ vs DBA/2).

Polyinosinic-polycytidilic acid (poly I:C) is known to augment NK activity (5) and was therefore tested for its effect on natural resistance in vivo. To determine whether poly I:C potentiated resistance by H-2 identical mice "syngeneic" with the leukaemia, experiments such as the following were done. Groups of 5 DBA/2J ($H-2^{d/d}$) and C3D2F$_1$ ($H-2^{k/d}$) were injected i.p. with either saline or 150 µg poly I:C 2.5 hrs before i.v. injection of 6 x $10^5$ $^{131}$IdUrd labelled L1210 cells. As shown in Table 1, poly I:C treatment caused a significant decrease in the number of tumour cells remaining in the spleens and lungs 22 hrs after tumour challenge in both "syngeneic" DBA/2J and the H-2 nonidentical C3D2F$_1$.

**Table 2.** Poly I:C is not Directly Cytotoxic to L1210 <u>in</u> <u>vitro</u>

| | | cells/ml$^a$ | viability | $^{125}$IUdR uptake CPM/$10^6$ cells |
|---|---|---|---|---|
| 100 µg Poly I:C/ml | 1 | 2.8 x $10^6$ | 100% | 37,765 |
| | 2 | 3.3 x $10^6$ | 100% | 36,669 |
| control | 1 | 2.4 x $10^6$ | 96% | 42,574 |
| | 2 | 2.8 x $10^6$ | 100% | 37,934 |

a) Cell culture inititated at $10^5$ cells/ml. Thirty hours later 0.5 µCi $^{125}$IUdR/ml was added to each culture. The readings were taken 48 hrs after culture initiation.

As shown in Table 2, we could find no direct effect of poly I:C on the survival or proliferation of L1210 in culture. This suggests, as do experiments to follow, that the decreased survival of L1210 in the spleens and lungs of poly I:C treated mice is mediated by potentiation of a host response.

**Table 3.** Pretreatment with Poly I:C Abrogates the Radiosusceptibility of Natural Resistance.

| Mice | Poly I:C | 800R | Per cent (± S.D.) of $^{131}$I-L1210 in: Spleen | Whole-body |
|---|---|---|---|---|
| CD2F$_1$ | - | - | 1.4 ± 0.1 | 20.5 ± 0.5 |
| | + | - | 1.2 ± 0.2 | 15.3 ± 3.0 |
| CBA/CaJ | - | - | 0.12± .02 | 10.3 ± 0.5 |
| | + | - | 0.08± .01 | 6.3 ± 0.9 |
| | - | + | 1.25± 0.4 | 22.0 ± 2.4 |
| | + | + | 0.06± .03 | 10.6 ± 2.0 |

All mice got 3 x $10^6$ $^{131}$I-L1210 i.v. on day 0. Poly I:C treatment consisted of ip injection of 130 µg poly I:C 17 hrs before irradiation and 22 hrs before tumour inoculation. The values shown are 3 days after tumour challenge.

One feature of H-2 associated natural resistance is that mice can be classified as radioresistant or radiosusceptible depending on the sensitivity of the rejection process to gamma irradiation (1). Mice of the C57BL family are radioresistant regardless of their H-2 haplotype, while other strains we have tested (eg., C3H, A, CBA) are radiosusceptible. The radioresistant phenotype is expressed in nonirradiated mice as a more rapid rejection process compared to radiosusceptible strains and as the ability to resist larger numbers of cells. Experiments such as that shown in Table 3 have demonstrated that poly I:C treatment renders radiosuceptible mice phenotypically radioresistant.

Table 4. Failure of Poly I:C to Augment Resistance in Irradiated, Silica-treated Mice

| Mice | Silica[a] | 800R[b] | Poly I:C[c] | Percent (± S.D.) $^{131}$I-L1210 in Spleen (day 0.9) |
|------|-----------|---------|-------------|------------------------------------------------------|
| CD2F$_1$ | - | - | - | 4.5 ± 0.7 |
|  | - | + | - | 5.0 ± 0.4 |
| CBA/CaJ | - | - | - | 0.4 ± 0.4 |
|  | - | + | - | 3.6 ± 0.4 |
|  | - | + | + | 1.4 ± 0.5 |
|  | + | + | - | 15.5 ± 4.9 |
|  | + | + | + | 18.2 ± 1.0 |

a) Silica, 5 mg i.v., 23 hrs before 4 x $10^6$ $^{131}$I-L1210
b) 800R 4 hrs before L1210
c) Poly I:C, 150 µg, 4 hrs before cells

The potentiating effect of poly I:C on natural killing in vitro has been shown to be mediated through stimulation of macrophages to produce interferon which in turn augments NK activity (6). Similarly, the reversal of radiosusceptibility seen in poly I:C treated mice is not seen in mice whose macrophages have been depleted by treatment with silica (Table 4). The role of interferon in these in vivo effects is yet to be determined. These experiments also indicate that poly I:C is not directly cytotoxic to L1210 in vivo.

An immediate question arising from these results is whether the potentiation of resistance by poly I:C treatment of radiosusceptible strains also reverses their poor resistance to Hh incompatible bone marrow grafts. Results such as those shown in Table 5 demonstrated that it does not.

Table 5. Treatment with Poly I:C does not Reverse the Susceptibility of Irradiated C3H/HeJ Mice to Allogeneic Bone Marrow Transplantation

| Recipient (900R day 0) | Poly I:C (150 ;g day -1) | $10^6$ BALB/c Bone Marrow Cells day 0 | Percent uptake of $^{125}$ IdUrd in Spleen (day 7) |
|---|---|---|---|
| BALB/c Cr | - | + | 0.61 ± .06 |
|  | + | + | 1.02 ± 0.1 |
|  | - | - | 0.02 ± .003 |
|  | + | - | 0.02 ± .002 |
| C3H/HeJ | - | + | 0.52 ± .08 |
|  | + | + | 0.58 ± 0.1 |
|  | - | - | 0.04 ‧ .003 |
|  | + | - | 0.05 ‧ .01 |

These results suggest that poly I:C may be potentiating an H-2 independent rejection system distinct from that of H-2 associated natural resistance or bone marrow graft rejection in irradiated mice. Recently, we have initiated experiments to study natural resistance to cell lines which are highly susceptible to NK activity in vitro. Using both YAC-1, which was a gift from Dr. G. Klein, and SL2.5, generously provided by Drs. D. Chow and A. Greenberg, we have found that although an effect of H-2 nonidentity is readily apparent in resistance, H-2 nonidentity is not a prerequisite for rejection nor does H-2 nonidentity between the host and graft guarantee that rejection will occur. An example is shown in Table 6. The mice were injected i.v. with 1.75 x $10^6$ $^{131}$I-SL2.5 cells ($H-2^{d/d}$) and the amount of remaining radioactivity in their spleens determined 19 hrs later.

Table 6. Natural Resistance in vivo against NK-Sensitive Cells

| Mice | H-2 | Radiation Sensitivity of H-2 Dependent Resistance (Test tumour) | NK Activity | Percent (±S.D.) of Remaining $^{131}$I-SL2.5 in spleen |
|---|---|---|---|---|
| DBA/2J | d | radiosusceptible (EL4) | low | 3.1 ± 0.75 |
| CD2F₁ | d | radioresistant (EL4) | high | 1.2 ± 0.3 |
| CBA/CaJ | k | radiosusceptible (L1210) | high | 0.3 ± 0.08 |
| C3H/HeJ | k | radiosusceptible (L1210) | low | 2.7 ± 0.6 |

Table 6 also shows the H-2 haplotypes, radiation sensitivity
of H-2 dependent resistance, and the NK activity of spleen
cells from nonimmunized mice in vitro.
    The ability to resist the NK sensitive cells showed a
strong correspondence with the NK activity of the strains of
mice tested. By monitoring the fate of $^{131}$IdUrd prelabelled
cells as described above, others have demonstrated in vivo
rejection of NK sensitive cell lines and interpreted the rejection as the in vivo manifestation of NK activity (13).
However, the results did not discriminate between H-2 dependent and independent natural resistance. Using tumour growth as the assay, Kiessling et al. (9) had previously demonstrated that the growth of NK sensitive lines correlates with
the host's NK potential, and our results, directly quantita-
ting killing of the tumour cells, indicate that natural
killing can indeed account for at least some of this retardation of tumour growth. However, NK-like cells which
recognize Hh-1 (H-2D) can also be measured in vitro (7),
and Kumar et al. (11) suggest that different effector cells
may be involved in lysis of EL4 (Hh-1 dependent lysis) and
YAC-1 (not H-2 dependent).
    The results presented in this report can be summarized
as follows:

1. There is an increase in the survival of leukaemia cells
   in the spleens of mice pretreated with either silica or
   $^{89}$Sr. This loss of resistance is seen both in mice H-2
   identical and in mice H-2 nonidentical with the grafted
   cells.
2. Poly I:C treatment potentiates H-2 independent resistance and permits resistance by irradiated radiosusceptible strains but does not have an augmenting effect on
   Hh-dependent resistance to bone marrow allografts.
3. The ability to resist NK-sensitive cell lines in vivo
   corresponds with the in vitro NK activity of the strains tested. However, the strain distribution of the
   radiosusceptibility of H-2 dependent natural resistance
   rejection potential does not correspond with in vitro
   NK activity (eg., Table 6).

These results suggest that an H-2 independent nonadaptive
resistance system can be quantitated in vivo as can H-2 dependent resistance against NK-insensitive and sensitive
cells. Isolation of the target structure for in vitro NK
activity showed that it was independent of known H-2 encoded
molecules (14). It remains to be determined whether H-2 independent resistance against NK-insensitive cells such as
L1210 is directed against a similar target antigen, and

whether H-2 dependent and independent rejection are mediated by the same effector cells in vivo.

## ACKNOWLEDGEMENT

Supported by the National Cancer Institute of Canada.

[1] Research Scholar of the National Cancer Institute of Canada Present address: The Jackson Laboratory, Bar Harbor, Maine 04609.

## REFERENCES

1. Carlson, G.A., and Wegmann, T.H. J.Immunol. 118:2130, 1977.
2. Carlson, G.A., Melnychuk, D., and Meeker, M.J. Int. J. Cancer 25:111, 1980.
3. Cudkowicz, G., and Bennett, M. J.Exp.Med. 134:83, 1971.
4. Cudkowicz, G., and Hochman, P.S. Immunol.Rev. 44:13, 1979.
5. Djeu, J.Y., Heinbaugh, J.A., Holden, H.T., and Herberman, R.B. J.Immunol. 122:175, 1979.
6. Djeu, J.Y., Heinbaugh, J.A., Holden, H.T., and Herberman, R.B. J.Immunol. 122:182, 1979.
7. Harmon, R.C., Clark, E.A., O'Toole, C., and Wixler, L.S. Immunogenetics 4:601, 1977.
8. Hofer, K.G., Prensky, W., and Hughes, W.L. J.Natl.-Cancer Inst. 43:763, 1969.
9. Kiessling, R., Petranyi, G., Klein, G., and Wigzell, H. Int.J.Cancer 15:933, 1975.
10. Kiessling, R., Hochman, P.S., Haller, O., Shearer, G.M. Wigzell, H., and Cudkowicz, G. Eur.J.Immunol. 7:655, 1977.
11. Kumar, V., Luevano, E., and Bennett, M. J.Exp.Med. 150:531, 1979.
12. Petranyi, G.G., Kiessling, R., and Klein, G. Immunogenetics 2:53, 1975.
13. Riccardi, C., Puccetti, P., Santoni, A., and Herberman, R.B. J.Natl.Cancer Inst. 63:1041, 1979.
14. Roder, J.C., Rosén, A., Fenyo, E.M., and Troy, F.A. Proc.Natl.Acad.Sci.USA 76:1405, 1979.
15. Snell, G.D. J.Natl.Cancer Inst. 21:843, 1958.
16. Bennett, M. J. Immunol. 110:510, 1973.

## DISCUSSION

**Kiessling:** I would like to ask about the radiosensitivity of the radiosusceptible strains reported by Carlson. How absolute is it? If one lowers the leukemia dose inoculum, will one then be able to detect rejection in those strains even after radiation?

**Carlson:** After irradiation, it seems there is a gradation, oversimplified as this may be. C3H and CBA mice are highly radiosusceptible and you wipe it out using as low a dose of cells as we can effectively monitor via $^{131}$I-IUdR. Furthermore, degrees of radioresistance are also expressed in terms of the ability to resist higher doses of cells. So there is a quantitative as well as a qualitative distinction. But at the extreme ends, where C57BL is extremely radioresistant and C3H is extremely susceptible, it does give the impression of being an absolute difference.

**Greenberg:** We have heard a lot about a variety of tumors that have been studied in these systems. I gather there seem to be assumptions about the H-2 identity of most of them. I wonder how carefully most workers screen their tumors for the antigens on them. Has Carlson done this?

**Carlson:** No, we know they are expressing the private antigens they are supposed to. We do not know if they are expressing inappropriate alloantigens. But one hypothesis which would be of interest, if natural resistance is a surveillance mechanism, is that an H-2-dependent system could be operating against an altered H-2. And this is, in my view, a distinct possibility. Of course, when I say syngeneic or H-2-identical, L1210 was induced in 1949 in DBA/2 and has been maintained separately over the intervening 30 years. So there would well be considerable drift between the tumors as used here; "syngeneic" should be in quotes.

**Greenberg:** Assuming that one has the right antigens, Carlson is still dealing with minor differences with the Balb-mouse with a DBA origin.

**Carlson:** I had forgotten the data on the DBA. The Balb/c x DBA hybrid behaves like a DBA unless one uses extremely low cell doses in which case one can measure non-H-2 resistance, such as Cudkowicz previously recorded for that combination.

**Greenberg:** Has Carlson any speculation to offer on what this non-NK mechanism is?

Carlson:   Greenberg means the H-2 dependent, which I would
say that is the classical hybrid resistance in bone marrow
allografting.

Greenberg:   And what of the H-2 independent mechanism?

Carlson:   I consider the H-2 independent to be NK cells.
Although it is not satisfactorily clarified, we have some
preliminary evidence that the final effector cell for both
the H-2 independent and the dependent rejection is the same.
But still there might be some intermediary, some induction
necessary in the H-2 dependent as opposed to the independent, for it to be expressed.

Cudkowicz:   I am trying to view Carlson's data, in a perhaps
more unified way.   Is it possible that what Carlson calls
radiosensitive is really a reflection of the patern of growth of the tumor in the various organs?   I say this because
both NK activity, whether it is against an H-2 compatible or
against an Hh-1 incompatible tumor, is really site-depen-
dent.   It is strong in the spleen, actually, strongest in
the spleen, and then it declines, as far as strength is concerned, in various other hemopoietic sites.   It is non-
existent in some organs such as liver or lungs.   So now what
one sees is this:   When one irradiates, proliferation of
cells is seen in sites where, in the non-irradiated mouse,
there is a regular T-cell mediated allograft response, which
is a non-irradiated mouse will keep the tumor in check in
those sites, let us say the liver.   When one irradiates, one
loses that component because it is radiosensitive and whatever is left, due to NK activity, is not strong enough to
matter, that is, unless one is looking in specific sites.
Would Carlson consider this a possibility?

Carlson:   It is possible, but we have shown, for example,
that in both non-irradiated and irradiated mice that there
is not a T-dependent mechanism that is causing this altered
distribution.   What we prefer to think, although your suggestion is a possibility analogous to what you and Hochman
have found, is that irradiation may initiate some suppressive mechanism that diminishes resistance in the radiosusceptible strains as opposed to the C57 family of mice.

Cudkowicz:   Now another distinction that Carlson makes that
I cannot endorse, is being modulated or non-modulated by interferon.   The resistance to Hh incompatibility marrow is
modulated by interferon.   You probably do not know about it
because it is not published information but Kaminsky will

communicate it at the FASEB meeting, 1980. It is modulated either when one stimulates or induces interferon with inducers, in which case one gets stronger resistance, or else abrogates it simply by injecting anti-interferon antibody. So that distinction does not really hold. I think one may have subtypes of NK cells (where NK is a general term) and Carlson has utilized the designation NK-like which further complicates the issue. But certainly, there may be subtypes of NK cells, some more and some less modulated.

Carlson: One thing we do find is an effect of poly I:C treatment with C3H and also CBA mice, and in the syngeneic recipient, the Balb, there was actually an increase. But it was the converse in the sense that, instead of increasing resistance, it actually increased the survival and proliferation of the engrafted cells.

NATURAL SURVEILLANCE OF NK-RESISTANT TUMORS.  THE ROLE OF
NATURAL ANTI-TUMOR ANTIBODY (NAb) AND MACROPHAGES (mph)

Arnold H. Greenberg, Donna A. Chow
and Liliana B. Wolosin

Department Pediatrics and Immunology
University of Manitoba
Manitoba Institute of Cell Biology
700 Bannatyne Avenue
Winnipeg R3E OV9, Canada

Since it has become abundantly clear over recent years
that the thymus-dependent immune system is not responsible
for the elimination of incipient tumors (20,23) the concept
of immunological surveillance has been restated in the hypothesis that T-independent anti-tumor effector mechanisms are
the important mediators (7,8).  Two main schools of thought
have emerged to champion either the NK cell (8,12,13) or the
macrophage (1,10,16) as the effectors of this alternative
immune surveillance mechanism.  Substantial evidence supporting a role for the NK effector cell has been described in
this symposium (12) and elsewhere (8,13).  Despite these encouraging results most investigators point out that not all
tumors are NK-sensitive (9), and that there is a discrete
organ distribution of NK cells which may mean that they play
an important but limited role in surveillance (13).  In this
regard, recent reports have suggested metastasis to the lung
may be controlled by NK cells (6).
    The investigators who have advanced the case of the
macrophage point to its potent (11,15), and selective (22)
lysis of tumor cells in vitro.  However, the requirement for
macrophage activation by adjuvants or intracellular parasites (11,18) weakens the argument that the mph is directly
involved in surveillance where neither the stimuli for activation, nor the time required to generate the response may
be available to the host during the critical early phase of
tumor growth.  Even if environmental stimuli can partially
activate mph's, in vitro evidence suggests a second signal
by lymphocyte factors is still required to see its full
lytic potential (4).  Despite these reservations it has been
demonstrated that mph's can be spontaneously activated in
vivo to directly lyse tumor cells (17).  That mph's play an
important role in surveillance is also quite evident from in
vivo experiments where the suppression of mph function is
associated with depressed surveillance of tumors (5,16).  In
work from this laboratory (5) we have pointed out that the

role of the mph may, in addition to its action as an effector cell, be more indirect than previously considered. This conclusion comes from the finding that although surveillance could be suppressed non-specifically by mph-ablating agents such as silica, the intravenous injection of soluble tumor membrane antigens could specifically interfere with the host's ability to eliminate small tumor inocula. This observation suggested the participation of an antigen specific receptor molecule in addition to the mph, and one candidate considered for this role was natural antibody (NAb). Natural anti-tumor antibodies are T-independent, specific and are capable of binding rapidly to the surface of injected tumors (24), characteristics which are well suited for a role in surveillance. In addition, evidence from other laboratories has implicated NAb in resistance to tumor growth (19).

In the present experiments we have chosen to approach the question of which natural effector mechanism, NK cells, NAb or activated mph, are relevant to surveillance by utilizing clones selected from three different tumors syngeneic to the DBA/2 mouse. These tumors demonstrated either high or low tumorigenicity when injected in small tumor doses of 10 to 100 cells, but were uniformly lethal in doses over $10^3$ cells (Table 1). One would reason that if the ability of the mouse to reject one of the clones more efficiently and the susceptibility of the clones to the putative natural surveillance mechanisms do not correlate, then it is unlikely that this effector could account for the more efficient surveillance of the clone.

Table 1. Correlation of <u>In Vivo</u> and <u>In Vitro</u> Parameters of Surveillance

| TUMOR | | IN VIVO | IN VITRO | | |
|---|---|---|---|---|---|
| | | | % Cytotoxicity ± S.E.M. | | |
| Clone | Inoculum | Tumor Frequency | NK (CBA spleen) | NAb (DBA/2) | C. Parvum activated macrophages (DBA/2) |
| L5178Y-F9 | 10 | 13.8 | 0.4 ± 0.4 | 21.5 ± 8.1 | 36.1 ± 7.8 |
| L5178Y-1 | 10 | 39.4 | 0.0 ± 0.0 | 5.3 ± 2.7 | 39.9 ± 3.6 |
| P815X2-18 | 10 | 14.1 | 0.0 ± 0.0 | 7.2 ± 7.1 | 31.9 ± 6.1 |
| P815X2-16 | 10 | 52.5 | 0.3 ± 0.5 | 7.5 ± 7.4 | 35.3 ± 5.5 |
| SL2-5 | 100 | 10.0 | 36.7 ± 9.2 | 37.2 ± 3.3 | 17.2 ± 3.9 |
| SL2-9 | 100 | 40.0 | 1.4 ± 0.4 | 49.1 ± 2.5 | 10.9 ± 1.5 |

The methods for measuring NK and NAb have been described in earlier publications (5,24). The lysis of tumor by C. parvum activated macrophages follows the method of Keller (J.Natl.Cancer Inst. 59:1751, 1977).

Two of the three pairs of clones (L5178Y and P815X2) were NK-insensitive, while the SL2 clones were selected so that one was susceptible to CBA and DBA/2 NK cells and the other was totally resistant (Table 1). The variation in tumorigenicity of the L5178Y and P815X2 could, therefore, not be related to NK cell mediated surveillance, while the SL2 clone 5 which was highly susceptible to NK cells was more readily rejected than its NK resistant sister clone.

In examining the sensitivity to syngeneic NAb, both pairs of P815X2 and SL2 clones were equally lysed and the decreased tumorigenicity of the P815X2-18 and SL2-5 could not be attributed to NAb. The tumorigenicity of the L5178Y clones, on the other hand, directly related to NAb binding, and therefore suggested the participation of these antibodies in the hosts ability to reduce the tumor frequency of the L5178Y-F9 clone.

Interestingly, the P815X2 clones, which are NK-insensitive cells, are killed equally by NAb and activated mph, a result which was not expected in view of the difference in tumorigenicity of these clones. This suggests either another, as yet unidentified, factor participating in the surveillance of these tumors, or that certain aspects of the action of these effector mechanisms in vivo are not detected in our in vitro assays. For example, the lack of correlation of complement-mediated NAb lysis with the fate of the other clones does not necessarily mean that NAb's do not participate in their surveillance, only that sensitivity to NAb is not sufficient to account for the difference in the observed tumor frequencies between the clones. The SL2 tumor clones, for instance, are able to bind NAb's quite well, and, in other studies, the frequency of P815X2-16 tumors was decreased by coating the cells with NAb before injection (D.A. Chow, L.B. Wolosin and A.H. Greenberg, manuscript in preparation).

Sensitivity to the C. parvum activated mph's appears to play no role in distinguishing the fate of these clones. if activated mph are not responsible for in vivo tumor lysis, could the observation that surveillance is mph-dependent be a reflection of their role as regulators rather than as effector cells? Although there is some evidence that the expression of NK cell activity is mph-dependent (14), we have been studying NK-resistant tumors so that mph regulation may be affecting another aspect of the anti-tumor surveillance. We, therefore, examined the possibility that mph controls NAb production by subjecting mice to treatments with macrophage stimulating and suppressive agents. Intraperitoneal injection of three reticuloendothelial activators, lipopolysaccharide (LPS),mycobacterium butyricum or proteose peptone produced polyclonal increases in serum NAb levels reaching maximum levels around day 5 after treatment (Table 2).

Table 2.  Stimulation of Serum Natural Antibody (NAb) by Reticulo-Endothelial Activators

| TUMOR CLONE | DAY | % NAb CYTOTOXICITY ± S.E.M. | | |
|---|---|---|---|---|
| | | LPS (20 ug) | Proteose Peptone (100 mg) | Mycobacterium Butyricum (0.1 ug) |
| P815X2-16 | 0 | 13.9 ± 1.3 | 14.0 ± 1.3 | 12.4 ± 1.4 |
| | 5 | 58.0 ± 8.2 | 32.9 ± 7.1 | 16.5 ± 4.3 |
| L5178Y-F9 | 0 | 6.8 ± 0.5 | 6.3 ± 3.1 | 3.4 ± 0.1 |
| | 5 | 41.2 ± 21.0 | 17.1 ± 1.5 | 12.5 ± 6.8 |
| YAC-1 | 0 | 18.6 ± 5.5 | 26.8 ± 11.0 | 13.6 |
| | 5 | 72.4 ± 15.6 | 41.6 ± 11.0 | 17.4 |

The regulation of NAb production by macrophages was also suggested by the obsevation that the intraperitoneal inject- ion of DBA/2 mice with silica resulted in a prompt decrease in serum NAb, which reached its nadir by day 5 and recovered to near normal levels by day 12.  In previous work from the laboratory we had demonstrated that these RES stimulants de- creased tumor frequencies, and silica significantly increa- sed the number of tumors observed under the identical ex- perimental conditions (5).  It is possible then, that for these NK-resistant tumors, mph's may be participating in sunveillance as a regulator of natural antibody.

Table 3.  Suppression of Serum Natural Antibody (NAb) by Silica

| Tumor Clone | Day | %NAb Cytotoxicity | %Inhibition of Cytotoxicity |
|---|---|---|---|
| YAC-1.3 | 0 | 70.6 ± 6.3 | -- |
| | 1 | 39.4 ± 0.7 | 44.2 |
| | 5 | 21.1 ± 2.7 | 70.1 |
| | 12 | 61.5 ± 1.2 | 12.9 |

Fumed silica (CAB-0-SIL) was injected i.p. in two 100 ug doses on day 0 and day 1.

In conclusion, the surveillance of nascent tumors appears to be mediated by more than one and possibly several T-independent 'natural' effector mechanisms which may include NK cells, natural antibodies and mph's. Which of these mechanisms is predominant most probably depends on the susceptibility of a given tumor, and the relative importance of each effector in the tissues at the site of origin of the malignancy. These factors, of course, are played out in a host in which other genetic variations may contribute to the tumors' fate, particularly in view of the fact that the expression of NK (21), NAb (2 and Wolosin, L.B., and Greenberg, A.H., manuscript in preparation), and macrophage (3) phenotypes are under genetic control. The role of the macrophage both as a regulator of NAb and NK function, as well as an effector cell, place it, not surprisingly, at the centre of the surveillance response to incipient tumors.

## ACKNOWLEDGEMENT

We wish to acknowledge the fine technical assistance of Mrs. E. Shewechuk and Mr. A. Chan, and thank Mrs. P. Emery for typing this manuscript. This work was supported by the MRC of Canada and the NCI of Canada.

## REFERENCES

1.  Adams, D.O., and Snyderman, P.  J.Natl.Cancer Inst. 62:1341, 1979.
2.  Ando, I., Erdei, J., Makela, O., and Fachet, J. Eur.J.Immunol. 8:101, 1978.
3.  Boraschi, D., and Meltzer, M.S.  Cell.Immunol. 45:188, 1979.
4.  Chapman, H.A., and Hibbs, J.B.  Science 197:279, 1977.
5.  Chow, D.A., Greene, M.I., and Greenberg, A.H.  Int.J.Cancer 23:788, 1979.
6.  Gorelik, E., Fogel, M., Feldman, M., and Segal, S. J.Natl.Cancer Inst. 63:1397, 1979.
7.  Greenberg, A.H., and Greene, M.I.  Nature 264:356, 1976.
8.  Haller, O., Hanssen, M., Kiessling, R., and Wigzell, H. Nature 270:609, 1977.
9.  Hansson, M., Karre, K., Bakacs, T., Kiessling, R., and Klein, G.  J.Immunol. 121:6, 1978.
10. Hibbs, J.B., lambert, L.H., and Remington, J.S. Science 177:998, 1972.

11. Hibbs, J.B., Lambert, L.H., and Remington, J.S. Nature 235:48, 1972.

12. Karre, K., Klein, G., Kiessling, R., Klein, G., and Roder, J. In Genetic Control of Natural Resistance to Infection and Malignancy. E. Skamene, P.A.L. Kongshavn, and M. Landy (eds). New York, Academic Press, 1980 (in press).

13. Kasai, M., LeClerc, J.C., McVay-Boudreau, L., Shen, F.W., and Cantor, H. J.Exp.Med. 149:1260, 1979.

14. Kiessling, R., Hochman, P.S., Haller, O., Shearer, G.M. Wigzell, H., and Cudkowicz, G. Eur.J. Immunol. 7:655, 1977.

15. Keller, R. J.Exp.Med. 138:625, 1973.

16. Keller, R. J.Natl.Cancer Inst. 57:1355, 1976.

17. Keller, R. Brit.J.Cancer 37:379, 1978.

18. Meltzer, M.S., Tucker, K.K., and Leonard, E.J. J.Natl.Cancer Inst. 54:1177, 1975.

19. Menard, S., Colnaghi, M.I., and Della Porta, G. Int.J.Cancer 19:267, 1977.

20. Moller, G., and Moller, B. Transplant. Rev. 28:3, 1976.

21. Petranyi, G.G., Kiessling, R., and Klein, G. Immunogenet. 2:53, 1975.

22. Piessens, W.F., Churchill, C.H., and David, J.R. J.Immunol. 114:293, 1975.

23. Rygaard, J., and Povlsen, C.O. Transplant.Rev. 28:43, 1976.

24. Wolosin, L.B., and Greenberg, A.H. Int.J.Cancer 23:519, 1979.

# DIFFERENTIAL TUMOR SUSCEPTIBILITY AND IMMUNE RESPONSIVENESS IN HRS/J MICE

David A. Johnson, H.G. Bedigian
and Hans Meier

The Jackson Laboratory
Bar Harbor, Maine 04609

The HRS/J inbred mouse strain, which carries the autosomal recessive gene for hairlessness (hr) on Chromosome 14,
is an interesting model for evaluating the role(s) of genetic and other factors in leukemogenesis.  It has previously
been reported that mice homozygous for this gene (hr/hr)
have a greater incidence of lymphoid leukemia (45% at 8-10
months) than do heterozygotes (hr/+;1% at 8-10 months) (7).
Studies made in an effort to determine the cause(s) of this
divergence in leukemia incidence have implicated genotype-
dependent differences in the immune systems (4,10) and
allelic disparities in endogenous murine leukemia virus
(MuLV) titers (4,5).  Hiai et al. (5) also reported finding
recombinant (MCF-type) MuLVs in preleukemic and leukemic
HRS/J mice.  Certain findings appear conflicting (4,5,7),
probably because markedly different assays and tissues were
used.  In this report we re-evaluate the expression of infection ecotropic (MuLV (type-C virus able to grow on mouse
cells but not on cells of other species) using the infectious center assay on SC-1 cells (8).  The quantity of group
specific MuLV viral antigen (p30) was also determined in the
serum of individual mice using the double antibody method
described (1) with Moloney leukemia virus p30 (generously
supplied by Dr. James N. Ihle of the Frederick Cancer
Research Center, USA) and goat anti-p30 (obtained through
Dr. Jack Gruber of the National Cancer Institute, office of
Program Logistics, USA).  Furthermore, we also found that
homozygous hairless mice are more susceptible to challenge
with a syngeneic tumor (designated HTU) than are heterozygous hairless mice.  We present data which indicate that
this difference in susceptibility is related to differences
in ability of these mice to respond immunologically to the
tumor.

Virus titers from spleens of 10 hr/hr and 10 hr/+ mice
were evaluated in the infectious center assays.  Mice 2.5, 4
and 9 months of age were tested.  The titers found ranged
from $2.4 \times 10^6$ to $4.5 \times 10^6$ infectious centers per $10^6$
cells.  Although there was a slight increase in titer with
age, there was no significant differences between homozygous

and heterozygous mice.

Serum levels of viral p30 antigen are known to relate to virus expression and therefore would be expected to parallel the results of the infectious center assays. The p30 radioimmune competition assays are reported as the amount of whole MuLV which would contain the detected amount of p30. Ten 2 month old hr/+ female mice contained an average of 2.15 ± 2.12 (99%) ug virus/ml serum while ten age and sex matched hr/hr mice contained 2.86 ± 1.38 (48%) ug virus/ml serum. This difference is not significant.

The results of these virus assays, then, are in agreement with the original complement fixation studies of Meier et al. (7) in that they indicate no significant difference in ecotropic leukemia virus expression between the homozygous and heterozygous hairless mice. These findings are consistent with the hypothesis that virus-related tumor induction occurs in these mice at identical rates. The observed differences in leukemia incidence may therefore result from secondary factors resulting in a differential ability of tumor cell clones to expand and eventually kill the animal. If this were the situation, one would expect that exposing homozygous and heterozygous mice to identical tumor cell challenges would result in an earlier death in the homozygotes. In order to test this hypothesis we developed a transplantable syngeneic tumor, designated HTU. This tumor arose spontaneously in a 7-month old HRS/J mouse which was diagnosed histologically as having leukemic infiltrates of the thymus, lymph nodes and spleen. Spleen cells from this mouse, when injected intraperitoneally (i.p.) into young adult HRS/J mice of either sex resulted in the development of similar leukemias three to four weeks later. When the mice were moribund, the enlarged spleens were removed, suspended in Hank's balanced salt solution and injected i.p. into additional recipient mice. The experiments described here were carried out using tumors which had been transplanted in this manner six times.

Massive spleen enlargement in HTU-inoculated mice was a consistent symptom of tumor development. We chose to evaluate tumor growth in preliminary experiments by measuring spleen wet weight 21 days after tumor inoculation since histologic examination indicated that tumor cells constituted the vast majority of spleen cells in both genotype by that time. The effects of varied HTU cell doses on this parameter are indicated on Figure 1. When zero or $1 \times 10^4$ HTU cells were injected, spleen wet weights averaged less than 0.2 g. When $5 \times 10^4$ cells were inoculated the spleens of both groups were greatly enlarged, hr/+ spleens weighing significantly less than hr/hr spleens. We concluded that

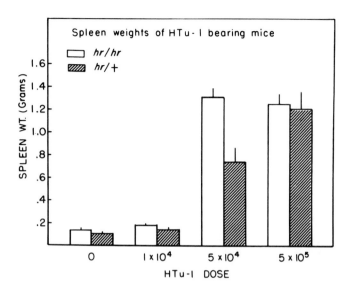

Figure 1.

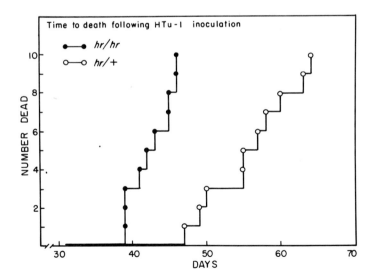

Figure 2.

tumor growth occurs more slowly in the hr/+ mice. The difference in growth rate could be overcome, however, by inoculating 5 x $10^5$ HTU cells which results in similarly high
spleen weights in both types of mice.

We next determined whether the reduced rate of tumor
growth in hr/+ mice would result in prolonged survival
following tumor challenge. Groups of age- and sex-matched
mice were inoculated with 5 x $10^4$ HTU cells and their survival was evaluated. The results are indicated on Figure 2;
they show that hr/+ mice survive significantly longer
(average 55.8 ± 5.7 days) after tumor inoculation than do
hr/hr mice (average 42.5 ± 2.9 days).

On explanation for the differential tumor growth observed is that the homozygous and heterozygous hairless mice
differ in their ability to mount an immune response against
tumor antigens. This would be consistent with the findings
of Heiniger et al. (3) regarding genotype-dependent differences in immune responsiveness in these mice. We therefore
immunized hr/hr and hr/+ mice with inactivated HTU cells in
an effort to accentuate any existing differences in immune
responsiveness.

Table 1.

| Group | Average Survival (days ± standard deviation) |
|-------|----------------------------------------------|
| hr/+ unimmunized | 35.4 ± 7.6 |
| hr/+ immunized | 51.7 ± 10.6 |
| hr/hr unimmunized | 29.45 ± 5.6 |
| hr/hr immunized | 37.1 ± 11.8 |

Groups of 15 hr/hr or hr/+ mice were inoculated with 1
x $10^7$ HTU cells which had previously been exposed to 5000 R
of gamma irradiation. Controls were injected with saline.
After two weeks the immunizations were repeated and after an
additional week all mice were challenged with 5 x $10^4$ viable
HTU cells. The average survival times are shown in Table 1.
Immuniation of hr/+ mice resulted in a significantly prolonged life relative to unimmunized hr/+ mice. Immunized
hr/hr mice lived slightly longer than unimmunized hr/hr mice
but this difference was not significant (confidence limits:
P < .02) indicating that these mice do not develop a

protective immune response to the tumor.

The results are consistent with the hypothesis that hr-/hr mice develop spontaneous leukemia at a higher rate than hr/+ because of differences in their ability to mount an immune response. The exact nature of this is not entirely clear at present. Heiniger et al. (3) found that the hr/hr mice were deficient in their secondary antibody response to tetanus toxoid. It would therefore be tempting to speculate that hr/hr mice have a defective immune surveillance mechanism (2) which allows more rapid tumor progression. On the other hand, Heiniger et al. (4) found that there was no significant difference between hr/hr and hr/+ mice with respect to their ability to respond to the mitogen phytohemagglutinin (PHA), thus indicating that the two genotypes have equally responsive cellular immune mechanisms. We have confirmed these observations (data not shown). The possibility that immunostumulatory mechanisms (for review see 6,9) may play a role in this system should therefore be borne in mind. It may be of some value to bear in mind that immune responses are highly specific in nature. It therefore follows that the overall responsiveness of an animal to unrelated antigens may be of less importance than the response to a particular antigen (in this case perhaps tumor- or leukemia virus-specific antigens). Thus, a mouse may have one kind of response to PHA or tetanus toxoid and have an entirely different level of response to other specific antigens. If an animal differs in its ability to respond to a particular antigen which happens to be an important determinant on a tumor cell, the result may be an altered ability to survive in the face of tumor challenge. With this in mind, we are continuing to investigate the role of the hr gene in leukemogenesis by examining its effect on the ability of mice to respond to tumor- and leukemia virus- specific antigens.

## ACKNOWLEDGEMENT

This research was supported, in part, by NCI research contract NO1 CP33255 and, in part, by NCI Young Investigator Research Grant R23-CA-25944.

## REFERENCES

1.    Benade L., Ihle, J., and Decleve, A. Proc.Natl.Acad.-Sci.USA 75:4553, 1978.

2.    Burnet, F.  Progr.Exper.Tumor Res. 13:1, 1970.
3.    Heiniger, H.J., Meier, H., Kaliss, N., Cherry, M.,
      Chen, H.W., and Stoner, R.D.  Cancer Res. 34:201, 1974.
4.    Heinigier, H., Huebner, R.J., and Meier, H.  J.Natl.-
      Cancer Inst. 56:5, 1976.
5.    Hiai, H., Morrissey, P., Khirooya, R., and Schwartz,
      R.S.  Nature 270:247, 1977.
6.    Lewis, M., Phillips, T., and Rowden, G.  In
      Immunological Tolerance and Enhancement.  F.P. Stuart
      and F.W. Fitch (eds).  Baltimore: University Park
      Press, p149, 1979.
7.    Meier, H., Myers, D., and Huebner, R.J.  Proc.Natl.-
      Acad.Sci. 63:759, 1969.
8.    Melief, C., Datta, S., Louie, S., Johnson, S., Melief,
      M., and Schwartz, R.  Proc.Soc.Exp.Biol.Med. 149:1015,
      1975.
9.    Prehn, R.T.  J.Natl.Cancer Inst. 59:1043, 1977.
10.   Reske-Kunz, A.B., Scheid, M., and Boyse, E.A.  J.Exp.-
      Med. 149:228, 1979.

# HYBRID RESISTANCE TO PARENTAL TUMORS: INFLUENCE OF HOST AND TUMOR GENOTYPE AND TUMOR DERIVATION

Gunnar O. Klein, George Klein
and Rolf Kiessling

Department of Tumor Biology
Karolinska Institutet
S-104 01 Stockholm 60
Sweden

## INTRODUCTION

The natural resistance found in unimmunized $F_1$ hybrid mice challenged with a threshold dose of transplantable tumor cells of parental origin was first described by Snell and Stevens (5). In spite of the fact that this hybrid resistance has been known for many years, the genetic regulation and the mechanism behind this phenomenon is still incompletely undertstood. In $F_1$ hybrids of unrelated strains of mice, the introduction of a fully new genome is likely to be able to introduce resistance in many different ways and it is conceivable that different mechanisms are active.

To get a more complete picutre of the phenomenon of hybrid resistance to parental tumors we have engaged in a broad project, at present involving about 70 tumors of varied genotypes. They belong to all three major tumor groups (lymphomas, sarcomas and carcinomas) and have various etiologies; spontaneous as well as virally and chemically induced tumors. They are all tested in a similar way by subcutaneous inoculation of a threshold dose giving less than 100% takes in the syngeneic strain of origin. This system is more likely to reflect the immunological defense against the early stages of tumor development than systems using very high cell doses which ultimately produce tumor formation and death in all inoculated animals.

We are particularly interested in the following questions:

1) Do different tumors that have originated in the same parental host genotype show the same hybrid resistance pattern, when tested in a spectrum of $F_1$ hybrids? Or may different patterns be dissected out dependent on histology or etiology of the tumor?

2) Is resistance linked to the major histocompatibility complex, H-2? If so, does the resistance associated with different haplotypes reflect alleles of the same, locus, or different H-2 linked loci?

GENETIC CONTROL OF NATURAL RESISTANCE
TO INFECTION AND MALIGNANCY

3)     Do   the   H-2   linked   genes   introduce   resistance
against tumors of all genotypes?
4)     What is the relationship between the non-H-2 background and the H-2 linked resistance genes?

## Assay System

For each tumor, syngeneic, $F_1$ hybrid, and backcross
mice were inoculated with the same number of cells subcutaneously.  The serially transplanted in vivo lines were used.
The dose was chosen to give less than 100% but more than 50%
progressively growing tumors in the syngeneic strain of
origin (usually $10^3$ cells).  Tumor growth was followed by
weekly palpation and the cumulative incidence of tumors was
recorded and presented as percentage tumor take.


## RESULTS

### 1)  Tumors of B6 Origin

a) Lymphomas, virally induced

Tumor take incidence after the inoculation of $10^3$ cells
of five different virally induced lymphomas was examined.
RBL-5 is a Rauscher virus induced, GIR II Graffi virus induced and ALC, P-52-127-166 and 136-3 are radiation leukemia
virus induced tumors.  They are showed essentially the same
pattern with a strong resistance in the hybrids B6 x DBA/2,
B6 x CBA, B6 x C3H, B6 x A.CA and B6 x A/Sn.  The $H-2^{b/b}$
homozygous hybrids B6 x A.BY and B6 x C57L showed no detectable resistance.  Interestingly, the B6 x A.SW hybrid was
slightly more susceptible than the B6 parental itself to 4
out of the 5 tumors (GIR II, ALC, P-52-127-166 and 136-3).
The clear resistance introduced by A/Sn and A.CA but not
with the A congenic strains A.SW and A.BY showed that this
resistance is associated with $H-2^a$ and $H-2^f$, respectively.

b)  Lymphomas, chemically induced

EL-4 is a benzypyrene induced lymphoma and J-80-19,
J-80-21 and J-80-22 are DMBA (dimethylbenzantracene) induced.  The pattern otained with chemically induced lymphomas
resembled that of the virally induced tumors in that the CBA
x B6, C3H x B6, DBA/2 x B6, A x B6 and ACA x B6 hybrids were
resistant, whereas the A.SW x B6 and A.BY x B6 were as susceptible as the parental B6.  We have previously reported

that EL-4 showed a pattern close to the one for the virally induced lymphomas but with the exception of a lack of resistance in A.CA x B6 (1). However, with further testing of this hybrid we have found it also to be resistant to EL-4. The A.CA x B6 was also resistant to all three DMBA tumors.

c)  Sarcomas, methylcholanthrene induced

We have previously reported the $F_1$ hybrid resistance pattern for one methylcholanthrene induced sarcoma, MC57X (1). This pattern was clearly different from the lymphoma pattern with resistance in all hybrids (also in A.SW x B6 and A.BY x B6) except the C57L x B6. The MC57X tumor was compared in this study to two other methylcholanthrene induced sarcomas MC57Y and MC57G. For these two latter tumors the hybrid resistance pattern was very close to the usual lymphoma pattern and no resistance was found in B6 x A.SW and B6 x A.BY.

d)  Backcross analysis

$H-2^d$ linkage of resistance was studied in the (DBA/2 x B6) x B6 backcross (Fig. 1). The $H-2^{d/b}$ heterozygotes were more resistant than the $H-2^{b/b}$ homozygous mice to the three lymphomas RBL-5 (2), P-52-127-166 and ALC. We have previously reported that tests with MC57X in this backcross did not show significant H-2 linkage of resistance (1). However, with further testing the slight difference between $H-2^{d/b}$ heterozygotes and $H-2^{b/b}$ homozygotes have become significant (p <0.05) to his methylcholantrene induced sarcoma as well.

The results with the (A/Sn x B6) x B6 backcross can be seen in Fig. 2. RBL-5, GIR II and P-52-127-166 were all clearly more resisted by the $H-2^{a/b}$ heterozygotes than by the $H-2^{b/b}$ mice.

Finally $H-2^k$ linked resistance was demonstrated in the (CBA x B6) x B6 backcross (to RBL-5 and ALC) (Fig. 3) and in the (C3H x B6) x B6 cross, (Fig. 4) (to EL-4 and ALC). The sarcoma MC57X tested in the (CBA x B6) x B6 backcross showed no detectable $H-2^k$ linkage of resistance.

e)  Summary of the findings with tumors of B6 origin

In general the same hybrids were resistant to all lymphomas tested irrespective of inducing agent. The resistance was shown to be associated with the following H-2 haplotypes: d, a, k and f. One methylcholantrene induced sarcoma showed a different pattern with resistance also in

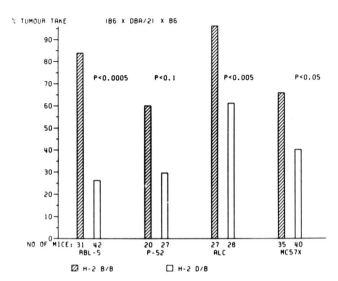

Figure 1. Percent tumor take incidence after s.c. inoculation of four different tumors of strain B6 origin in (DBA/2 x B6) x B6 backcross mice. H-2 homozygous mice, - shaded bars. H-2 heterozygous mice, - open bars. The statistical significance of the difference in take incidence in heterozygotes compared to homozygotes is indicated in the figure ($X^2$-test).

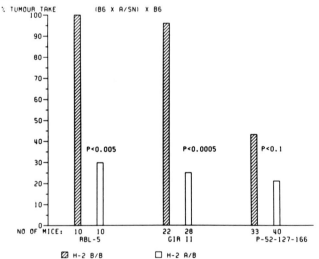

Figure 2. Percent tumor take incidence after s.c. inoculation of three lymphomas of strain B6 origin in (A/Sn x B6) x B6 backcross.

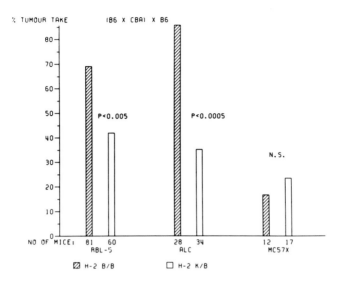

**Figure 3.** Percent tumor take incidence after s.c. inoculation of three tumors of B6 origin in (CBA x B6) x B6 backcross mice.

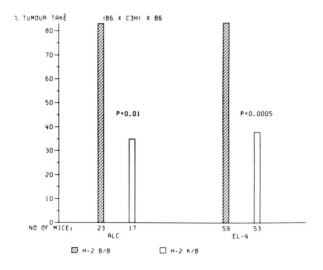

**Figure 4.** Percent tumor take incidence after s.c. inoculation of two lymphomas of strain B6 origin in (C3H x B6) x B6 backcross mice.

the B6 x A.BY and B6 x A.SW hybrids and little evidence for H-2 linkage of resistance except for a week linkage to H-2$^d$. Two other methylcholantrene induced B6 sarcomas showed a hybrid resistance close to the lymphoma pattern.

## Tumors of A/Sn origin

### a) Lymphomas

YAC is a Moloney lymphoma which has been studied in detail for hybrid resistance and *in vitro* sensitivity to the action of natural killer cells. The byrids with CBA, C3H, DBA/2, B6 and C57L were found to be highly resistant and the resistance was found to be linked to H-2$^b$ in the (B6 x A/Sn) x A/Sn and (C57L x A/Sn) x A/Sn backcrosses (3). In this study, resistance to the YAC lymphoma was compared with that to the YAD (also a moloney lymphoma but in contrast to YAC very insensitive to NK-activity), NSA1 (also a Moloney lymphoma), and GAB (Gross virus lymphoma). These lymphomas showed the same pattern as YAC except for YAD which grew equally well in all hybrids.

### b) Carcinomas

Hybrid resistance tests to the spontaneous mammary car- cinomas S3A and TA3/St together with the undifferentiated polyoma tumor SESO-C15 was studied. All tests hybrids were resistant to S3A while A.CA x A/Sn lacks resistance to the TA3 carcinoma. For SESO-C15 B6xA/Sn and C57L x A/Sn were the only hybrids which showed any resistance.

### c) Backcross analysis

In Fig. 5 the results of tests with the lymphoma NSA12 and the carcinoma S3A in the (C57L x A/Sn) x A/Sn are pre- sented. For NSA1 the H-2 heterozygotes are more resistant than the H-2$^{a/a}$ homozygotes as has previously been shown for YAC. In contrast the H-2$^b$ haplotype has absolutely no influence on the resistance against S3A, despite the clear resistance of the C57L x A/Sn hybrid (1/15 in tumor take compared to 28/29 for the A/Sn parental strain).

### d) Summary of the findings with tumors of A/Sn origin.

A strong hybrid resistance was found to the lymphomas with the exception of the NK-insensitive YAD. In spite of the H-2$^b$ linkage of resistance shown in backcross studies with C57L and B6, the A.BY strain (also H-2$^b$ but congenic with A/Sn) failed to introduce resistance. This suggests

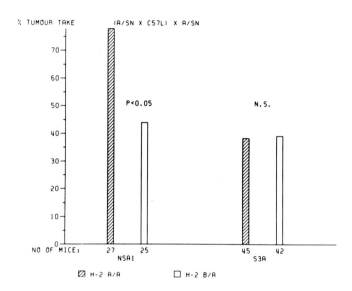

Figure 5. Percent tumor take incidence after s.c. inoculation of one lymphoma NSA 1 and one carcinoma in (C57L x A/Sn)
x A/Sn backcross mice.

that the H-2$^b$ linked gene is outside H-2 but still on
chromosome 17, or alternaively that the non H-2 background
of C57L or B6 is necessary for the expression of the H-2$^b$
linked resistance gene. No H-2 linked resistance gene was
found to exert influence on the resistance against the carcinomas tested.


DISCUSSION

A certain pattern of hybrid resistance to lymphomas of
one genotype exists so that some hybrids are resistant to
all lymphomas of that genotype. Exceptions may be found as
the NK-insensitive YAD lymphoma to which no hybrid was found
to be resistant. The etiology of the lymphoma has no influence on the resistance pattern.
Most sarcomas we have tested (in B6 and other strains,
data not shown) have a different hybrid resistance pattern

than the lymphomas but there are some methylcholantrene induced sarcomas that show a hybrid resistance close to the
lymphoma pattern.

The spontaneous mammary carcinoma often show very
little hybrid resistance and for the tumors where a strong
hybrid resistance have been found, the pattern have been
different from the lymphoma pattern.

H-2 linkage of resistance can be demonstrated to most
lymphomas. Resistance to B6-lymphomas was associated with
the following H-2 haplotypes: d, a, k and f. Resistance to
strain A/Sn-lymphomas was linked to H-2$^b$ as demonstrated
in the (C57L x A/Sn) x A/Sn and (B6 x A/Sn) x A/Sn backcrosses. The H-2$^{b/a}$ hybrid A.BY x A/Sn was however not
resistant to A/Sn-lymphomas which suggests that the H-2$^b$
linked gene may be localized outside H-2 on chromosome 17 or
alternatively, that the H-2 associated gene require a certain non H-2 background present in C57L and B6 but not in
A/Sn.

In contrast to what was found for the lymphomas only
weak H-2 linkage of hybrid resistance could be detected to
the sarcomas and no H-2 linkage at all was found in strong
hybrid resistance to mammary carcinomas.

We have found a clear association of hybrid resistance
to every tested H-2 haplotype in at least one combination.
It is not clear whether these resistance factors are alleles
of the same locus or different H-2 linked loci. However, a
haplotype that can introduce resistance in a given strain-
tumor combination does not always confer resistance to lymphomas of other strain origins. Several explanations for
this must be considered. Firstly, it is important ot remember that these resistance genes are dominant (by definition
of the hybrid resistance test). This means that e.g. for B6
tumors, A.BY and C57L (H-2$^b$) cannot contribute with more
H-2 associated resistance genes when crossed to B6 (H-2$^b$).
Secondly, the H-2 associated genes may depend on non H-2
background genes for full penetrance as was suggested above
for the lack of resistance in A.BY x A/Sn. Thirdly, the
action of resistance factors introduced by H-2 linked genes
may be dependent of the tumor at the level of H-2, Hh or
more unique tumor specific antigens. Finally the action of
"suppressor genes" may influence resistance, which might explain the higher susceptibility in certain F$_1$-hybrids compared to the parental strain.

A close similarity of the genetics of natural killer
cell activity and hybrid resistance to lymphomas of the
strains B6 and A/Sn exists. This together with the fact tha
the hybrid resistance have been shown to be thymus independent for a few lymphomas of these strains (4; and Klein et

al. manuscript in preparation) suggests that hybrid resistance against lymphomas is mediated largely if not entirely by NK-cells.

## ACKNOWLEDGEMENT

This investigation wa supported by Grant No. 2 RO1 CA 14054-07A1 and No. 1 RO1 CA 14054-C7, awarded by the National Cancer Institute, DHEW, and by grants from the Swedish Cancer Society.

## REFERENCES

1. Klein, G., Klein, G.O., Karre, K., and Kiessling, R. Immunogenetics 7:391, 1978.
2. Klein, G.O., Klein, G., Kiessling, R., and Karre, K. Immunogenetics 6:561, 1978.
3. Kiessling, R., Petranyi, G., Klein, G., and Wigzell, H. Int.J.Cancer 15:933, 1975.
4. Kiessling, R., Petranyi, G., Klein, G., and Wigzell, H. Int.J.Cancer 17:1, 1976.
5. Snell, G.D., and Stevens, L.C. Immunology 4:366, 1961.

## DISCUSSION

Participant: Klein said he had different H-2 haplotypes associated with resistance in the heterozygotes. Why does he call those high resistance alleles, rather than interpreting them, e.g., as Hh-dependent hybrid resistance, where they are recognizing H-2 non-identical cells rather than an influence of H-2 on the killer activity of his effectors? It is possible that the H-2 homozygous cells do express a recessive hemopoietic histocompatibility antigen and, just being H-2 heterozygous, these animals are now recognizing the recessive antigen?

Klein: Yes, that is a possible explanation but, in those cases where we have tested NK activity in parallel, this high NK activity is not seen to be dependent on the genotype of the targets. We can even use human targets and the same hybrids are highly reactive.

# PRELIMINARY ANALYSIS OF HYBRID RESISTANCE TO HISTOCOMPATIBLE P815 UTILIZING BONE MARROW AND THYMUS EPITHELIUM RADIATION CHIMERAS

R. Michael Williams, Blair M. Eig[1]
and Daniel E. Singer[2]

from
Section of Medical Oncology
Department of Medicine and the Cancer Center
Northwestern University
Chicago, Illinois

## INTRODUCTION

According to the classical laws of transplantation, parental tissue grafts should grow equally well in both the inbred strain of origin and in F1 hybrids between that strain and other allogeneic strains. However, as early as 1958, Snell demonstrated that a C57BL mouse lymphoma grew more successfully in C57BL mice than in F1 hybrids between C57BL and other strains (9). This phenomenon of hybrid resistance has since been observed in other tumor (4,5) and hematopoietic (1,2) transplantation systems.

The F1 offspring between DBA/2 mice ($H-2^d$) and other allogeneic strains have been shown to exhibit hybrid resistance to the DBA/2 mastocytoma P815 (11). In this paper we report our preliminary investigations into the cellular mechanism of hybrid resistance to P815 through the production of bone marrow and thymic chimeras between DBA/2 mice and the markedly resistant [C57BL/6 x DBA/2] F1 hybrid ($H-2^{b/d}$).

## MATERIALS AND METHODS

Female DBA/2, C57BL/6J, and (C57BL/6J x DBA/2J)F1 (hereafter called B6D2F1) were obtained from the Jackson Laboratory. Bone marrow chimeras were produced according to an established protocol (12). Recipient mice were irradiated (1000 rad) and reconstituted with $20 \times 10^6$ bone marrow cells. Where indicated the donor cells were treated with two cycles of AKR anti-C3H antiserum (anti-Thy 1.2) and mouse-absorbed rabbit serum as a course of complement. Thymic chimeras were produced according to Zinkernagel's protocol (13). Following irradiation and bone marrow reconstitution, each thymectomized recipient received six irradiated thymus lobes implanted subcutaneously in the left flank.

Chimeras were allowed approximately two months recuperation after which time the peripheral blood was verified to be of donor genotype by ability or inability to absorb anti-H-2$^b$ antibody. Experimental groups to be directly compared were injected subcutaneously in the foot with 10$^6$ P815 cells from the same tumor ascites preparation. Median survival times were determined to be that day on which the $\frac{(n + 1)}{2}$th mouse expired and p-values were determined by the log rank test (7).

RESULTS

Comparison of survival of DBA/2 and B6D2F1 mice following injection of P815 repeatedly shows the hybrid to be the longest lived. In a representative experiment depicted in Figure 1, B6D2F1 mice had a median survival time (MST) of 23.5 days compared to 16 days for DBA/2 mice injected with the same preparation of tumor.

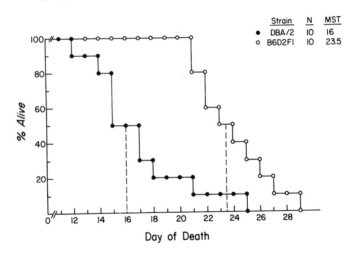

**Figure 1.** Survival of DBA/2 and B6D2F1 following injection of P815.

This tumor dose was chosen to assure that all mice from both groups would die in a reasonably short time. Our purpose was to determine whether or not survival between two groups was significantly different, so the statistical approach favored by most biostatisticians who specialize in survival analysis was utilized. In this case the p-value was .0045

ence in survival between these groups by chance is less than
1%. It is important to note that we were interested only in
the fact of a real difference in an objective parameter
(survival) analyzed by including all the data points (i.e.
requiring 0% survival in both groups), not in the absolute
magnitude of the MST. Accordingly, the absolute MST's from
separate experiments cannot be legitimately compared.

Table 1. Median survival time[1] of bone marrow recipient
chimeras injected with P815:[2] Role of bone marrow genotype
and effect of treatment with anti-Thy1.2 plus complement

| Exp. | Recipient Genotype | Bone Marrow Genotype | | | | |
|------|-----|---------|---------|---------|---------|---|
| | | Untreated | | Anti-Thy1.2 + C' Treated | | |
| | | B6D2F1 | DBA/2 | B6D2F1 | DBA/2 | p |
| 1 | DBA/2 | 20(11) | 15(12) | | | .0005 |
| 2 | DBA/2 | 19(7) | | 17(8) | 16(9) | see foot-note 3 |
| | B6D2F1 | | | 21(10) | 17(15) | .0029 |

[1]In days. N given in parentheses.
[2]Recipient mice were irradiated with 1000 rads and reconstituted with 20 x 10[6] bone marrow cells (either treated with
anti-Thy1.2 plus complement or untreated, as indicated).
Following at least three weeks recuperation, chimeras were
injected subcutaneously in the left hind footpad with 10[6]
P815 cells on day 0.
[3]For comparison of untreated B6D2F1→DBA/2 chimeras, p=.0427.
For comparison of treated B6D2F1→DBA/2 and treated DBA/2→-
DBA/2 chimeras, p=.0896.

The capacity of untreated B6D2F1 bone marrow to transfer hybrid resistance is demonstrated in the first experiment presented in Table 1. The DBA/2 chimeras reconstituted
with B6D2F1 bone marrow lived 33% longer (MST of 20 days)
than those reconstituted with DBA/2 bone marrow (MST of 15
days) following the injection of P815. In a second experiment the capacity of B6D2F1 bone marrow, both with and without anti-Thy 1.2 treatment, to confer resistance was tested
(Table 1, and experiment 2). In this case, the anti-Thy 1.2
treated B6D2F1 cells provided the DBA/2 recipients with only
a 6% increase in survival time (MST of 17 days) over the

treated DBA/2 bone marrow (MST of 16 days). In the same experiment, untreated B6D2F1 bone marrow was able to transfer
a higher level of resistanc to DBA/2 recipients (MST of 19
days).

Transfer of DBA/2 susceptibility to P815 into irradiated B6D2F1 recipients with DBA/2 bone marrow is also demonstrated in Table 1. B6D2F1 mice reconstituted with DBA/2 bone
marrow had a 19% shorter survival time (MST of 17 days) than
those which were reconstituted with B6D2F1 bone marrow (MST
of 21 days), following the injection of tumor. The data
presented in Table 1 also show that some form of hybrid resistance remains in the lethally irradiated B6D2F1 recipient. B6D2F1 recipients had a 24% longer survival time
(MST of 21 days) than their DBA/2 counterparts (MST of 17
days) when both were reconstituted with the same anti-Thy
1.2 plus complement treated B6D2F1 bone marrow (p = .0041).
This residual host resistance was less impressive when the
reconstituting bone marrow came from DBA/2 donors in that
DBA/2→B6D2F1 chimeras (MST of 17 days) lived only slightly
longer than DBA/2→DBA/2 chimeras (MST of 16 days;p = .0891).

Table 2a presents the role of the bone marrow genotype
in the generation of hybrid resistance in bone marrow and
thymic chimeras. Transfer of the most pronounced resistance
to P815 occurred in those DBA/2 which received B6D2F1 bone
marrow and a B6D2F1 thymus (MST of 19 days, as compared to
DBA/2 which received DBA/2 bone marrow and a B6D2F1 thymus,
MST of 14 days). The difference in median survival between
DBA/2 reconstituted with B6D2F1 (MST of 16 days) or DBA/2
(MST of 14 days) bone marrow was less dramatic when they
were implanted with a DBA/2 thymus. Finally, when no thymus
was present in the DBA/2 recipients, it appears that little
or no hybrid resistance was transferred by B6D2F1 bone marrow (MST of 14 days).

Table 2b presents the role of the recipient genotype in
the generation of hybrid resistance in these same chimeras.
A hybrid host effect is present in the B6D2F1 which received
B6D2F1 bone marrow and no thymus (MST of 19 days) as compared to the DBA/2 which received B6D2F1 bone marrow and no
thymus (MST of 14 days). However, this effect begins to
disappear when, along with the B6D2F1 bone marrow, a DBA/2
thymus is transferred to the B6D2F1 (MST of 18 days) and to
the DBA/2 (MST of 16 days) recipients. The hybrid host effect is no longer demonstrable when a B6D2F1 thymus is transplanted along with the B6D2F1 bone marrow into B6D2F1 and
DBA/2 recipients. The data from Tables 2a and 2b suggest
that in order to optimally transfer hybrid resistance to
P815, the B6D2F1 thymus is required in addition to B6D2F1
bone marrow that was previously depleted of adult T cells.

Table 2.  Median survival time[1] of bone marrow and thymic recipient chimeras injected with P815[2].

a.  Role of bone marrow genotype (recipient and thymus constant)

|  | | Bone Marrow Genotype | | |
| Recipient Genotype | Thymus Genotype | B6D2F1 | DBA/2 | p[3] |
| DBA/2 | no thymus | 14(13) | no data | - |
| DBA/2 | DBA/2 | 16(15) | 14(9) | .0121 |
| | p=.0190 | | | |
| DBA/2 | B6D2F1 | 19(15) | 14(5) | .0045 |

b.  Role of recipient genotype (bone marrow and thymus constant)

|  | | Recipient Genotype | | |
| Bone Marrow Genotype | Thymus Genotype | B6D2F1 | DBA/2 | p |
| B6D2F1 | no thymus | 19(14) | 14(13) | <.0001 |
| B6D2F1 | DBA/2 | 18(15) | 16(15) | .0251 |
| B6D2F1 | B6D2F1 | 17.5(14) | 19(15) | .7532 |

[1] In days.  N given in parentheses.
[2] Thymectomized recipient mice were irradiated with 1000 rads and reconstituted with $20 \times 10^6$ anti-Thy 1.2 plus complement treated bone marrow cells.  Mice were then given subcutaneously in the flank six 1000 rad irradiated thymic lobes (in selected cases, no thymic lobes were implanted).  Following a two month recuperation, chimeras were injected subcutaneously in the left hind footpad with $10^6$ P815 cells on day 0.
[3] Except when indicated, p-value are for comparisons between adjacent columns.


DISCUSSION

Since Snell first described the phenomenon of enhanced resistance by F1 hybrids to parental tumors (9), the mechanism of this apparent violation of the "classic" laws of transplantation has been the subject of considerable speculation and some controversy (5,8).  We began to investigate this question because the apparent H-2 dependence could involve immune response gene phenomena in tumor resistance

(10). The initial genetic data (11) appeared paradoxical
because they implicated both more than one H-2 gene and H-2
dependent immune suppression in a response which was presumably directed to a simple yet undefined tumor associated
antigen. There was also evidence of an influence by non H-2
genes. Subsequent studies of immune response gene control
of antibody responses to random polymers (3) and our own
data utilizing mutants at $H-2K^b$ and $I-A^b$ (Melvold, R,
and Williams, R.M., this volume) support the conclusion that
several, at least three, genes could be involved in determining resistance. Thus, it is not surprising that the
present data generated with B6D2F1 and DBA/2 mice, which
differ by multiple loci, could support many interpretations
concerning mechanism.

     In addition to the normal situation we investigated
bone marrow and thymus epithelium chimeras in which all but
one component was held constant. When binary genotype comparisons between F1 and parental were made for recipient,
thymus epithelium, and bone marrow, the B6D2F1 was superior
in nearly every case. The only exception was the inability
to demonstrate superiority of the F1 hybrid recipient genotype when both bone marrow and thymus epithelium were of
hybrid genotype (Table 2b, last line, p= .7532). This could
mean that the survival advantage of the B6D2F1 genotype depends entirely on bone marrow derived cell dependent phenomena. These could be partly thymus independent as seen when
irradiated recipients have no thymus (Table 2b, line 1, p
<.0001). The effect might be augmented by DBA/2 and B6D2F1
thymus to the extent that no additional host genotype effect
is observable when both hybrid bone marrow and thymus are
utilized. It seems plausible that some T-cell dependent
activity can participate in resistance since anti-Thy 1.2
treatment of B6D2F1 bone marrow diminished the resistance in
non-thymectomized DBA/2 recipients (Table 1, experiment 2).

     Several questions remain unanswered in this system.
For example, presence of thymus may actually decrease resistance through suppressor mechanisms and we have not characterized the T-cell function of these chimeras. The present
experiments can serve as models, but clear cut answers to
most of our questions will probably require that these
studies be done in models which differ by only a single
gene.

## ACKNOWLEDGEMENT

     Supported by NIH Grant CA27599 and a grant from the
Leukemia Research Foundation.

## REFERENCES

1.  Cudkowicz, G.   In The Proliferation and Spread of Neoplastic Cells.   21st Ann. Symposium on Fundamental Cancer Research, Houston. p.662, 1967.
2.  Cudkowicz, G., and Stimpfling, J.H.   Nature 204:450, 1964.
3.  Dorf, M.E., Stimpfling, J.H., and Benacerraf, B. J.Exp.Med. 141:1459, 1975.
4.  Hellstrom, K.E.   Int.J.Cancer 1:349, 1966.
5.  Hellstrom, K.E., and Hellstrom, I.   Progr.Exp.Tumor Res. 9:40, 1967.
6.  Melvold, R.W., and Williams, R.M.   1980 (this volume).
7.  Peto, R., and Peto, J.   J.Roy.Stat.Soc.A. 135:185, 1972.
8.  Sanford, B.H., and Soo, S.F.   J.Natl.Cancer Inst. 46:95, 1971.
9.  Snell, G.D.   J.Natl.Cancer Inst. 21:843, 1958.
10. William, R.M.   Fed.Proc. 32:880, 1973.
11. Williams, R.M., Dorf, M.E., and Benacerraf, B.   Cancer Res. 35:1586, 1975.
12. Sprent, J., von Boehmer, H., and Nabholz, M. J.Exp.Med. 142:321, 1975.
13. Zinkernagel, R.M., Callahan, G.N., Althage, A., Cooper, S. Klein, P.A., and Klein, J.   J.Exp.Med. 147:882, 1978.

[1] Present address:   c/o Student Affairs Office, Harvard Medical School, 25 Shattuck St., Boston, Massachusetts.

[2] Present address:   Department of Medicine, Massachusetts General Hospital, Fruit St., Boston, Massachusetts.

# GENETIC CONTROL OF NATURAL RESISTANCE TO GRAFT VERSUS HOST-ASSOCIATED SUPPRESSION OF T CELL-MEDIATED LYMPHOLYSIS

Gene M. Shearer, Richard P. Polisson,
Matthew W. Miller and Elena Cudkowicz
Immunology Branch
National Cancer Institute
Bethesda, Maryland 20205

A number of studies have shown that the injection of parental T lymphocytes into $F_1$ hybrid mice can lead to the rapid onset of depressed immune potential (3,6,7,10,11). Such immune depression is associated with the development of a graft vs. host (GVH) reaction, and has been shown to be due to suppressor cells found in the lymphoid tissue of the injected $F_1$ animals (9,11). We have recently described a similar observation in which the ability of spleen cells from $F_1$ mice injected with parental T cells to generate in vitro T cell-mediated lympholysis (CML) responses to trinitrophenyl-modified syngeneic (TNP-self) or allogeneic cells is abrogated or severely reduced (13). This depression of CML potential was found to be associated with the onset of a GVH reaction, and was also shown to be due to suppressor cells, some of which have the potential to kill F cells, and some of which do not. We also observed that immunosuppression and the GVH reaction were not equally inducible in $F_1$ mice by injection of lymphocytes from each parent (13). For example, intravenous injection of (C57BL/10 x B10.A)$F_1$ (abbreviated (BxA)$F_1$) mice with $2 \times 10^7$ B10.A (abbreviated A) parental spleen cells abrogated the host $F_1$ spleen cells in vitro CML potential to TNP-self and alloantigens. This effect could be detected within 4 days and persisted for at least 21 days. In contrast, the CML potential of spleen cells from (BxA)$F_1$ injected with $2 \times 10^7$ C57BL/10 (abbreviated B) spleen cells was not affected. The present report: (a) summarizes the basic phenomenon and illustrates the differential patterns of suppression observed in four $F_1$ strain combinations; (b) demonstrates that $F_1$ mice are resistant to induction of GVH-associated CML suppression by H-2$^b$ parental spleen cells; (c) provides mapping results which indicate that the $F_1$ resistance involves recognition by radiosensitive cells of homozygous parental H-2D$^b$ alleles; and (d) discusses the possible implications of the similarities between resistance of $F_1$ to parental induced GVH and resistance to infection and malignancy.

The protocol which is described in detail elsewhere (13) is briefly summarized as follows: Groups of mice were injected intravenously with $20 \times 10^6$ viable spleen cells

from either parent A or B or from the $F_1$. Seven or 14 days
later, spleen cells from the inoculated $F_1$ mice were sensitized <u>in</u> <u>vitro</u> with irradiated, trinitrophenyl-modified
syngeneic spleen cells to generate cytotoxic T lymphocyte
(CTL) responses against TNP-self. After five days, the
cultures were tested for CTL activity using TNP-modified
blast targets in a 4-hour $^{51}$Cr-release assay.

The basic observation of depressed CML potential in
$(BxA)F_1$ mice following injection of A spleen cells, but not
after injection of B spleen cells is summarized in Fig. 1.

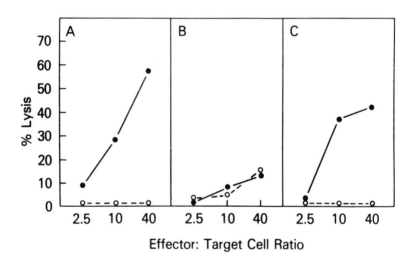

Fig. 1. Cell-mediated cytotoxic potential to TNP-self using
spleen cels from $(BxA)F_1$ mice; (A) uninjected;(B) injected
14 days earlier with 2 x $10^7$ B10.A spleen cells; or (c) injected 14 days earlier with 2 x $10^7$ B10 spleen cells. Effector cells were generated by sensitization with TNBS-modif-
ied (●--●) or unmodified (O---O)$F_1$ spleen cells, and assayed
on TNBS modified PHA-stimulated $F_1$ splenic blasts.

The CML potential of spleen cells from $F_1$ mice injected
seven days earlier with A splen cells was completely abrogated (Fig. 1A), whereas the cytotoxic activity of cells
from $F_1$ injected with B spleen cells was unaffected (Fig.
1B). This indicates either that the ability of B to recognize <u>H-2</u>$^a$ antigens is much weaker than the ability of A to

recognize $H-2^b$ antigens expressed by the $F_1$, or that there is selective resistance of the $F_1$ host against engraftment of B but not of A parental lymphocytes. Results to be published elsewhere demonstrate that : (a) the ability of B and A spleen cells to recognize $H-2^a$ and $H-2^b$ alloantigens respectively on $F_1$ lymphocytes, as demonstrated by in vitro CML responses is about equal; (b) $F_1$ mice can be rendered CML unresponsive by injecting larger numbers of B spleen cells (e.., 40-60 x $10^6$); and (c) pre-injection of $F_1$ mice with small numbers of B spleen cells results in susceptibility of $F_1$ mice to immunosuppression induced by a second injection of B lymphocytes. These findings indicate that the failure of B spleen cells to induce CML unresponsiveness in $F_1$ hosts is due to resistance of the $F_1$ mice against B parental lymphocytes.

Natural resistance of $F_1$ mice to $H-2^b$ parental hemopoietic grafts (1,2), and $F_1$ anti-$H-2^b$ parental CML potential (12) has been known for sometime. Mapping studies indicated that the homozygous $H-2^b$ allele recognized by the $F_1$ in resistance to marrow grafts (1) as well as for $F_1$ anti-parental CTL targets (8) mapped to the D region of the H-2 complex. The possibility that $F_1$ resistance to $H-2^b$ parental-induced GVH-associated CML suppression is due to a similar or an identical natural resistance phenomenon was investigated by genetic experiments. First, we tested whether a number of different $F_1$ mouse strains would exhibit selective resistance to CML suppression induced by $H-2^b$ parental spleen cells. The results, published in detail elsewhere (13), and summarized in Table 1, indicate that

**Table 1.** Selective resistance of $F_1$ mouse strains to immunosuppression by $H-2^b$ but not by non-$H-2^b$ parental spleen cells.*

| $F_1$ host mice | Parental spleen cells injected | CML potential suppressed |
|---|---|---|
| (C57BL/10 x B10.A)$F_1$ | C57BL/10 | No |
|  | B10.A | Yes |
| (C57BL/10 x B10.BR)$F_1$ | C57BL/10 | No |
|  | B10.BR | Yes |
| (C57BL/6 x DBA/2)$F_1$ | C57BL/6 | No |
|  | DBA/2 | Yes |

*$F_1$ mice were injected intravenously with 20 x $10^6$ parental spleen cells. Seven to 14 days later, spleen cells from the injected $F_1$ mice were tested for suppression of CML potential against TNP-self and allogeneic cells.

resistance was detected only against $\underline{H-2^b}$ parental spleen
cells. Second, (BxA)$F_1$ host mice were injected with spleen
cells from parental and B10 congenic recombinant mice, and
the CML potential of the injected $F_1$ mice was determined 14
days later. This experiment was designed to map the $\underline{H-2^b}$
allele recognized by the (BxA)$F_1$. The recombinant strains
were chosen such that there could not be recognition by the
$F_1$ host of H-2 antigens expressed by the recombinant mice
(i.e., no HVG), but such that there would be recognition by
the injected recombinant cells of an entire H-2 haplotype
expressed by the $F_1$. This maximizes the potential for a GVH
reaction, if resistance is not operating.

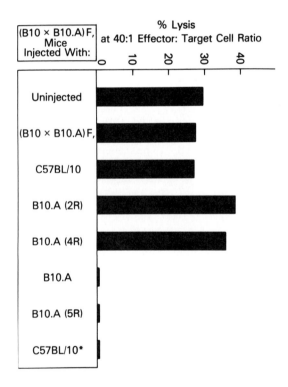

Fig. 2. Cell-mediated cytotoxic potential to TNP-self using
spleen cells from (BxA)$F_1$ mice injected 14 days earlier with
20 x 10$^6$ parental or B10.A recombinant spleen cells. *Injection with 40 x 10$^6$ B parental spleen cells. Effector
cells were generated and assayed as in Fig. 1.

The data summarized in Fig. 2 for one effector:target cell ratio illustrate that the $F_1$ was resistant to B10, B10.A-(4R), and B10.A(2R), but not to B10.A or B10.A(5R). These results indicate that resistance of (BxA)$F_1$ mice to GVH-associated CML suppression is due to recognition of homozygous H-2D$^b$. (See Table 2 for mapping of the H-2 alleles). These findings indicate that $F_1$ natural resistance to hemopoietic grafts and parental-induced CML suppression and $F_1$ anti-parental CML activity are immunogenetically similar.

Table 2. Mapping of homozygous H-2$^b$ allele recognized by (BxA)$F_1$ in resistance to GVH-associated CML suppression.

| Host H-2 region | Donor H-2 region | Donor Strain | $F_1$ resistant (R) or susceptible (S) |
|---|---|---|---|
| K I S D<br>A B J E C | K I S D<br>A B J E C | | |
| b b b b b b b b<br>k k k k k d d d | b b b b b b b b | C57BL/10 | R |
| | k k k k k d d d | B10.A | S |
| | k k b b b b b b | B10.A(4R) | R |
| | k k k k k d d b | B10.A(2R) | R |
| | b b b k k d d d | B10.A(5R) | S |

Although the above genetic study indicates that there are similarities between $F_1$ resistance to parental hemopoietic grafts and to parental induced CML suppression, at least one difference between the two phenomena exists. $F_1$ resistance to hemopoietic grafts can be overcome by inoculating an excessive number of H-2$^b$ marrow cells, i.e., in the range of $1 \times 10^6$ (1). $F_1$ resistance to CML suppression can also be overcome, but the range for saturation is around $40 \times 10^6$ (see Fig. 2). Thus, approximately 40-fold more cells are required to saturate natural resistance for CML suppression than that for hemopoietic grafts. This indicates that there could be selective resistance for a small subpopulation of H-2$^b$ parental lymphocytes (possibly those which express receptors for anti-$\underline{H-2}^a$ activity), and/or that the resistance to CML suppression is much stronger than the resistance to hemopoietic grafts.

One difference in the experimental protocols between these two resistance models is that the $F_1$ hosts were irradiated prior to marrow grafting, whereas the $F_1$ mice were not irradiated. In order to test whether resistance to CML suppression was radiosensitive, (BxA)$F_1$ mice were exposed to 850 R whole body x-rays and injected with B or A parental spleen cells. Seven days later, the suppressive potential of the parental repopulated $F_1$ spleens was tested by co-culture with normal $F_1$ spleen cells which were simultaneously sensitized to TNP-self. The findings, summarized briefly in Table 3, and shown in detail elsewhere, indicate that $F_1$ natural resistance to parental B spleen cells, as assessed by CML suppression, is sensitive to 850 R. Thus, it appears that the difference between the number of $\underline{H-2}^b$ parental cells required to overcome $F_1$ resistance to hemopoietic grafts and to CML suppression can be accounted for, at least in part, by the existence of a potent radiosensitive component of $F_1$ resistance to GVH-associated CML suppression. Studies are in progress to determine whether this radiosensitive component of resistance is mediated by T-lymphocytes, and whether it represents the in vivo counterpart of $F_1$ antiparental CML activity demonstrated in vitro (12).

Table 3. Comparison of suppressor cell function in the spleens of irradiated and unirradiated (BxA)$F_1$ mice injected with B or A spleen cells.*

| Status of $F_1$ host | $F_1$ host injected with: | Suppressor cell activity detected in host spleens |
|---|---|---|
| unirradiated | A | yes |
|  | B | no |
| irradiated** | A | yes |
|  | B | yes |

*Detailed results are to be published elsewhere[1].
**$F_1$ mice were exposed to 850 R whole body x-rays injection of parental spleen cells.

This conference is concerned with natural resistance to infection and malignancy, and has not directly addressed the issue of the graft vs. host reaction, nor the immunosuppression that frequently accompanies it. Yet, immunosuppression associated with GVH renders the individual more

susceptible to infection (5,14) as well as to spontaneously
appearing tumors (4). However, the most important observation of this study is <u>not</u> the association of GVH and immunosuppression, but rather the demonstration of natural resistance to GVH-associated immunosuppression - and the realization that this natural resistance resembles, both genetically and mechanistically, many of the natural resistance systems described for infection and malignancy. We postulate
that the example of natural resistance discussed in this
conference show a common mechanism of surveillance and protection against infection and malignancy, as well as for
GVH-associated immunosuppression (see Table 4 for model).

Table 4. Model of natural resistance surveillance system
(NRSS)

---

NRSS can be challenged by:

1. Infection

2. Graft versus host reaction

3. Spontaneous neoplasms

Input:          1.    2.    3.

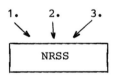

Outcome:        1 + 2 = severe graft versus host
                        and/or infection

                2 → 3   spontaneous neoplasms

---

We interpret: (a) the findings that natural resistance to
hemopoietic and tumor grafts (1) as well as to GVH (this
study) can be saturated or over-ridden by excessive cell
numbers; (b) the long-known observations that the severity
of GVH disease often parallels susceptibility to opportu-
nistic infections (5,14); and (c) that GVH disease is frequently followed by the appearance of spontaneously arising
tumors (4), to mean that each of these insults are competing
for a common natural resistance system. This natural resistance probably has both radioresistant and radiosensitive
components, and unlike the more conventional immune systems

appears to have limited potential for priming and memory. That a common natural resistance system with limited overall capacity for surveillance may exist, and that its efficient function may be susceptible to the competing effects of these seemingly independent insults should underscore an attitude of caution for clinical approaches to tumor therapy and hemopoietic transplantation, and may eventually point to cause and effect relationships in certain types of spontaneous neoplastic transformation.

## REFERENCES

1.  Cudkowicz, G. "Natural Resistance Systems Against Foreign Cells, Tumors, and Microbes". G. Cudkowicz, M. Landy, G.M. Shearer (eds). Academic Press, New York, p. 3, 1978.
2.  Cudkowicz, G., and Bennet, M. J.Exp.Med. 134:1513, 1971.
3.  Elie, R., and Lapp, W.S. Cell.Immunol., 1976.
4.  Gleichman, E., Gleichman, H., and Wilke, W. Transpl.-Rev. 31:156, 1976.
5.  Glucksberg, H., Storb, R., Fefer, A., Buckner, C.D., Neiman, P.E., Clift, R.A., Lerner, K.G., and Thomas, E.D. Transplantation 18:295, 1974.
6.  Howard, J.G., and Woodruff, M.F.A. Proc.R.Soc.Lond.-B.Biol.Sci. 154:532, 1961.
7.  Lapp, W.S., and Moller, G. Immunology 17:339, 1969.
8.  Nakamura, I., and Cudkowicz, G. Eur.J.Immunol. 9:371, 1979.
9.  Pickel, V., and Hoffman, M.K. J.Immunol. 118:653, 1977.
10. Shand, F.L. Immunology 29:953, 1975.
11. Shand, F.L. Immunology 31:943, 1976.
12. Shearer, G.M., and Cudkowicz, G. Science 190:890, 1975.
13. Shearer, G.M., and Polisson, R.P. J.Exp.Med. 151:20, 1980.
14. Thomas, E.D., Storb, R., Clift, R.A., Fefer, A., Johnson, F.L., Neiman, P.E., Lerner, K.G., Glucksberg, H., and Buckner, C.D. N.Eng.J.Med. 292:832, 1975.

## DISCUSSION

Kirchner: I do not seem to recall Shearer saying anything about the nature of the suppressor cell.

Shearer: I did not simply because that would be beyond the

scope of this meeting. But we are working on that. There
are two, possibly at least three, types. There is a killer
cell which obviously hits the alloantigens on the $F_1$ but
there are other cells that cannot account for that. We do
not know what proportion of the suppressor cells are of $F_1$
origin and what proportion are of parental origin.

Kirchner: We have data showing that tumor-bearing animals
have very strong suppressor cytotoxic responses and we would
attribute this to the presence of macrophages. Lapp has
similar data.

Shearer: Considered as a function of time, we do not know
whether we are dealing with macrophages or T cells. Even
now we do not know in functional terms what the cell types
are, or if they are of parental or $F_1$ origin. We do know
that they cannot be accounted for exclusively by killer
cells hitting the alloantigen expressed on the $F_1$.

Hormaeche: Has Shearer ever actually tested resistance to
infection experimentally in his chimeras? I was asking
Howard about some of his earlier work where he found that
animals undergoing GVH disease were more resistant. At the
time it was interpreted as macrophage activation.

Shearer: We have not ascertained resistance to infection,
but hope to do so later on.

Hormaeche: Shearer mentioned that resistance to GVH suppression was radiosensitive. Has he tested any other recipient strains outside of the B10 family?

Shearer: Yes, but this can get rather confusing; I think
that here one is dealing with the resistance genes. The
moment we bring in backgrounds such as C3H, we get into more
difficulties. We have gone over to nude mice now where,
despite resistance appearing to be radiosensitive, the nude
animal proves very resistant to inoculation of B10 or B6
cells. But the moment we bring in the C3H background, we
move into an entirely different situation. It is not clear
whether this is a T cell or an NK cell. We know in one defined situation it is radiosensitive but we know that, using
those same cells in a nude $F_1$, the nude expresses resistance.

Lapp: We appreciate that an animal undergoing a GVH reaction will not respond with either cell mediated or humoral
immune responses. An H-2 difference between donor and re-

cipient is not a prerequisite for obtaining GVH-induced immunosuppression. My own feeling is that this is an important point. We have shown, with Kirchner, that there is an increase in interferon production in the course of a GVH reaction. We have also shown there is an increase in prostaglandin as well, and that macrophage-mediated prostaglandin is probably an early GVH effect that could account for suppression of both cell mediated and humoral immune responses. We have been looking at NK cell activity as well, and one sees a marked increase in NK cell activity in the early phase of the reaction, which then recedes by day 12-15 post-GVH induction.

Winn: During the time the animals are unable to mount a good allogeneic response in vitro, what would happen if a skin graft were applied?

Shearer: We have not yet done this particular test.

Winn: So you really do not know how severe the in vivo depression is.

Shearer: No, but I would say, if these animals will not respond to alloantigens (and those curves are flat at an effector target cell ratio of 4:1), they are pretty much immunoincompetent.

# GENETIC CONTROL OF NATURAL RESISTANCE TO TUMOR GROWTH

Chairman's Summary

Henry J. Winn

Transplantation Unit, Department of Surgery
Massachusetts General Hospital
Boston, Mass. 02114

There is considerable and well-documented variation in the susceptibility of different groups of animals and man to the induction of cancer by chemical, physical and biological agents, and much of this variation has been shown to be under genetic control. Where such differences have been subjected to close study they have been found to be associated with such things as differences in the ability to convert inactive chemical agents to carcinogens, differences in ability to resist infection, or differences in other less well defined predisposing factors. There is, for example, a curious and unexplained relationship between the various alleles at the agouti locus in the mouse and the incidence of spontaneously occurring or chemically induced pulmonary tumors. Also, it has been suggested that malignant transformation may in some instances entail the occurrence of two independent mutations and that individuals who inherit one mutant gene are, thereby, more likely to develop neoplastic disease.

All of these examples represent, to some extent at least, genetically controlled variations in the susceptibility of individuals to the induction of neoplastic transformation, and their practical and conceptual significance is widely acknowledged. However, they are not here considered to come under the heading of genetically controlled natural resistance to cancer. Rather, we have considered under that heading those genetically regulated factors that provide resistance to the growth and spread of cells already transformed to the neoplastic state.

Most tumor biologists believe that there are multiple mechanisms that influence the growth and development of malignant tumors and that many of them are, in a broad sense, genetically regulated. However it has been difficult, in most cases impossible, to identify these mechanisms precisely or to undertake a formal analysis of the genes that regulate them. Moreover, many of them do not involve active or aggressive resistance to malignancy and are, therefore, not considered here as contributing to natural

resistance to cancer. The subject of genetic control of
immune responsiveness to tumors was also thought to fall
beyond the purview of this Conference, since the very concept of "natural" resistance excludes specific adaptive
mechanisms.

When, in fact, one reflects on the constitutive mechanisms that might provide for active resistance to neoplastic disease, it is difficult to come up with anything
other than the recently discovered natural killer cells,
consequently this formed the principal subject of discussion
during this aspect of the Conference.

The effects of natural killer cells were initially
observed in conjunction with studies on the tumoricidal
effects of lymphoid cells that had been prepared from puta-
tively immune donors. Cells from nonimmune control donors
frequently caused lysis of variable but generally small
numbers of tumor cells and this puzzling background activity
was traced to the action of a minor population of lymphoid
cells that have been classified as non-T, non-B, non-
adherent cells. The discovery of a system of alloantigens
that appears to be restricted in distribution to NK cells
helped to establish them as a unique population within the
lymphoreticular tissues and it provided a means of isolating
and characterizing this new class of cells.

Interest in NK cells grew rapidly and they have now
become the subject of study in numerous laboratories. A
very large body of literature dealing with them is steadily
accumulating and it would be surprising had not our knowledge of them expanded greatly by the time these proceedings
are published. Accordingly, only the major conclusions
reached by the participants are here briefly summarized. It
is recognized, of course, that much of the evidence supporting these conclusions has come from studies carried out not
only by the conference participants but by other investigators in various laboratories world-wide.

First, as already indicated, there is no longer any
question of the existence of NK cells as a distinctive definable subpopulation of lymphoreticular cells. There are
several observations that support this view but the disclo-
sure of NK cell specific antigens is especially convincing.
This does not, of course, mean that the biological function
of these cells is to provide protection against malignant
tumors. Indeed, the tumoricidal activity of these cells may
turn out to be fortuitous property providing little if any
positive selective value to their bearers.

NK cells are heterogenous, a view first put forth on
the basis of observations that normal spleen cells that had
been incubated at 37°C for 12 hours were no longer able to

kill YAC cells, whereas their action on other tumor cells remained undiminished. The possibility that a single cell type had lost the ability to kill one but not another target was not excluded but is now made very unlikely by reports made at this Conference. Treatment of spleen cells with anti-NK sera and C abrogated the ability of these cells to kill YAC but not their ability to destroy other tumor cells. Anti-NK sera were not effective without C, indicating that a sub-population of cells had been destroyed. Furthermore, treatment of mice with $^{89}$Sr led to a loss of toxicity for YAC with little effect on natural killing of several other tumors. Finally, spleen cells of beige mice have greatly diminished natural toxicity for YAC but essentially normal levels of activity against other types of tumor cells. The significance of this heterogeneity is not understood but it is relevant to considering the nature and function of NK cells and their relationships to other cells of the lympho-reticular system.

NK cells, at least those that kill YAC cells, are also the cells that mediate ADCC. There are several lines of evidence that support this conclusion, and there are no experimental data that conflict with it. This finding should provide new approaches to exploring the tumoricidal properties of the NK cell. It is intriguing, for example, that it can kill some types of tumor cells only in the presence of antibody and others in its absence. Yet among mice of various inbred strains there seems to be no association between these two attributes. There seems also to be an association between NK activity and the phenomenon of hybrid resistance but this association is poorly defined, and the poor definition may be a reflection of the heterogeneity of NK cells. Nevertheless, this association deserves close study for it may touch on a major function of NK cells, viz regulation of the activities of other lymphoreticular cells.

Finally, there is evidence for some association between NK cells and the thymus. It has been claimed that there is an inverse relationship between thymic activity and NK activity, a point which is perhaps best illustrated by the high levels of NK activity found in congenitally athymic mice. It has also been claimed that natural killing can be reduced by treatment of cells with anti-Thy-1 and C, and in fact that has now been established with monoclonal reagents. The reduction in activity that is effected by monoclonal anti-Thy-1 is, however, never complete, indicating the presence of two cells populations. In any case the significance of Thy-1 on NK cells is difficult to evaluate. It could indicate on the one hand that NK cells are part of the T-cell lineage, - it has suggested for example that they are pre-T cells - or on the other hand that the Thy-1 antigen is more widely distributed on cell types than has been previously thought. Here, again, the availability of antisera specifically reactive with NK cells should help in sorting out these relationships.

Genetic control of NK activity undoubtedly occurs at many functional levels but is perhaps best seen in the case of beige mice in which there is a marked reduction of activity and in nude mice in which there is consistent elevation of activity. Genetic regulation in these cases, and more especially in other less dramatic instances, is difficult to study because of the strong influence of environmental factors on NK activity. It is well known, for example, that activity is strikingly affected by the age and general state of health of the cell donors. Still it is clear that NK activity is regulated in mice by genes associated with the MHC as well as by other independently segregating genes. The action of these genes is entirely unknown and it is by no means clear that they are involved principally or only in the function of NK cells.

The specificity of NK cells is poorly defined and even now seems to be very complicated. Recognition of the heterogeneity of NK cells and their association with ADCC may provide leads to further analysis of this problem but it does not seem likely that the issue will be resolved in the near future.

The activity of NK cells _in vivo_ clearly needs further consideration. There is no question that implants of mixtures of tumor cells and NK cells grow less well than do implants of tumor cells alone or tumor cells mixed with other kinds of lymphoid cells. But the extent to which NK cells influence the growth and spread of malignant cells that arise _de novo_ remains quite unknown.

# THE GENETIC BASIS OF MACROPHAGE COLONY FORMATION

Carleton C. Stewart, Emil Skamene*
and Patricia A.L. Kongshavn*

Section of Cancer Biology
Mallinckrodt Institute of Radiology
Washington University School of Medicine
St. Louis, Missouri 63110

*Montreal General Hospital Research Institute
1650 Cedar Avenue
Montreal, Quebec H3G 1A4, Canada

Bradley and Metcalf (1) showed that bone marrow cells will form colonies of granulocytes and macrophages when cultured in 0.3% agar medium with colony-stimulating (CSF). Virolainen and Defendi (2) reported that peritoneal macrophages elicited with starch would proliferate extensively when cultured in the presence of L-cell conditioned medium. They termed the active factor in the L-cell conditioned medium "macrophage growth factor" (MGF). Lin and Stewart (31) found that peritoneal exudate cells elicited with thioglycollate medium would form colonies containing only macrophages when cultured at low density in agar medium supplemented with L-cell conditioned medium. Stewart et al. 94) reported that colonies of mononuclear phagocytes would also form in medium containing no agar. Finally, Stanley et al. (5) showed that MGF was identical to subclass of CSF found in L-cell conditioned medium.

In subsequent studies, it has been shown that murine macrophages from the bone marrow and spleen, monocytes from the peripheral blood, elicited macrophages from the peritoneal and pleural cavities, alveolar, lymph node and thymic macrophages, and Kupffer cells from the liver will form colonies when cultured either in agar-containing or liquid medium, providing MGF is present (6,7). The frequency of the colony forming progenitor cells from various murine sources is summarized in Table 1.

When bone marrow cells are cultured, about 0.3% of cells form large colonies by day 7, with a mean diameter of 2.7 ± 0.7 mm. By day 14 the number of colonies has increased to 1.9% of plated cells. These new colonies, however, are only 1.1 ± 0.1 mm in diameter. Since approximately 3% of marrow cells are mononuclear phagocytes (8), nearly all bone marrow mononuclear phagocytes are capable of surviving

Table 1.  Colony Formation of Mononuclear Phagocytes

| Source | Colonies per 1,000 cells* | |
|---|---|---|
| | Day 7 | Day 14 |
| Bone marrow | 3.4 ± 0.5 | 29 ± 12 |
| Peripheral blood | none | 68 ± 11 |
| Spleen | 0.1 | 7.0 ± 1.0 |
| Peritoneal cells | none | 2 ± 0.5 |
| Peritoneal exudate cells | none | 156 ± 25 |
| Alveolar lavage | none | 90 ± 5 |

*Cells were obtained from $C_3Hf/AN$ female mice 8-12 weeks old.

and forming colonies in vitro. The progenitor cells of the large bone marrow colonies which form by day 7 are nonadherent cells, while the progenitors for the small colonies are adherent cells. As the nonadherent bone marrow progenitor cells proliferate, their progeny become adherent cells which also continue to proliferate.

When peritoneal cells are grown in culture medium containing MGF, they, too, will form colonies. In agar-containing medium, colonies of 50 or more cells are not found until day 21. When liquid culture is used, however, the lag period is much shorter so that by day 10, clusters have increased to more than 50 cells and by day 14 colonies have an average diameter of about 1 mm and contain over 500 cells. Colonies will continue to enlarge over the next week, and then stop growing. While it has been difficult to subculture these cells because they cannot be easily removed from the culture dishes, we found that each progenitor could produce at least 25,000 progeny (9).

Like cells from the peritoneal cavity, peripheral blood mononuclear cells and alveolar cells exhibit the longer lag period and no colonies can be found before day 10. The colony-forming cells, found in the adherent fraction, consist only of macrophages.

We have interpreted these observations to mean that the most immature progenitors in the mononuclear phagocyte series (the nonadherent progenitors) are characeized by a high proliferative potential. (They form large colonies on day 7). The more mature adherent progenitors found in the bone marrow and peripheral tissues are characterized by a longer lag period prior to proliferating and a lower proliferative potential. (They form smaller colonies on day 14).

Like bone marrow, spleen cells also contain nonadherent progenitors which form large colonies containing several thousand cells by day 7. The frequency, however, of these colony-forming cells is only about one per ten thousand spleen cells. The majority of spleen-derived colony-forming cells, like those derived from other peripheral tissues, are characterized by the longer lag period. It is not surprising that the spleen is similar to the bone marrow, because it too is a source of hematopoietic cells.

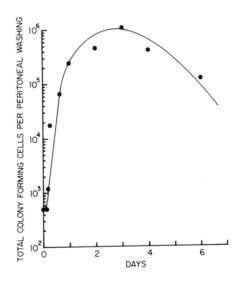

Figure 1. Peritoneal colony forming cells elicited with thioglycollate medium. $C_3Hf/AN$ mice were injected with 1.5 ml thioglycollate medium and, as a function of time, the peritoneal exudate cells were harvested from 3 mice and pooled. The yield of cells and the fraction that would form macrophage colonies were determined. We determined the total number of colony-forming cells per peritoneal washing by multiplying the yield by the fraction of cells forming colonies. From Stewart et al. (4).

Resident peritoneal cells contain a very low frequency of colony-forming cells (0.2%). As shown in Figure 1, after injection of thioglycollate medium, the plating efficiency of colony-forming cells increases dramatically, reaching a maximum on day 3. At this time 10%-20% of cells will form colonies of macrophages. One likely explanation of these results is that a low fraction of resident peritoneal cells have the ability to proliferate; i.e., the population is primarily senescent. Injection of a phlogogenic agent into the peritoneal (or pleural) cavity causes a dramatic influx of progenitors. Since all blood monocytes which survive will form colonies, it is likely that monocytes are the immediate precursor cells.

Table 2. Effect of Age on Colony Formation of Peritoneal Exudate Cells

| Age (Weeks) | Cells/Exudate* $(X\ 10^{-6})$ | Colonies Thousand Cells |
|---|---|---|
| 1 | 2.4 ± 0.6 | 18.2 ± 4.5 |
| 3 | 2.8 ± 0.8 | 39.3 ± 10.4 |
| 5 | 8.2 ± 0.9 | 36.0 ± 15.5 |
| 8 | 7.3 ± 2.9 | 42.5 ± 8.2 |
| 15 | 7.5 ± 3.0 | 35.2 ± 7.8 |
| 25 | 6.9 ± 2.9 | 38.6 ± 10.1 |
| 40 | 6.7 ± 1.8 | 35.7 ± 9.4 |
| *wk control | 2.3 ± 1.2 | <0.1 |

*AKR female mice 3 days after 1.5 ml thioglycollate medium, i.p. Cells were grown in agar growth medium. From Lin et al. (10).

Lin et al. (10) have studied the colony-forming potential of peritoneal exudate cells obtained from mice of different ages. Using AKR female mice and peritoneal cells obtained three days after injection of 1.5 ml of thioglycollate medium, they found no substantial difference in colony-forming ability (Table 2) after mice reached the age of 5 weeks.These cells were grown in agar growth medium instead of liquid growth medium. It has been our consistent experience that fewer colonies form in agar-containing medium than in medium without agar. The reasons for this finding are not known.

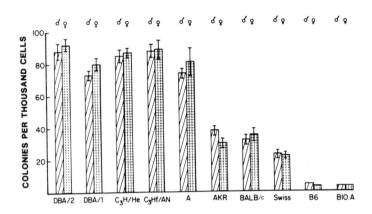

<u>Figure 2.</u>  Strain variation in colony formation in agar cul-
ture.  Peritoneal cells were harvested three days after  ip
injection of thioglycollate medium and incubated 28  days  in
agar growth medium.  Colonies were counted <u>in situ</u> under  a
dissecting microscope.  From Lin et al. (10).

Figure 2 summarizes the colony-forming ability of peritoneal exudate cells elicited with thioglycollate medium from
several diferent strains of mice.  Cells from DBA, C3H and A
strain mice have a high frequency of colony-forming cells;
AKR, Balb/C and Swiss outbred mice produce cells exhibiting
an intermedium frequency, while cells from C57BL/6 (B6) and
B10.A mice have a low plating efficiency.  Cells from male
and female mice, however, were not different in their ability to form colonies.
    The yield of peritoneal cells from C57BL mice after in-
jection of thioglycollate medium is generally very high (>2
x $10^7$ cells), while the yield from the other mouse strains
is lower (<2 x $10^7$ cells).  In addition, C57BL mice tend to
exhibit several superior host defense functions, one of
which is their ability to control infection with <u>Listeria</u>
<u>monocytogenes</u> (12,13,14).  As a result, we have investigated

in more detail the genetic differences between a high (A) and low (B10.A) strain, for colony formation.

We noted a considerable degree of variability among different experiments when performing assays on individual mice. Accordingly, we developed a procedure to minimize the number of manipulations required to initiate cultures of bone marrow and peritoneal exudate cells. For bone marrow cells the femur was removed and flushed with 1 ml α-MEM culture medium (11). We added 0.2 ml of this cell suspension to 2 ml growth medium. The growth medium was α-MEM supplemented with 10% fetal bovine serum, 5% horse serum, and 10% L-cell conditioned medium. To make an additional dilution, we put 0.1 ml of the suspension in 7 ml of growth medium and plated 3 ml of this cell suspension into two 35 mm culture dishes. After all the cultures had been placed in the incubator, the concentration of cells in each suspension was determined by the pronase cetrimide procedure (4,11). After 7 days of incubation the cultures were fixed and stained with methylene blue and the colonies were counted under a dissecting microscope. We prepared peritoneal cells similarly after harvest, using 5 ml α-MEM to lavage the cavity except that we prepared an additional 1:10 dilution prior to staining and colony-counting.

We have found that peritoneal cells harvested from B10.A mice were severely aggregated. This made it difficult to get accurate hemocytometer or electronic particle counts. Cetrimide, which liberates nuclei for counting, was not completely effective in breaking up these larger aggregates. Accordingly, we plated 1 ml of stock peritoneal cells on a 35 mm culture dish and allowed them to adhere for one hour. During this time the cells would migrate out of the aggregates onto the dish's surface. When these dishes were treated with cetrimide, nuclei from individual mononuclear phagocytes were obtained and counted. These determinations produced cell counts 10%-30% higher than their freshly counted aggregated counts.

The results of these studies are summarized in Table 3, where the data are expressed as the number of colonies per 1,000 cells cultured. For bone marrow we selected 5.5 colonies to separate the high responder A strain mice from the low responder B10.A strain mice. While there were 3 of 18 A strain mice with less than 5.5 colonies (5.4, 5.3 and 5.2 colonies per 1,000 cells), the average was 6.2 colonies per 1,000 cells. For B10.A mice, none showed more than 5.5 colonies and the average was $4.0 \pm 0.5$. Thus, no overlap of low responder into the high responder mouse category was observed, but 17% of high responder samples overlapped into the higher end of the low responder cutoff. The F1 mice

Table 3. Genetics of Macrophage Colony Formation by Bone Marrow Cells

| Strain | N* | % | Colonies per 1,000 cells | |
|--------|----|----|-----|-----|
| A | 15 | 83 | >5.5 | 6.2 ± 0.7 |
|  | 3 | 17 | <5.5 | —— |
| B10.A | 0 | 0 | >5.5 | —— |
|  | 5 | 100 | <5.5 | 4.0 ± 0.5 |
| $F_1$ | 1 | 6 | >5.5 | —— |
|  | 17 | 94 | <5.5 | 3.5 ± 0.6 |
| $F_2$ | 11 | 28 | >5.5 | 7.2 ± 0.2 |
|  | 28 | 72 | <5.5 | 4.1 ± 0.2 |
| $F_1$ X A | 22 | 52 | >5.5 | 9.6 ± 0.7 |
|  | 20 | 48 | <5.5 | 2.5 ± 0.3 |

*Number of mice

behaved most like the B10.A parent, as 94% of mice yielded cells which produced less than 5.5 colonies per 1,000 cells; the average was 3.5 colonies per 1,000 cells. When cells from F2 mice were tested, 28% of mice yielded cells giving rise to more than 5.5 colonies, while 72% gave rise to less than 5.5. colonies. When the F1 mice were backcrossed with the A strain parent, half the progeny yielded a high number of colonies (mean of 9.6), like the A parent, and half were like the B10.A parent (mean of 2.5).

A similar trend was observed when peritoneal cels were tested; the results are summarized in Table 4. For this study 90 colonies per 1,000 cells was used as the cutoff. Some overlap was again noted as cells from one B10.A mouse formed more than 90 colonies and cells from two A strain mice formed less than 90 colonies. The mean number of colonies from A strain mice was 162 per 1,000 cells and from B10.A mice, 58 colonies per 1,000 cells. When the F1 mice were tested, the mean was 57 colonies, characterizing this mouse as resembling its B10.A parent. When the F2 mice were tested, cells from 23% of mice formed an average of 205 colonies per 1,000 cells. When cells from the backcross mice were tested, about half were like the A strain parent (138 colonies per 1,000) and half were like the B10.A parent (45 colonies per 1,000 cells).

Table 4.  Genetics of Macrophage Colony Formation by
Peritoneal Exudate Cells

| Strain | N* | % | | Colonies per 1,000 cells |
|--------|----|----|----|--------------------------|
| A | 18 | 90 | >90 | 162 ± 38 |
|   | 2 | 10 | <90 | —— |
| B10.A | 1 | 10 | >90 | —— |
|   | 9 | 90 | <90 | 58 ± 6 |
| $F_1$ | 1 | 10 | >90 | —— |
|   | 0 | 90 | <90 | 57 ± 12 |
| $F_2$ | 9 | 23 | >90 | 205 ± 36 |
|   | 31 | 77 | <90 | 26 ± 7 |
| $F_1$ X A | 20 | 51 | >90 | 138 ± 11 |
|   | 19 | 49 | <90 | 45 ± 6 |

*Number of mice.

These results collectively suggest that the quantitative trait of high plating efficiency for macrophage colony
formation in A/J mice (or alternatively, of its inhibition
in B10.A mice) is under control of a single, dominant gene.
B10.A strain mice as well as other inbred strains derived from C57BL background exhibit enhanced resistance to
infection with Listeria monocytogenes as compared to A strain mice which are relatively sensitive to this infection
(12,13).   This enhanced resistance, also genetically-con-
trolled, appears to be due to the superior ability of C57BL
mice to produce and mobilize adequate numbers of young mononuclear phagocytes very promptly at the site of infection
(15).    The above data for colony formation thus appears to
show just the opposite effect.  The formation of mononuclear
phagocyte colonies in vitro by C57BL strain cells is low.
Accordingly, we tested chimeric mice for their ability to
form colonies;  the data are summarized in Table 5.  When A
strain mice were reconstituted with bone marrow from B10.A
mice, the cells obtained responded like cells from the B10.A
mouse, i.e., colony formation was low.  When B10.A mice were
reconstituted with bone marrow from A strain mice, the cells
responded like those from A strain mice, i.e., colony formation was high.  These results show that, whereas resistance

to infection with Listeria is a property of the host environment (15), colony formation is a property of the cells.

Table 5. Macrophage Colony Formation from Mouse Chimeras

| Strain | | Colonies per 1,000 Cells | |
| --- | --- | --- | --- |
| Donor | Recipient | Bone Marrow | Exudate |
| A control | | 6.2 | 162 |
| A | A | 7.2 | 96 |
| B10.A | A | 2.0 | 63 |
| | | | |
| B10.A control | | 4.0 | 58 |
| B10.A | B10.A | 2.8 | 89 |
| A | B10.A | 6.4 | 137 |

There are two potential explanations for the low plating efficiency of cells from B10.A mice: first, the frequency of colony-forming cells within the population is low
or, second, the frequency of colony-forming cells is identical among the various mouse strains, but the ability of the
cells to form colonies is environmentally compromised within our culture system. Chen and Lin (16) have provided some
insights into the answer. They showed that cells from
C57BL/6 mice were considerably more sensitive to an inhibit-
or found in L-cell conditioned medium than were the cells
derived from the C3H mouse strain. They have called this
inhibitor "colony inhibitory factor" (CIF). When CIF is removed, the frequency of colony-forming cells is the same in
both C57BL/6 and C3H mice. Yen and Stewart (17) have recently shown that an inhibitor of colony formation is present in the peritoneal cavity of C3H mice. Whether this endogenous inhibitor is identical to CIF needs to be determined.

With these observations in mind, we have formulated a
tentative model to describe the chimera studies. Cells from
A strain mice are less sensitive and can, therefore, proliferate to high numbers either in vitro or in vivo. In the
B10.A strain mouse, the tissue levels of CIF are much less
than in the A strain mouse. Thus, in the B10.A mouse both A
cells and B10.A cells proliferate extensively in response to
pathogenic stimuli such as Listeria. The greater number of
cells produced provide a high degree of resistance to the
infection. In contrast, when cells with exquisitely high
sensitivity to inhibitor (B10.A cells) are placed in a host

environment having high endogenous inhibitor activity (A mouse), these cells are unable to proliferate extensively. Thus, the host response to infection would be seen as environmentally determined while proliferation of progenitor cells would be seen as a cell-dependent phenomenon resulting from their relative sensitivity to the inhibitor. Experiments are in progress to test this hypothesis.

In summary, our results clearly show that colony-forming ability may be regulated by a single gene which likely controls the sensitivity of cells to an inhibitor which has yet to be identified. This sensitivity of cells to the inhibitor appears to be dominant. It remains to be shown, however, if the concentration of endogenous inhibitor varies among animal strains.

## REFERENCES

1.  Bradley, T.R., and Metcalf, D.  Aust.J.Exp.Biol.Med.-Sci. 44:287, 1966.
2.  Virolainen, M., and Defendi, V.  In Growth Regulating Substances for Animal Cells in Culture. V. Defendi and M. Stokes (eds). Philadelphia: Wistar Institute, p67, 1967.
3.  Lin, H-L., and Stewart, C.C.  Nature (NB) 243:176, 1973.
4.  Stewart, C.C., Lin, H., and Adles, C.  J.Exp.Med. 141:-1114, 1975.
5.  Stanley, E.R., Cifone, M., Heard, P.M., and Defendi, V. J.Exp.Med. 143:631, 1976.
6.  Stewart, C.C.  In Mononuclear Phagocytes: Functional Aspects. R. Van Furth, and Z. Cohn (eds). Boston: N.V. Nyhoff, 1980 (in press).
7.  Stewart, C.C., Yen, S-E., and Senior, R.M.  In Manual of Macrophage Methodology: Collection, Characterization and Function. H.B. Herscowitz, H.T. Holden, J.A. Bellanti, and A. Gaffar (eds). New York: Marcel-Dekkar, 1980 (in press).
8.  van Furth, R., and Diesselhoff-Den Dulk, M.M.C. J.Exp.Med. 132:813, 1970.
9.  van der Ziest, B.A.M., Stewart, C.C., and Schlesinger, S. J.Exp.Med. 147:1253, 1978.
10. Lin, H-L, Kuhn, C., and Stewart, C.C.  J.Cell.Physiol. 96:133, 1978.
11. Stewart, C.C.  In Methods for Studying Mononuclear Phagocytes. D.O. Adams, H. Koren, and P. Edelson (eds). New York: Academic Press, 1980 (in press).
12. Cheers, C., and McKenzie, I.F.C.  Infect.Immun. 19:755, 1978.

13. Skamene, E., Kongshavn, P.A.L., and Sachs, D.H.
    J.Infect.Dis. 139:228, 1979.
14. Skamene, E., and Kongshavn, P.A.L. Infect.Immun. 25:-
    345, 1979.
15. Kongshavn, P.A.L., Sadarangani, C., and Skamene, E.,
    this volume.
16. Chen, D-M and Lin, H-S. Fed.Proc. 30:452, 1980.
17. Yen, S-E., and Stewart, C.C. J.Cell.Physiol., 1980
    (submitted).

## DISCUSSION

O'Brien: Has Stewart had occasion to look at cell surface receptors, for example, on any of these macrophage colonies? Is he selecting by this procedure a particular subpopulation of macrophages?

Stewart: O'Brien has identified a very interesting aspect one can explore via these colonies; that is, to pose questions about sub-popultions - whether the heterogeneity of function is within the cells in a given colony, where one cell does one thing and one another, or whether all members of a colony represent a single macrophage function - one colony secreting elastase, another secreting plasminogen activator and so forth. We have done considerable work in this area. The story is that all the cells in a colony are the same - there is no discernible heterogeneity among the cells in a given macrphage colony. However, when one looks at Ia, for example, only about 10% of colonies express Ia but a single colony all the cells express Ia. So we are, in fact, looking at a function which is delegated only to certain sub-sets of progenitor cells. If one explores tumoricidal activity, there would seem to be no heterogeneity in function among colonies.

# AN LPS RESPONSIVE CELL IN C3H/HeJ MICE: THE PERITONEAL EXUDATE-DERIVED MACROPHAGE COLONY-FORMING CELL (M-CFC)

T.J. MacVittie and S.R. Weinberg

Experimental Hematology Department
Armed Forces Radiobiology Research Institute
Bethesda, Maryland 20014

## INTRODUCTION

The C3H/HeJ mouse is a substrain particularly noted for its resistance to the many diverse biologic effects of bacterial lipopolysaccharide (LPS) experienced by many other strains (1,5,6,7,14,17,18,20,22). In addition to decreased lethality and selective in vitro macrophage unresponsiveness, the hematopoietic system of C3H/HeJ is markedly unresponsive to LPS in terms of decreased radiosensitivity (21), plasma colony stimulating activity (CSA) levels (1,18) and splenic stem (FU-S) and granulocyte-macrophage progenitor cells [GM-(FC)] (1,3,13) than the responsive C3HeB/FeJ strain.

An in vitro colony-forming cell specific for the formation of macrophages has been detected within the murine marrow, extramedullary organs (11,12,19) and tissue spaces (4,-8,9,10). The ubiquitous nature of this macrophage colony-forming cell (M-CFC) and the specific nature of its progeny prompted us to investigate its temporal pattern of induction within the peritoneal cavity of C3H/HeJ mice relative to their counterpart C3HeB/FeJ in response to an i.p. injection of LPS-W.

## MATERIALS AND METHODS

Cell Suspensions, In Vitro Culture Technique. Femoral bone marrow (BM), spleens (SPL), peripheral blood leukocytes (PBL), and thymus (T) were obtained from 8- to 12-week-old male or female mice of the strains C3Heb/FeJ and C3H/HeJ (Jackson Labs., Bar Harbor, Maine). Cell suspensions were prepared as previously described (MacVittie, 79). Peritoneal exudates (PEC) were induced by injection of 10 ug of lipopolysaccharide-W, E. coli (016:B6, Difco Labs, Detroit, Michigan), in 0.5 ml pyrogen-free saline.

The double-layer agar culture technique used for detection of M-CFC has been described previously (11). Pregnant mouse uterine extract (PMUE) and mouse L-cell-conditioned medium were used as sources of CSA. Colony morphology and

identification of cell types were carried out as described
previously (12).

RESULTS

M-CFC Content in Control C3Heb/FeJ and C3H/HeJ Mice.  Shown
in Table 1 are the relative and absolute M-CFC values for
normal BM. SPL, T, PBL, and PEC in C3HeB/FeJ and C3H/HeJ
mice.   The C3H/HeJ mice had significantly (p <0.01 to
<0.005) higher values in every organ as well as peripheral
blood and peritoneal cavity.  All organ cellularities were
equivocal between the paired strains.  It is of particular
interest that the resident C3H/HeJ PEC suspension contained
a 16-fold greater number of M-CFC than did its counterpart
C3HeB/FeJ.

Table 1.   M-CFC:  Concentration and Total Number per Organ
of Control C3Heb/FeJ and C3H/HeJ Mice.

|      |       | BM | SPL | PBL | PEC | T |
|------|-------|-----|-----|-----|-----|---|
| FeJ | conc. | 599.0+84.0 | 37.0+ 8.0 | 303.0+63.0 | 3.2+1.5 | 1.3 +0.3 |
|      | organ | 86.0+11.7 | 53.8+ 6.6 | 14.1+ 0.9 | 0.1+0.03 | 1.23+5.5 |
| HeJ | conc. | 1074.0+156.0 | 73.0+13.0 | 507.0+51.0 | 52.0+9.0 | 3.7 +0.5 |
|      | organ | 144.8+ 15.7 | 100.9+13.2 | 21.1+ 2.6 | 1.6+0.1 | 3.13+0.08 |

Concentration of M-CFC per $10^5$ nucleated cells, 8-10 replicate determinations.  Organ values ± SEM (x $10^3$) BM, SPL, T
indicate values per femur, spleen, and thymus, respectively.
PEC and PBL are values per peritoneal cavity and ml of blood
leukocytes.

LPS-Induced Cellular Response in the Peritoneal Cavity.
Total nucleated exudate cells in C3Heb/FeJ increased gradually to peak values at 72 hr after LPS-W (Table 2).  The
C3H/HeJ mice showed a significantly greater (P <0.001) cellular response than the C3Heb/FeJ at 6, 24, and 48 hr after
LPS-W.  Examination of the cells responding to LPS-W revealed a biphasic response in the C3H/HeJ strain.  The first
phase was an early phase in which neutrophils peaked at 6 hr
through 24 hr after LPS and then markedly decreased by 48
hr.  The second phase was marked by a significant rise in
macrophages, which peaked at 72 hr.  C3Heb/FeJ showed a
monophasic response in both cell types, although the macrophage response was significantly greater than that of the
neutrophils (Table 2).

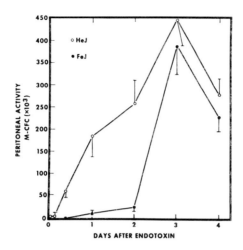

<u>Figure 1.</u>    Total  M-CFC  detected  in  peritoneal  cavity  of
C3Heb/FeJ  and  C3H/HeJ  mice  following  an  i.p.  injection  of
LPS-W, <u>E. coli</u>.

<u>LPS-Induced  M-CFC  Response  in  the  Peritoneal  Cavity</u>.    The
concentration  and  total  number  of  M-CFC  increased  markedly
in  the  peritoneal  exudate  of  both  paired  strains  in  response
to  the  i.p.  injection  of  LPS-W  (Table  3,  Fig.  1),  although  a
marked  contrast  is  noted  between  the  strains  during  the  initial  48  hr.    The  CH/HeJ  M-CFC  increased  in  concentration
from  73  per  $10^5$  to  a  peak  value  of  4807  per  $10^5$  cells  at  48
hr,  representing  a  66-fold  increase.    This  resulted  in  a  10-
fold  advantage  in  the  absolute  number  of  M-CFC  in  the  PEC  of
C3H/HeJ  mice  over  C3Heb/FeJ  (Fig.  1).    This  is  in  spite  of
the  dramatic  176-fold  increase  in  M-CFC  concentration  in  the
C3Heb/FeJ  over  the  same  48-hr  period.    It  required  an  additional  24  hr  for  the  C3Heb/FeJ  to  catch  the  C3H/HeJ  in  relative  number  of  M-CFC  and  hence  approach  a  comparable  absolute  number  of  M-CFC  by  72  hr  after  injection  of  LPS-W
(Fig.  1).

DISCUSSION

In  view  of  the  high  potential  for  involvement  of  macrophages  in  the  many  diverse  biologic  reactions  to  endotoxin
and  the  well  documented  unresponsiveness  of  macrophages  as
well  as  granulocyte-macrophage  progenitor  cells  from  C3H/HeJ
strain  mice  to  these  reactions,  we  measured  the  response  of

Table 2. Total Cells (TNC), Neutrophils (N), and Macrophages (Mφ) in Peritoneal Exudate Following an I.P. Injection of LPS-W in C3Heb/FeJ and C3H/HeJ Mice

| | | 0 | 3 | 6 | 24 | 48 | 72 | 96 |
|---|---|---|---|---|---|---|---|---|
| | | | | Hours After LPS LPS-W | | | | |
| TNC[1] | FeJ | 4.10 ± 0.8 | 0.9 ± 0.2 | 1.5 ± 0.3 | 2.2 ± 0.7 | 3.4 ± 0.2 | 12.4 ± 3.2 | 9.9 ± 2.1 |
| | HeJ | 4.20 ± 0.6 | 0.7 ± 0.2 | 3.8 ± 0.6[2] | 6.8 ± 0.8[2] | 8.9 ± 1.2[2] | 13.0 ± 2.4 | 12.2 ± 1.8 |
| N | FeJ | | 0.16 ± 0.1 | 0.47 ± 0.2 | 1.14 ± 0.3 | 1.60 ± 0.3 | 2.48 ± 0.7 | 1.98 ± 0.2 |
| | HeJ | | 0.31 ± 0.1 | 2.90 ± 0.7[2] | 2.58 ± 0.8[2] | 0.23 ± 0.1 | 0.26 ± 0.1 | |
| Mφ | FeJ | 3.30 ± 0.8 | 0.41 ± 0.1 | 0.45 ± 0.2 | 0.95 ± 0.3 | 1.76 ± 0.6 | 9.72 ± 0.4 | 7.72 ± 1.4 |
| | HeJ | 3.30 ± 0.6 | 0.10 ± | 0.59 ± 0.2 | 3.45 ± 0.7[2] | 7.83 ± 1.1[2] | 11.44 ± 0.8 | 11.10 ± 2.1 |

[1] TNC, N, and Mφ values (x $10^6$) harvested per mouse.
[2] Values are significantly different from respective counterpart at P <0.001.

Table 3.  Concentration of M-CFC (±SEM) Per $10^5$ Nucleated Peritoneal Exudate Cells
With Time After LPS Injection

Hours After LPS-W

| | 0 | 3 | 6 | 24 | 48 | 72 | 96 |
|---|---|---|---|---|---|---|---|
| FEJ | 5±2 | 0 | 14±3 | 282±104 | 881±162 | 3158±822 | 2283±532 |
| HeJ | 73±19 | 57±6 | 1400±48 | 3537±662 | 4807±1200 | 3955±1031 | 2455±685 |

an in vitro colony-forming cell specific for macrophages to an intraperitoneal injection of LPS-W in both C3HeB/FeJ and C3H/HeJ mice.

Our studies have shown that the C3H/HeJ strain contains a significantly greater number of macrophage colony-forming cells in the hematopoietic organs, peripheral blood, thymus, and peritoneal cavity and that in response to endotoxin, the peritoneal exudate is characterized by a more accelerated rise in content of M-CFC within initial 48 hr after injection. At 48 hr, the C3H/HeJ PEC contained 257,000 M-CFC versus 25,000 M-CFC for the C3Heb/FeJ. Peak values, however, were comparable at 72 hr in both strains. This is probably the result of a marked rise in migration and proliferation of M-CFC in the C3Heb/FeJ.

Concomitant with the marked rise in absolute values of M-CFC in the C3H/HeJ is a biphasic increase in neutrophils and macrophages. This response confirmed that reported by Sultzer and Goodman (20) and Moeller et al (15). The C3H/HeJ responded more quickly, eliciting an early polymorphonuclear increase within 6 hr, followed by a rapid decrease to negligible numbers within 48 hr. A rapid rise in macrophages ensued. Sultzer and Goodman (20) concluded that the C3H/HeJ is not a low responder in terms of the peritoneal inflammatory response. We have also shown that it is capable of an accelerated response in terms of the peritoneal exudate-derived M-CFC. The control data also indicated a significantly greater number of M-CFC in other organs and tissue spaces also affected by endotoxin. The bone marrow and extramedullary organs and tissue spaces appear to be primed in this respect for a rapid increase in systemic M-CFC.

The diversity of the LPS-induced activities affected by this mutation have recently been shown to include many aspects of the hematopoietic response (2,3,13). The cellular effect is most evident in the splenic tissue where endogenous CFU, exogenous CFU-s, and GM-CFC are all significantly diminished in their characteristic in vivo response to endotoxin. Recent experiments analyzing the temporal response to endotoxin of the M-CFC in bone marrow, spleen, and peripheral blood of C3H/HeJ mice have shown significant differences from the response of their earlier progenitors, the CFU-s and GM-CFC (unpublished observations). These various populations of M-CFC (BM,SPL, PBL,PEC) are markedly responsive during the initial 48 hr following endotoxin challenge. The exact relationship between the M-CFC, the response of the hematopoietic and mononuclear phagocyte system to endotoxin, and the defective cellular mechanism in C3H/HeJ mice remains to be determined.

## ACKNOWLEDGEMENT

The authors gratefully acknowledge the excellent technical assistance of Ms. Emmeline G. McCarthy and Mr. James L. Atkinson as well as the professional and editorial assistance of Dr. S.J. Baum and Ms. Judith Van Deusen in the preparation of this manuscript.

## REFERENCES

1. Apte, R.N., Hertogs, C.F., and Pluznik, D.H. J. Reticul.Soc. 26:491, 1979.
2. Apte, R.N., and Pluznik, D.N. J.Cell.Physiol. 89:313, 1976.
3. Bogs, S.S., Boggs, D.R., and Joyce, P.A. Blood, 1980 (in press).
4. Chu, J.Y., and Lin, H. J.Reticul.Soc. 20:299, 1976.
5. Doe, W.F., and Henson, P.M. J.Immunol. 123:2304, 1979.
6. Glode, M.L., Mergenhagen, S.E., and Rosenstreich, D.L. Infect.Immun. 14:626, 1976.
7. Kurland, J.I. In Experimental Hematology Today. S.J. Baum, and G.D. Ledney, (eds). New York: Springer Verlag, p47, 1978.
8. Lin, H. Blood 49:593, 1977.
9. Lin, H., Kuhn, C., and Kuo, T.T. J.Exp.Med. 142:877, 1975.
10. Lin, H., and Stewart, C.C. Nature 243:176, 1973.
11. MacVittie, T.J., and McCarthy, K.F. J.Cell.Physiol. 92:203, 1977.
12. MacVittie, T.J., and Porvaznik, M. J.Cell.Physiol. 97:305, 1978.
13. MacVittie, T.J., and Weinberg, S.R. In Experimental Hematology Today. S.J. Baum and G.D. Ledney (eds). New York: Springer Verlag, 1980 (in press).
14. McGhee, J.R., Michalek, S.M., Moore, R.N., Mergenhagen, S.E., and Rosenstreich, D.L. J.Immunol.122:2052, 1979.
15. Moeller, G.R., Terry, L., and Snyderman, R. J.Immunol. 120:116, 1978.
16. Rosenstreich, D.L., Glode, M.L., Wahl, L.M., Sandberg, A.L., and Mergenhagen, S.E. In Microbiology. D. Schlesinger (ed). Washington, D.C.: American Society of Microbiology, p314, 1977.
17. Rucco, L.P., and Meltzer, M.S. J.Immunol. 120:329, 1978.
18. Russo, M., and Lutton, J.D. J.Cell.Physiol. 92:303, 1977.

19. Stanley, E.R., Chen D-M, and Lin, H-S. Nature <u>274</u>:168, 1978.

20. Sultzer, B.M., and Goodman, G.W. In Microbiology. D. Schlesinger (ed). Washington D.C.: American Society of Microbiology,p304, 1977.

21. Urbaschek, R., Mergenhagen, S.E., and Urbaschek, B. Infect.Immun. <u>18</u>:860, 1977.

22. Vogel, S.N., and Rosenstreich, D.L. J.Immunol. <u>123</u>:2842, 1979.

## DISCUSSION

<u>Eisenstein</u>: I gather that MacVittie has worked with LPS prepared by the phenol water procedure. Were he to use TCA-LPS, a product that retains the endotoxin protein, in the assay where he found differences, for example in the spleen assay for colony-forming units, would he then be able to make the HeJ mice respond?

<u>MacVittie</u>: We have not done that but I suspect one could so so.

ACTIVITY OF MACROPHAGE CELL LINES IN SPONTANEOUS AND LPS,
LYMPHOKINE OR ANTIBODY-DEPENDENT KILLING OF TUMOR TARGETS

Peter Ralph, Ilona Nakoinz, Jane E.R. Potter,*
and Malcolm A.S. Moore
Sloan-Kettering Institute for Cancer Research
Rye, New York 10580

*Present address:  Jackson Laboratory, Bar Harbor, Maine

INTRODUCTION

The mechanism of macrophage toxicity to target organisms is still controversial.  In different systems evidence
has been obtained for the role of oxygen radicals, enzymes,
high and low molecular weight toxins, and other effector
systems.  Macrophage lines derived from tumors or long-term
cultures of normal cells manifest most of the functions of
normal mononuclear phagocytes (4,5,6,11).  We show here that
macrophage lines can be stimulated to kill tumor cells by a
variety of methods.  Several different toxic mechanisms must
be operative in these studies.

METHODS AND MATERIALS

Sources of macrophages.  Mouse macrophage cell lines
have been described previously (4,5,6,11) (Table 1). MSL23
is a macrophage line adapted to culture from a tumor induced
in a CAL-20 mouse by Abelson leukemia virus provided by M.
Potter, National Cancer Institute, Bethesda, Maryland.  M9-
78 is a DBA/2 cell line from a tumor arising after injection
of 40-day cultures of adherent peritoneal cells treated with
3-methylcholanthrene;  it has Fc receptors but no T, B or
macrophage-specific characteristics (3).  J774.16C3C was
selected by G. Damiani for low NBT reduction by NBT suicide,
and another clone J774.2 is also essentially negative for
NBT reduction (2).  Both have undetectable $O_2^-$ production
to the medium in contrast to J774.1 (B.R. Bloom and R.B.
Johnston, unpublished).
Normal peritoneal cells were obtained from 12-15 month
old C3H/Anf mice (Cumerbland View Farms, Clinton, Tennessee)
because they were available.
Cytotoxic assays.  $4 \times 10^3$ target cells were mixed with
20x cell line effector cells or 40x normal peritoneal cells
listed above in 0.2 ml incubations in round-bottom wells (1-
-220-24x, Dynatech Labs, Alexandria, Va.).  After 20 hr culture, 0.1 ml supernatant was measured for released radio-

## TABLE 1

### Murine Macrophage-Related Cell Lines[a]

| Line | Strain | Etiology | Fc | C | LZ | Latex | Ab-RBC φ | K |
|------|--------|----------|-----|-----|-----|-------|---------|-----|
| M1 | SL | S | (-) | - | - | (-) | - | - |
| WEHI-3 | C | Oil | + | + | (+) | + | - | - |
| SKW2 | C | A-MuLV | + | + | + | + | | |
| LS23 | CAL-20 | M-MuLV | + | + | + | + | + | (+) |
| P388D₁ | DBA/2 | S? | + | + | + | + | + | (+) |
| J774 | C | Oil | + | + | + | + | + | (+) |
| PU5-1.8 | C | S | + | + | + | + | + | (+) |
| RAW264 | BAB/14 | A-MuLV | + | + | + | + | + | + |
| M9 | DBA/2 | MCA | + | - | - | - | - | - |

[a] C = BALB/c strain;   S = spontaneous;   A = Abelson, M-MuLV = Moloney murine leukemia virus;   MCA = methyl-cholanthrene, see Methods and Materials;   Fc and C = receptors for immunoglobulin and complement;   LZ = lys-ozyme;   latex phagocytosis (φ); antibody-dependent sheep RBC phagocytosis (Ab-RBC φ) and killing (K).

activity. Mouse targets M1 myeloblastic leukemia (Y. Ichikawa, Kyoto Univ.; 6), 18-8 Abelson virus-induced pre-B leukemia (C. Scher, Harvard Medical School; 14), EL4 T leukemia (7) and human CEM T leukemia (11) were prelabelled with $^{125}$IUdR, and human U937 monocyte line (6) with $^{51}$Cr. 4 x 10⁴ $^3$H-thymidine-labeled SV-3T3 (transformed mouse fibro-blasts, A. Demsey, Sloan-Kettering Institute) were incubated 44 hr with 12x effector cells in 1 ml wells (76-033-05), Linbro Scientific, Hamden, Conn.) according to Ruco and Meltzer (12). The different labeling methods were chosen for low background release by targets. LPS (S. typhosa W0901, Difco) was added to cultures usually at 20 µg/ml and lymphokine at 10% v/v (PPD stimulation of BCG immune spleen cells (12).

1:50 Heat-inactivated rabbit anti-BALB/c spleen or goat
anti-human brain sera were used to sensitize $2 \times 10^5$ target
cells/ml (20 min room temperature, wash 2x). Medium used
was RPMI 1640 + 5% heat-inactivated fetal calf serum. Cytotoxicity is shown as % label released minus background release, substituting unlabeled targets for effector cells
(plus appropriate stimulating agents). Background values
ranged from 5% to 15%, changing less than 2 percentage
points by inclusion of stimulating agents.

## RESULTS

Spontaneous and stimulated toxicity to M1 targets.
Figure 1 shows that macrophage line J774.1 kills about 25%
M1 targets "spontaneously" with lower cytotoxicity apparent
with RAW264.10 and peritoneal cells. In 2/3 experiments,
conditioned medium from J774 significantly killed M1. Inclusion of LPS in the 20-hr assay caused another 15-30% targets to be killed by all the effectors tested except the
immature WEHI-3 line. This parallels the LPS induction of
myeloid colony-stimulating factor (CSF) (9) and prostaglandin (4) in these lines. LPS concentrations as low as 1
ng/ml significantly stimulated J774 cytotoxicity (Fig. 2).
Antibody-dependent cellular cytotoxicity (ADCC) ranged from
10-35% for macrophage line effectors, except WEHI-3.
Lymphokine gave a moderate increase in cytotoxicity for
macrophage lines RAW264 and LS23, but not J774 or WEHI-3.

Sensitivity of SV-3T3, 18-8 and U937 to macrophage line
toxicity. J774 exhibited considerable spontaneous killing
of 18-8 targets (Fig. 3). Other effectors tested also showed moderate spontaneous lysis of 18-8, including nonmacro-
phage line M9-78. This line kills a variety of solid tumor
targets and some leukemias (P815, L1210) in a different
pattern from typical $NK_L$-sensitive targets (3). It did
not lyse M1 targets and was not affected by LPS, lymphokine
or antibody stimulants of toxicity. These stimulating
agents caused a moderate enhancement in killing of 18-8
targets by some of the macrophage lines.

The highest spontaneous toxicity for U937 targets was
mediated by M9 (Fig. 4). J774 killing was especially stimulated by lymphokine, PU5-1.8 by LPS and antibody, and RAW264
by antibody. In a study of lymphokine-activated lysis of
nonhemic tumor targets, only J774, PU5-1.8, RAW264, and
P388D$_1$ were stimulated to kill SV-3T3 in a 40-hr assay
(Fig. 5). Protection of SV-3T3 label release was demonstrated by RAW264 and P388D$_1$ in the absence of lymphokine.
Lymphokine-induced lysis of SV-3T3 occurred at less than

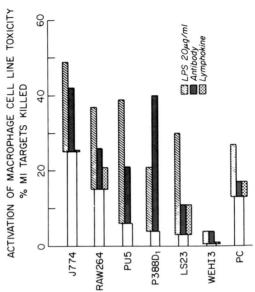

<u>Figure 1.</u>   Macrophage cell line toxicity to M1 targets.   20x
cell line  or  40x  peritoneal  cells  cultured  with  [125]IUdR-
labeled M1 targets 18 hr.

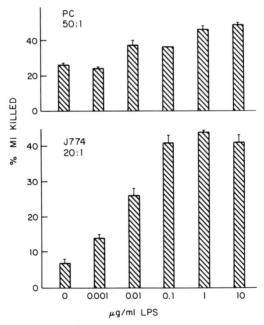

<u>Figure 2.</u>   LPS  concentration  to  stimulate  J774  killing  of
M1.    LPS   added   to   the   assay   as   in   Fig. 1.    Macrophage
toxicity ± S.E.M.

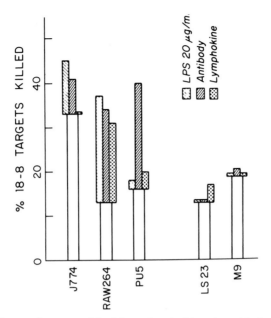

**Figure 3.** Macrophage cell line toxicity to 18-8 targets. Assay as in Fig. 1.

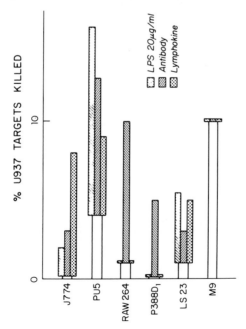

**Figure 4.** Macrophage cell line toxicity to U937 targets. Assay as in Fig. 1.

0.5:1 ratio of effector-to-target cells for RAW264 (2 x $10^4$-/ml), whereas normal peritoneal cells required 10-fold higher numbers for comparable killing (unpublished).

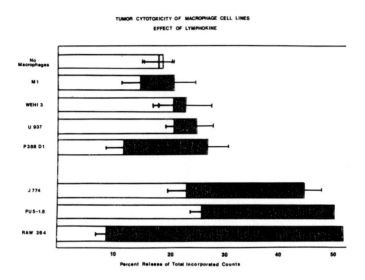

<u>Figure 5.</u>  Lymphokine-induced lysis of SV-3T3 targets.  12x cell line effectors cultured with $^3$H-thymidine-labeled SV-3T3 40 h ± 10% lymphokine (shaded).  Label release ± S.E.M.

<u>Cytotoxicity by $O_2^-$ negative macrophage lines.</u>  One of the mechanisms proposed for macrophage toxicity is superoxide anion production.  Two clones of J774 lacking NBT reduction (2) and $O_2^-$ generation during PMA stimulation (R. Johnston and B.R. Bloom, unpublished) were tested.  Table 2 shows that these clones kill M1 spontaneously and with LPS and tumor promoter phorbol myristic acetate (PMA) stimulation similarly to the standard J774.1.  In ADCC, the 16C3C clone was considerably superior to J774.1.  There was no difference among these three clones in antibody-dependent

phagocytosis and lysis of sheep RBC (unpublished).  PMA also induces myeloid colony-stimulating factor in macrophage cell lines correlated with growth inhibition (10), in contrast to its mitogenic differentiation-inhibiting effects on epithelial cells.

TABLE 2

Tumor Toxicity Mediated by $O_2^-$ Negative Variants of J774

|  | Line | NBT | % Lysis of M1 Targets | | | |
|---|---|---|---|---|---|---|
|  |  |  | - | + LPS | + Ab | + PMA |
| Exp. 1 | J774.1 | + | 5 ± 0.5 | 24 ± 0 | 10 ± 0.5 | 7 ± 0.5 |
|  | J774.2 | - | 5 ± 0 | 13 ± 2.0 | 11 ± 1.0 | 8 ± 0 |
|  | J774.16C3C | - | 6 ± 0 | 19 ± 0.5 | 41 ± 3.5 | 9 ± 2.0 |
| Exp. 2 | J774.1 |  | 9 ± 0.5 | 43 ± 0.5 | 12 ± 0.5 | 24 ± 1.5 |
|  | J774.2 |  | 9 ± 0 | 29 ± 2.0 | 11 ± 1.0 | 25 ± 0.5 |
|  | J774.16C3C |  | 6 | 23 ± 1.0 | 39 ± 5.0 | 17 ± 4.0 |

20 hr [125]IUdR release, 20:1 effector-to-target ratio, 2 µg/ ml LPS, 1 µg/ml PMA in Exp. 1, 2 µg/ml PMA in Exp. 2.  $O_2^-$ production measured as nmol ferricytochrome C reduced per mg protein during zymosan or PMA stimulation (16).

## SUMMARY OF RESULTS

We have previously ranked macrophage cell lines for their ability to ingest and lyse antibody-coated sheep RBC and to mediate ADCC against EL4 lymphoma targets (7).  A summary of effector mechanisms is given in Figure 6.  The immature lines M1 and WEHI-3 are inactive.  PU5 and RAW264 are generally active in most forms of cytotoxicity.  Other lines show intermediate effects.  However, the pattern is very complex depending on choice of target, effector cell, and method of inducing lysis.

Antibody-dependent killing of U937 and M1 by RAW264 is similar (9% vs. 11%), but U937 is not killed by LPS (0%) or lymphokine (0%) stimulation, whereas M1 is (22% and 6%). Thus, U937 is suceptible to lysis by antibody but not by two other methods even though the RAW264 effector is capable of cytotoxicity to different targets using all three agents. Since RAW264 kills some M1 targets spontaneously, LPS and lymphokine may enhance this toxicity to M1 by a lytic mechanism to which U937 is not susceptible. As another example, LS23 kills 18-8 spontaneously (13%) but not M1 significantly (4%), yet LPS induces lysis of M1 (18%) but not of 18-8 (0%). This clearly suggets that at least two lytic mechanisms are operable.

Spontaneous cytotoxicity and that stimulated by various agents have also been described by other investigators (1,13,15).

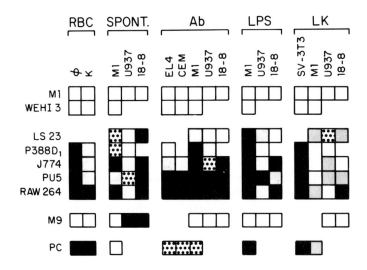

Figure 6. Summary of macrophage line cytotoxic effects. Open square <2% killing of targets, dotted 2-4%, shaded lines 4-10%, solid >10%. Open areas = no sufficient data. RBC φ and K refer to antibody-dependent phagocytosis and killing of sheep RBC.

CONCLUSIONS

1.  Macrophage cell lines can be used to study cytotoxic mechanisms, stimulated by antibody, lymphokine, microbial factors, etc., in the guaranteed absence of other cell types.

2.   Variants can be selected lacking a proposed toxic mec-
     hanism, and then analyzed for remaining lytic ability.
3.   As with microbes, tumor targets vary in susceptibility
     to killing by different mechanisms.

We have begun using inhibitors of macrophage cytotoxicity to study the lytic mechanism (8). Esterase inhibitor
TLCK and in most cases trypan blue will block tumor lysis at
nontoxic concentrations. The general protease inhibitor
trasylol had variable effects. These combined approaches
will yield model systems for molecular understanding of
macrophage activation steps and lytic mechanisms.

## ACKNOWLEDGEMENTS

We thank those mentioned for sharing cell lines or
tumors and M. Ito, M. Meltzer and B.R. Bloom for advice and
encouragement.
Supported by grants CA243000 and T32 CA09149 from the
National Institutes of Health, IM-216 from the American
Cancer Society, and the Gar-Reichman Foundation.

## REFERENCES

1.   Askamit, R.R., and Kim, K.J.   J.Immunol.   122:1785,
     1979.
2.   Bloom, B.R., Diamond, B., Muschel, R., Rosen, N.,
     Schneck, J., Damiani, G., Rosen, O., and Scharff, M.
     Fed.Proc. 37:2765, 1978.
3.   Kerbel, R.S., Roder, J.C., and Pross, H.F.   Submitted
     for publication.
4.   Kurland, J.I., Pelus, L., Ralph, P., Bockman, R.S., and
     Moore, M.A.S. Proc.Natl.Acad.Sci.USA. 76:2326, 1979.
5.   Morahan, P.S. J.Reticul.Soc. 27:223, 1980.
6.   Ralph, P.   In "Mononuclear Phagocytes - Functional
     Aspects", R. van Furth (ed.). The Hague: Martinius
     Nijhoff, 1979 (in press).
7.   Ralph, P., and nakoinz, I.   J.Immunol. 119:950, 1977.
8.   Ralph, P., and Nakoinz, I.   Ce..Immunol. 50:94, 1980.
9.   Ralph, P., Broxmeyer, H., and Nakoinz, I.   J.Exp.Med.
     146:611, 1977.
10.  Ralph, P., Broxmeyer, H., Nakoinz, I., and Moore,
     M.A.S.  Cancer Res. 38:1414, 1978.
11.  Ralph, P., Ito,M., Broxmeyer, H.E., and Nakoinz, I.
     J.Immunol. 121:300, 1978.
12.  Ruco, L.P., and Meltzer, M.S. Cell.Immunol. 41:35,

1978.

13.  Russel, S.W., Gillespie, G.Y., and Pace, J.L.  Submitted for publication.

14.  Siden, E.J., Baltimore, D., Clark, D., and Rosenberg, N.E.  Cell 16:389, 1979.

15.  Taniyama, T., and Holden, H.T.  Cell.Immunol. 48:369, 1979.

16.  Johnston et al.  J.Exp.Med. 148:115, 1978.

## DISCUSSION

Kirchner:  My query relates to interferon.  Can macrophage-mediated killing be augmented by interferon?  Does Ralph know of any work where these macrophage lines were used as producers of interferon, in response to different stimuli?

Ralph:  The answers to both questions is yes, in work coming from Holden and Herberman's group.  At least one macrophage cell line has been shown to produce interferon following stimulation with poly I:C.  Interferon has indeed been shown to increase certain types of macrophage killing.

Kirchner:  Does Ralph envision interferon playing a role in some of the reactions he has been studying?  Let us assume that LPS can induce interferon in some of the cell lines and that this interferon actually is increasing the reaction?

Ralph:  Yes, and as I understood from several earlier reports, studies with anti-interferon will probably help sort this out.

Hormaeche:  Ralph indicated that, as with microbes, different cell targets vary widely in their susceptibility to macrophage cytotoxicity.  Could Ralph tell us by what means these different lines kill microbes?

Ralph:  My understanding is that there is a good evidence for certain parasites being killed by macrophage hydrogen peroxide or by the superoxide anion, whereas others are not. I was seeking to make the point that there must be several, different, mechanisms of killing.  This is obviously the emergence of another more complex problem.  It can be approached by the use of inhibitors, such as anti-interferon. We have also used TLCK, an esterase inhibitor, which blocks almost all of these reactions.  Trypan blue in non-toxic concentrations blocks most of these reactions.  Looking for soluble effectors is another facet of this problem.

Kirchner:    In  tissue  culture  work,  mycoplasmas  generally
make for serious problems.  Is that the case also for those
working with macrophage lines?   Or do the macrophages take
care of the mycoplasmas?

Ralph:   The mouse lines that I have been studying, which include  myeloma  and  T-lymphomas  as  well  as  macrophages,  are
quite  free  of  mycoplasmas.   I  do  a  lot  of  work  with  human
cell  lines  and  invariably  mycoplasmas  are  present  in  them.
I  do  not  think  that  mouse  macrophages  are  clearing  mycoplasmas because I do not find them in lymphoid lines either.
It just seems to be less of a problem in mouse work.

Cudkowicz:   Does  Ralph  know  if  some  of  these  lines  would
exert  a  suppressor  influence  on  cytotoxicity  by  normal
macrophages or other effectors of cytotoxicity?

Ralph:    They  certainly  produce  lots  of  prostaglandin  in
physiological  amounts  that  can  be  shown  to  suppress  other
things in culture such as mitogen responses of lymphocytes,
colony-forming  assays  etc.    They  are  active  metabolically
and  they  create  an  acid  environment  in  media  very  quickly.
There  have  been  reports  that  they  make  certain  enzymes
(e.g. arginase) that are toxic for other systems.

Cudkowicz:   Is  there  any  particular  distribution  of  these
properties in one or the other line?

Ralph:   Every  line  except  for  the  two  very  immature  ones  I
mentioned make prostaglandins and CSF (a variety of CFS's,
actually) so they have counter-balancing effects.  But other
types of inhibitors have not been studied in any detail.

Cudkowicz:   Does  Ralph  know  whether  anyone  has  used  these
cells as antigen-presenting cells, let us say in CML or in
proliferative responses?

Ralph:   Yes,  it  has  been  studied,  with  respect  to  Ia  antigen.   Some  cell  lines  have  clearly  been  shown  to  have  Ia,
which  should  be  a  prerequisite  for  antigen  presentation.   I
have provided Ron Schwartz with many cell lines and he has
looked at additional ones as well;  and in his assay none of
the typically macrophage-like cell lines can present antigen
in an Ia-restricted manner to T cells.  Thus, so far we have
not encountered that kind of macrophage in any cell line.

# MACROPHAGE CELL LINE MUTANTS DEFICIENT IN PHAGOCYTOSIS HAVE REDUCED PINOCYTIC ACTIVITY

Allen J. Norin,
Montefiore Hospital and Medical Center
Albert Einstein  College of Medicine

Macrophages, depending on their state of acivation may display a variety of altered physiologic properties as compared to normal macrophages.  In this context one might expect that murine macrophages activated in vivo by bacteria or lectins would have different physiological characteristics as compared to thioglycolate elicited macrophages or resident macrophages since the former cells have microbicidal and tumoricidal ability (2,3).  Accordingly, I measured the pinocytic ability of macrophages obtained from mice treated IP with either concanavalin A (con A), thioglycolate broth or normal saline.  I found that con A activated cells pinocytized 8 to 10 times as much horse radish peroxidase (HRPO) per 100 µg cellular protein in an hour as resident macrophages (Table 1).

## Table 1
Pinocytic and Phagocytic Ability of Adherent Peritoneal Cells Obtained From Normal Mice and Mice Treated With Thioglycolate Broth or Concanavalin A

| TREATMENT | PINOCYTOSIS ng HRPO/100 ug protein/hr | PHAGOCYTOSIS $^{51}$Cr cpm/100 ug protein |
|---|---|---|
| Normal Saline | $100 \pm 14$ | $2,648 \pm 856$ |
| Thioglycolate Broth | $200 \pm 46$ | $24,564 \pm 3,856$ |
| Concanavalin A | $1,047 \pm 135$ | $11,303 \pm 2,199$ |

CBA mice were injected IP with 2 ml of thioglycolate broth (Difco), 2 ml Con A (1.5 mg/ml, Miles) or 2 ml normal saline.  Peritoneal cells were harvested 6 days later, washed in Hank's buffer and 1ml (RPMI 1640 medium plus 20% fetal calf serum) was plated at $1 \times 10^6$ cells/ml in plastic petri dishes (Nunc).  Non-adherent cells were removed after 2 hours.  The adherent cells were incubated overnight after which 1 mg/ml HRPO (Sigma) was added.  The procedure for analysis of internalized HRPO has been previously described (6).  Phagocytosis was measured in overnight cultures by the method of Ruco and Meltzer (5).  Each experimental value is the mean of 4 plates ± the standard deviation.

GENETIC CONTROL OF NATURAL RESISTANCE
TO INFECTION AND MALIGNANCY

Thioglycolate stimulated cells pinocytosed only 2 times as much HRPO per 100 μg protein per hour as resident cells. Since thioglycolate elicited cells have about twice as much protein per $10^6$ cells as resident cells the difference in pinocytosis on a per cell basis is 3 to 4 fold. Edelson et al (1), found a 5 fold increase in pinocytosis per $10^6$ cells after thioglycolate stimulation. Interestingly, the difference in surface area of a thioglycolate elicited cell is about 4 times that of a resident cell. Con A activated peritoneal cells have about 15% less protein than thioglycolate stimulated adherent cells so that the difference in pinocytosis probably reflects a difference in the activity of the cell membrane. Thioglycolate elicited macrophages phagocytized more opsonized sheep red blood cells (E-IgG) than con A activated cells or resident cells (Table 1). This data is consistent with the proposal that the pinocytic ability of macrophages correlates with their cidal ability.

### Table 2
Pinocytosis of Horse Radish Peroxidase by a Macrophage-Like Cell Line and Variants Deficient in Phagocytosis

| CELL LINE | PINOCYTIC ACTIVITY ng HRPO/100 ug protein/hr |
|-----------|----------------------------------------------|
| J 774.2 | $290 \pm 53$ |
| 3.4 N | $99 \pm 19$[a] |
| Cat 55 | $121 \pm 16$[b] |

Cell lines were cultured similar to the method of Muschel et al. (4). Cells were plated at $5\times10^5$/ml and analyzed for pinocytosis after 18 hours as described in Table 1. The experimental values are the mean of 4 plates ± the standard deviation. [a] Significant at $\alpha = 0.01$ compared to J 774.2; [b] significant at $\alpha = 0.05$ compared to J 774.2

I further studied the process of pinocytosis in macrophage-like cell lines. Since phagocytosis and pinocytosis involve the plasma membrane, I compared the pinocytic ability of a phagocytic cell line, J 774.2, to that of two phagocytic deficient variants, 3.4 N and Cat 55. The variants were cloned after treatment with the mutagen N methyl N' nitrosoguanidine by Muschel et al. (4). The 3.4 N cell line

readily phagocytizes latex beads but phagocytizes only 20%
of the IgG coated SRBCs compared to J 774.2. The phagocytic
deficiency can be corrected in part by incubation for at
least 8 hours in media containing 8Br-cAMP (B. Bloom, personal communication and Muschel et al. 4). The Cat 55 cell
line was derived from 3.4 N by further mutagenesis and selection in medium with 8Br-cAMP. Cat 55 is unable to phagocytize latex beads and E-IgG. The defect is not corrected
by addition of 8Br-cAMP. I found that both variant cell
lines had significantly lower levels of pinocytosis compared
to the parent cell line. The pinocytic ability of 3.4 N was
not significantly different than that of Cat 55 (Table 2).

Table 3
Effect of Culture on Pinocytic Activity

| CELL LINE | 24 HOURS | | 72 HOURS | |
|---|---|---|---|---|
| | PINOCYTIC ACTIVITY | PROTEIN | PINOCYTIC ACTIVITY | PROTEIN |
| J 774.2 | 268 $\pm$ 10 | 92 $\pm$ 10 | 338 $\pm$ 4 | 49 $\pm$ 1 |
| Cat 55 | 61 $\pm$ 7 | 147 $\pm$ 12 | 54 $\pm$ 7 | 132 $\pm$ 27 |

Cells were cultured and analyzed as described in Table 2 except that plates were inoculated with $8 \times 10^5$/ml. Differences
in pinocytic activity and protein for J 774.2 at 24 hours
and 72 hours are significant at $\alpha = 0.01$. Pinocytic activity was measured in ng HRPO/100 ug protein/hr. Protein is
in units of µg/ml.

    Phagocytic proficient cells grew slower and did not
reach as high a cell density as the phagocytic variants.
Pinocytic levels were greater in J 774.2 cultures plated at
near confluency and analyzed 72 hours later than cultures
studied after 24 hours (Table 3). The amount of protein per
dish was less at 72 hours than at 24 hours indicating the
lose of viable cells. This affect was not seen with Cat 55.
These results suggest that "old" J 774.2 cells attain a
higher level of pinocytosis or that cells which died off
more readily at confluency have a lower level of pinocytosis.
    Since addition of 8Br-cAMP to 3.4 N cultures stimulated
phagocytosis I tested the effect of the cyclic nucelotide on
pinocytosis. Surprisingly, incubation in medium with 8Br-

cAMP significantly reduced the pinocytic ability of both the
variant cell lines.  Cultures of J 774.2 incubated with 8Br-
cAMP had an increased level of pinocytosis though this difference was not statistically significant (Table 4).  Incubation of J 774.2 with 8Br-cAMP has been shown to slightly
increase phagocytosis (4).

Table 4.
Effect of 8Br-cAMP on Pinocytic Activity

| EXPT. | CELL LINE | UNTREATED | | 8Br-cAMP | |
| --- | --- | --- | --- | --- | --- |
| | | PINOCYTIC ACTIVITY | PROTEIN | PINOCYTIC ACTIVITY | PROTEIN |
| | J 774.2 | 305 $\pm$ 16 | 47 $\pm$ 5 | 343 $\pm$ 25 | 56 $\pm$ 7 |
| A | Cat 55 | 119 $\pm$ 12 | 108 $\pm$ 21 | 48 $\pm$ 4 | 120 $\pm$ 22 |
| | 3.4 N | 136 $\pm$ 6 | 85 $\pm$ 13 | 102 $\pm$ 20 | 88 $\pm$ 12 |
| | J 774.2 | 37 $\pm$ 2 | 116 $\pm$ 3 | 38 $\pm$ 2 | 122 $\pm$ 13 |
| B | Cat 55 | 39 $\pm$ 6 | 134 $\pm$ 18 | 28 $\pm$ 2 | 160 $\pm$ 6 |
| | 3.4 N | 35 $\pm$ 1 | 172 $\pm$ 18 | 26 $\pm$ 1 | 186 $\pm$ 17 |

Macrophage cell lines were cultured and analyzed as described in Table 2.  8Br-cAMP, 0.5 mM, was added 2 hours before
addition of HRPO.  Pinocytic activity is in ng HRPO/100 µg
protein/hr.  Protein is in µg/ml.  Experiment B was performed about 3 months after continuous culture of the cells used
in experimental A.

The cells from experiment A were maintained in continuous culture for two and a half months and then restudied
(experiment B).  All three cell lines gave lower levels of
pinocytosis compared to the original experiment.  8Br-cAMP
had no effect on J 774.2 but there was a small but significant effect on Cat 55 and 3.4 N.  The three cell lines grew
to a higher cell density than the initial cultures.  The J
774.2 cell line also looses its ability to phagocytize E-IgG
upon continuous culture probably due to the loss of chromosomes that are not essential for cell growth (B. Bloom,
personal communication).

These studies suggest that the processes of pinocytosis
and phagocytosis overlap in part.    However, the alternate
effects of 8Br-cAMP on phagocytosis and pinocytosis on 3.4 N
cells are not clear.   A more complete characterization of
the variants studied in this report and the isolation and
characterization of additional variants should be helpful in
obtaining a better understanding of differentiated functions
in macrophages.

### ACKNOWLEDGEMENTS

I thank Dr. Barry Bloom for providing the cell lines
and for this helpful suggestions.   I also thank Ms. mary
Short, Mr. Jeffrey Miller and Ms. Sarah Weinshel for their
technical assistance.   This work was supported, in part, by
USPHS grants HL17417 and CA22088 and the Manning Foundation.

Address all correspondence to:
Dr. Allen J. Norin
Department of Surgery, Rm C416
Montefiore Hospital and Medical Center
111 East 210th Street
New York, New York 10467

### REFERENCES

1.   Edelson, P.J., Zwiebel, R., and Cohn, Z.   J.Exp.Med.
     142:1150, 1975.
2.   Mackaness, G.B.   J.Exp.Med. 116:381, 1962.
3.   Meltzer, M.S., Tucker, R.W., Sanford, K.K., and
     Leonard, E.J.  J. Natl.Cancer Inst. 54:1177, 1975.
4.   Muschel, R.J., Rosen, N., and Bloom, B.R.   J.Exp.Med.
     145:175, 1977.
5.   Ruco, L.P., and Meltzer, M.S.   J.Immunol. 120:1054,
     1978.
6.   Steinman, R.M., and Cohn, Z.A.   J.Cell.Biol. 55:186,
     1972.

# MACROPHAGE ACTIVATION FOR TUMOR CYTOTOXICITY: GENETIC INFLUENCES ON DEVELOPMENT OF MACROPHAGES WITH NONSPECIFIC TUMORICIDAL ACTIVITY

Monte S. Meltzer, Luigi P. Ruco, Diana Boraschi,
Daniela N. Mannel and Michael C. Edelstein
Immunopathology Section, Laboratory of Immunobiology
Immunology Program
National Cancer Institute
National Institutes of Health
Bethesda, Maryland 20014.

Development of macrophages with nonspecific microbicidal and/or tumoricidal activity ("activated macrophages") at sites of immune responses follows completion of a series of interrelated reactions (6,7,14,16). Each reaction requires the simultaneous presence of effective activation signals and competent mononuclear phagocytes. The reaction sequence for macrophage activation can be conceptually divided into three phases:

(1) The first phase involves recruitment and differentiation of blood-derived mononuclear phagocytes into inflammatory macrophages. The immediate precursor cells for activated macrophages are neither blood monocytes nor resident tissue macrophages but rather are the blood-derived cells which accumulate nonspecifically at sites of inflammation.

(2) Inflammatory macrophages are uniquely responsive to certain macrophage activation factors released from antigen-stimulated lymphocytes (lymphokines). Interactions between inflammatory macrophages and lymphokine activation signals constitute the second phase of macrophage activation and generate noncytotoxic intermediate cells, primed macrophages (12,14).

(3) The third and final phase of macrophage activation occurs as lymphokine-primed macrophages respond to any of several other activation signals (lymphokine-derived stimuli different from priming signals, stimuli derived from bacteria or from tumor cells) to develop complete tumoricidal activity. It should be noted that while these final activation signals or trigger signals are fully active on lymphokine-primed cells, they cannot directly activate inflammatory macrophages (13,14).

This series of reactions required for tumoricidal activity is analogous to similar reaction sequences documented with other macrophage functions: secretion and release of fibrinolytic activity, $H_2O_2$ or lymphocyte activation factor and C3b receptor-mediated phagocytosis (5,8,9). The cellular intermediates and stimuli for each of these macrophage functions, however, are very different.

Definition of strains of mice with genetic defects in development of macrophage cytotoxic activity provided a useful resource for characterization of the macrophage activation sequence. A survey of 27 mouse strains for development of activated tumoricidal macrophages during infection with viable <u>Mycobacterium</u> <u>bovis</u>, strain BCG revealed three groups with macrophage defects (1) (Table-1). This report will discuss genetic analysis of cytotoxic defects in two of the three groups: C3H/HeJ and A/J mice.

Table-1. Genetic variation in development of macrophage tumoricidal activity among mouse strains.

| RESPONSIVE | VARIABLE | NONRESPONSIVE |
|---|---|---|
| C3H/HeN | BALB/cAnN | A/J |
| AKR/N | A/WySnJ | A/HeJ |
| CBA/CaHN | AL/N | A/HeN |
| CBA/N | RIII/AnN | |
| C3Heb/FeJ | | C3H/HeJ |
| C57L/N | | C57BL/10ScCR |
| C57BL/6N | | C57BL/10ScN |
| C57BL/10SnJ | | |
| C57BL/10J | | P/J |
| DBA/1JN | | P/JN |
| DBA/2N | | |
| NZB/N | | |
| NZW/N | | |
| NIH Swiss (outbred) | | |
| B10.A/SgSnJ | | |

Peritoneal exudate macrophages from individual mice (3-60 mice/strain) inoculated intraperitoneally 7-10 days previously with viable BCG were adjusted to equal macrophage concentrations and assayed for tumoricidal activity by release of $^{3}$HTdR from prelabeled tumor target cells at 48 hours.

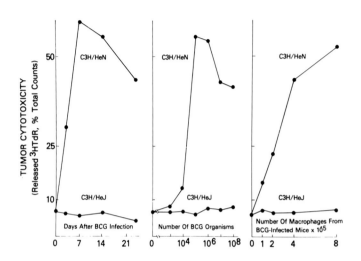

Figure-1. Tumor cytotoxicity by macrophages from BCG-infected C3H/HeN and C3H/HeJ mice.

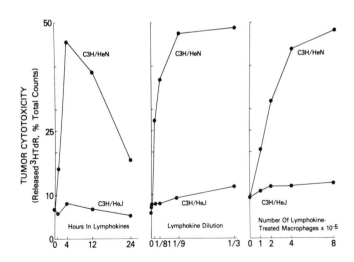

Figure-2. Tumor cytotoxicity by lymphokine-treated macrophages from C3H/HeN and C3H/HeJ mice.

C3H/HeJ and other (C57BL/10ScN) strains with abnormal responsiveness to the lipid A region of bacterial endotoxic lipopolysaccharides (LPS) fail to develop activated tumoricidal macrophages during intraperitoneal infection with BCG (Figure-1). Varying time of macrophage collection after BCG infection, number of BCG organisms in the infectious inoculum or numbers of macrophages from BCG-infected mice added to tumor target cells did not evoke cytotoxic activity. Macrophages from C3H/HeJ mice treated with killed Corynebacterium parvum or pyran copolymer, in vivo treatments which activate responsive C3H/HeN macrophages, were also not cytotoxic. Macrophage tumoricidal activity also did not develop after in vitro treatment of C3H/HeJ cells with lymphokines (Figure-2). Increasing time of macrophage incubation in lymphokines, concentration of lymphokines or numbers of lymphokine-treated macrophages added to tumor cells did not evoke tumoricidal activity (11).

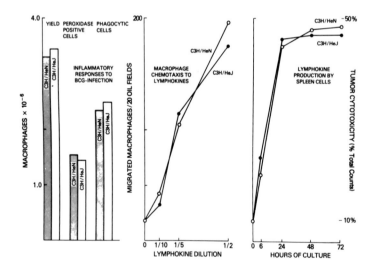

Figure-3. Inflammatory responses to BCG infection, macrophage chemotaxis in vitro and production of macrophage activation factors with cells from C3H/HeN and C3H/HeJ mice.

The tumoricidal defect of macrophages from C3H/HeJ mice was highly selective (Figure-3): inflammatory responses to BCG infection (macrophage yield, peroxidase cytochemistry and phagocytic responses) in C3H/HeJ and C3H/HeN mice were indistinguishable; macrophage responses to chemotactic lymphokines in vitro were also normal. Moreover, production of macrophage activation factors by antigen-stimulated spleen cells of C3H/HeJ mice was entirely normal. Thus, LPS-unresponsive C3H/HeJ macrophages possess a profound and selective defect in tumoricidal capacity following in vivo or in vitro treatments not directly dependent upon bacterial endotoxins (11,13).

Under certain conditions, however, macrophages from C3H/HeJ mice could become cytotoxic; macrophages primed by in vivo immune reactions initiated by BCG infection or injection of T cell mitogens or specific antigens, but not cells from irritant-induced inflammatory exudates, developed full tumoricidal capability after further exposure in vitro to a second activation or trigger signal (Table-2).

Table-2.    Tumor  cytotoxicity  by  macrophages  from BCG-infected  C3H/HeJ  mice  treated  in  vitro  with  LPS  or lymphokines.

| Macrophages treated with: | Tumor cytotoxicity by macrophages from C3H/HeJ mice treated with: | | |
| --- | --- | --- | --- |
| | SALINE | BCG | Con A |
| MEDIUM | 6 | 8 | 5 |
| LPS (2 ug/ml) | 6 | 46 | 35 |
| with polymyxin B | 8 | 10 | 7 |
| LYMPHOKINES (1/5) | 6 | 52 | 28 |
| with polymyxin B | 7 | 54 | 29 |

Adherent PC from treated mice were incubated in LPS or lymphokines for 4 hours. Cultures were washed and incubated with [3]HTdR prelabelled tumor target cells. Cytotoxicity was estimated at 48 hours by measurement of [3]HTdR release and expressed as a percentage of total counts.

These trigger signals include µg/ml concentrations of LPS
and certain factors in lymphokine supernatants.  It should
be noted that the effect of LPS but not that of lymphokines
was abrogated by polymyxin B, an antibiotic that binds to
lipid A.  This polymyxin B effect suggests that at least two
different factors can provide trigger signals for macrophage
cytotoxicity (13).

   C3H/HeJ mice are resistant or poorly responsive to all
known in vivo and in vitro effects of lipid A:  spleen cells
from this strain fail to proliferate in vitro in response to
LPS;   this spleen cell defect reflects a mutation in a
single gene, the Lps gene on chromosome 4 (17).  To define
the  genetic  relationship  between  defects  in  macrophage
tumoricidal capacity and in spleen cell responsiveness to
LPS, we examined both cell functions in C3H/HeJ x F₁(C3H/HeJ
x C3H/HeN) backcross mice (Table-3).  Macrophages from individual mice were treated with lymphokines, washed and assayed for tumor cytotoxicity.  Spleen cells from each of
these mice were simultaneously assayed for proliferative responses to LPS.  Lymphokine-treated macrophages from C3H/HeN
mice were tumoricidal in vitro; spleen cells from these mice
were strongly responsive to LPS.  In contrast, both macrophage and spleen cell responses were absent or minimal with
cells  from C3H/HeJ mice.  Lymphokine-induced  macrophage
tumoricidal responses and LPS-induced spleen cell proliferative responses of cells from F₁ hybrids were intermediate to
responses of cells from the two parental strains.  Among 19
C3H/HeJ x F₁ backcross mice, there was a strict correlation
between macrophage tumoricidal and spleen cell proliferative
responses.  For these responses, the correlation coefficient
was 0.97 (level of significance 0.001).  This analysis suggests that the gene for control of one or more essential reactions in development of nonspecific macrophage cytotoxic
activity is either closely linked or identical to the Lps
gene.  That macrophages from 6 other mouse strains with the
defective Lps gene also fail to develop normal tumoricidal
activity, supports this conclusion (15).

   Results with the C3H/HeJ strain suggest that LPS responsiveness and macrophage cytotoxic activity are somehow
related.  The nature of this relationship remains to be established.  However, immunotherapy of murine fibrosarcomas
with viable BCG, a reaction dependent upon development of
activated tumoricidal macrophages at the tumor site, was
less effective in both genetically unresponsive C3H/HeJ mice
and in normally responsive C3H/HeN mice made tolerant to LPS
by daily intravenous injections of lipid A (7,10) (Table-4).

Table-3.   Backcross   linkage   analysis   of   lymphokine-induced
macrophage  cytotoxic  activity  and  LPS-induced  spleen  cell
proliferation.

| Source of cells: | Tumor cytotoxicity (% total counts) | Spleen cell proliferation (LPS-treated/control) |
|---|---|---|
| C3H/HeN mice | $42 \pm 3$ | $14 \pm 1$ |
| C3H/HeJ mice | $6 \pm 1$ | $1 \pm 0$ |
| $F_1$(C3H/HeJ x C3H/HeN) hybrid mice | $22 \pm 2$ | $7 \pm 2$ |
| C3H/HeJ x $F_1$ backcross | | |
| | 18 | 5 |
| | 17 | 5 |
| | 30 | 10 |
| RESPONSIVE (8/19) | 24 | 7 |
| | 21 | 13 |
| | 25 | 8 |
| | 22 | 6 |
| | 21 | 9 |
| | 9 | 1 |
| | 6 | 1 |
| | 9 | 1 |
| NONRESPONSIVE (11/19) | 7 | 1 |
| | 5 | 1 |
| | 6 | 1 |
| | 6 | 1 |
| | 7 | 1 |
| | 5 | 1 |
| | 7 | 1 |
| | 5 | 1 |

Table-4.    Effect  of  LPS  tolerance  on  BCG-mediated  tumor regression.

| Mice | CONTROL | BCG-TREATED | % CURE |
|------|---------|-------------|--------|
| | | Tumor-free/total mice for: | |
| Expmt.#1. | | | |
| C3H/HeN | 0/6 | 14/20 | 70% |
| C3H/HeN(tolerant) | 0/5 | 0/20 | 0% |
| C3H/HeJ | 0/6 | 4/16 | 25% |
| Expmt.#2. | | | |
| C3H/HeN | 0/7 | 10/14 | 70% |
| C3H/HeN(tolerant) | 0/9 | 0/17 | 0% |
| C3H/HeJ | 0/9 | 1/16 | 6% |
| Expmt.#3. | | | |
| C3H/HeN | 0/5 | 12/19 | 63% |
| C3H/HeN(tolerant) | 0/5 | 0/20 | 0% |
| C3H/HeJ | 0/6 | 4/19 | 20% |

Mice with 5 day intradermal fibrosarcoma transplants were treated by intralesional injection of viable BCG organisms or diluent.  Certain animals were made tolerant to LPS (defined by hypothermia reactions) by daily intravenous injections of LPS from the R595 mutant of Salmonella minnesota for 10 consecutive days.  All animals were observed for 90 days.

The macrophage tumoricidal defect of A/J mice was very similar to the C3H/HeJ defect.  Cells from BCG-infected A/J mice or A/J macrophages treated in vitro with lymphokines were not cytotoxic over a wide range of experimental conditions (Figures 4 and 5).

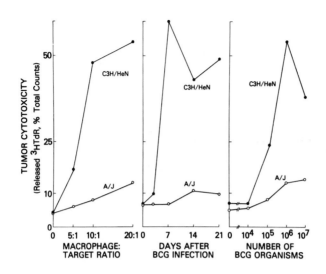

Figure-4.  Tumor cytotoxicity by macrophages from BCG-infected C3H/HeN and A/J mice.

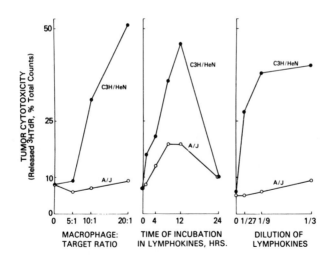

Figure-5.  Tumor cytotoxicity by lymphokine-treated macrophages from C3H/HeN and A/J mice.

Events in early stages of macrophage activation were normal: inflammatory responses to BCG infection were intact;
production of macrophage activation factors by antigen-
stimulated A/J spleen cells were also normal. A/J mice,
like C3H/HeJ mice, appear to have a genetic inability to
complete final responses required for expression of cytotoxic activity by lymphokine-primed cells. Again, macrophage cytotoxic activity can develop if additional trigger
signals are provided in vitro (Table-5). Thus, except for
the concentration of LPS needed to deliver trigger signals
(C3H/HeJ macrophages require μg/ml concentrations whereas
A/J macrophages need only pg to ng/ml levels), the macrophage cytotoxic defect of A/J mice is phenotypically identical to that of C3H/HeJ mice (2,3).

Table-5. Tumor cytotoxicity by macrophages from BCG-infected A/J mice treated in vitro with a variety of trigger
signals.

| Macrophages treated | Tumor cytotoxicity by macrophages from: | |
| --- | --- | --- |
| in vitro with: | CONTROL MICE | BCG-INFECTED MICE |
| MEDIUM | 5% | 14% |
| LYMPHOKINES | 6% | 57% |
| LPS | 7% | 54% |
| PHA | 7% | 52% |
| Con A | 8% | 63% |

Adherent PC from BCG-infected and control A/J mice were
treated in vitro with any of a variety of agents for 4
hours. Cultures were washed and assayed for tumoricidal
activity by release of $^3$HTdR from prelabeled tumor target
cells at 48 hours. Cytotoxicity was expressed as a percentage of total counts.

It is possible that the macrophage cytotoxic defect of
A/J mice may also reflect a genetic mutation at the Lps
locus. Consistent with this possibility is the observation
that spleen cell proliferative responses to LPS, responses
controlled by the Lps gene, were defective with both C3H/HeJ
and A/J mice (Figure-6).

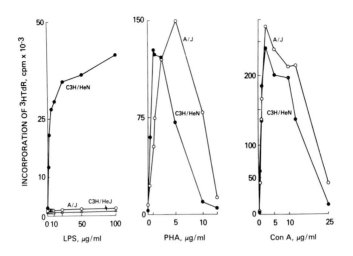

Figure-6. Proliferative responses to LPS, PHA, and Con A of spleen cells from C3H/HeN, C3H/HeJ and A/J mice.

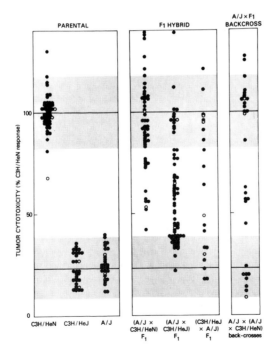

Figure-7. Genetic analysis of the macrophage tumoricidal defect of A/J mice.

Unlike C3H/HeJ mice, however, responses of A/J mice to the
lethal toxicity of LPS in vivo and of A/J macrophages to the
direct toxicity of LPS in vitro, responses also controlled
by the Lps gene, were normal (3,4). The macrophage cytotoxic defect of A/J mice must then either represent a previously undescribed allelic change at the Lps locus (a Lps allele different from that of C3H/HeJ mice) or genetic mutations at entirely different loci.

To resolve these alternative possibilities, we examined
macrophage cytotoxic responses in $F_1$ hybrids of A/J and C3H-
/HeN or C3H/HeJ mice and in A/J x $F_1$ (A/J x C3H/HeN) backcross mice. Results of this examination are summarized in
Figure-7. Tumoricidal reactions of macrophages from BCG-infected C3H/HeN mice were defined as responsive; reactions
of cells from BCG-infected C3H/HeJ mice were defined as nonresponsive. The mean ± 2 SD (95% confidence limits) for 57
responder and 34 nonresponder mice are designated by shaded
areas. These areas do not overlap. No tumoricidal activity
was evident with macrophages from any of 30 BCG-infected A/J
mice. Mouse-to-mouse variation within responder or nonresponder parental strains was very small. In contrast, cytotoxic responses of cells from BCG-infected $F_1$ hybrids were
heterogeneous and scattered over a wide range. Heterogeneity among the $F_1$ hybrids was not due to experiment-to-exper-
iment variation: variation throughout the response
range was evident within a single experiment (Figure-7),
open circles). Heterogeneity was also not due to sex
chromosome-linked factors: responses by male and female $F_1$
hybrids or the response distribution of (A/J x C3H/HeJ)$F_1$
versus (C3H/HeJ x A/J)$F_1$ hybrids were identical. Despite
this heterogeneity, macrophages from BCG-infected (A/J x
C3H/HeN)$F_1$ hybrid mice consistently exhibited strong tumoricidal activity: cells from 38 of 51 mice were fully responsive; responses of cells from the remaining 13 mice
were also positive but intermediate to responder and non-
responder reactions. No responses fell within the non-
responder range.

Tumoricidal responses of cells from BCG-infected $F_1$
hybrids of nonresponder A/J and C3H/HeJ parental mice were
of special interest: About one third of 88 mice were nonresponsive; responses of cells from the remaining mice were
scattered throughout responder and intermediate ranges.
That macrophage cytotoxic defects of unresponsive A/J and
C3H/HeJ parents were corrected in their $F_1$ hybrids strongly
suggests that defects in these strains were sequelae of entirely different genes. Moreover, the heterogeneity of
these responses suggests that control of the A/J macrophage
defect is polygenic.

Table-6. Backcross linkage analysis of lymphokine-induced macrophage cytotoxic activity LPS-induced spleen cell proliferation and macrophage sensitivity to toxic effects of LPS.

| Source of cells: | Tumor cytotoxicity | LPS toxicity to macrophages | LPS-induced spleen cell proliferation |
|---|---|---|---|
| PARENTS | | | |
| C3H/HeN | $100 \pm 3$ | $100 \pm 3$ | $100 \pm 7$ |
| C3H/HeJ | $16 \pm 2**$ | $15 \pm 1**$ | $14 \pm 3**$ |
| A/J | $21 \pm 2**$ | $96 \pm 2$ | $19 \pm 3**$ |
| $F_1$ HYBRIDS | | | |
| A/J x C3H/HeN | $91 \pm 8$ | $88 \pm 3$ | $62 \pm 4$ |
| A/J x C3H/HeJ | $60 \pm 9$ | $82 \pm 3$ | $12 \pm 4**$ |
| A/J x $F_1$(A/J x C3H/HeN) | | | |
| BACKCROSSES | | | |
| | 57 | 100 | 26** |
| | 100 | 72 | 63 |
| | 99 | 91 | 13** |
| | 104 | 74 | 48 |
| | 60 | 82 | 23** |
| | 68 | 96 | 15** |
| | 83 | 96 | 73 |
| | 76 | 90 | 57 |
| | | | |
| | 24** | 96 | 24** |
| | 9** | 87 | 66 |
| | 15** | 98 | 56 |

**NONRESPONDER

Analysis of macrophage tumoricidal responses among A/J x (A/J x C3H/HeN) backcross mice also suggested polygenic control. If differences between nonresponsive A/J mice and responsive C3H/HeN mice were due to effects of a single gene, then 50% of backcross mice should have the A/J parental trait. Among 50 backcross mice, however, 11 or 22% failed to develop tumoricidal macrophages during BCG infection (4). Thus, genetic control of the A/J macrophage defect was clearly polygenic and probably secondary to two different genes (predicted nonresponder percentage for backcross mice would be 25%).

It was also of interest to characterize the defect in spleen cell proliferation to LPS among A/J x (A/J x C3H/HeN) backcross mice and determine its relationship to the macrophage cytotoxicity defect. Analysis of these two responses among backcross mice, however, showed a clear dissociation (Table-5). Cells from BCG-infected parental, $F_1$ hybrid and A/J x $F_1$ backcross mice were simultaneously tested for macrophage cytotoxicity, macrophage sensitivity to LPS and LPS-induced spleen cell proliferation, responses all controlled by the Lps gene. Only macrophages from C3H/HeJ mice were resistant to toxicity of LPS in vitro. Spleen cell proliferative responses to LPS among A/J x $F_1$ backcross mice did not correlate with and segregated independently of both macrophage cytotoxic activity and macrophage sensitivity to the toxic effects of LPS. No differences were detected between male and female $F_1$ hybrid mice.

Among 15 A/J x (A/J x C3H/HeN) backcross mice, spleen cells from 8 (53%) animals were unresponsive to mitogenic effects of LPS. Thus, differences in spleen cell responsiveness to LPS between A/J and C3H/HeN mice were probably due to a single codominant autosomal gene. Although the spleen cell proliferative defect was not corrected in (A/J x C3H/HeJ)$F_1$ hybrids, that this trait segregates from macrophage sensitivity to LPS in vitro suggests the gene is not at the Lps locus.

We have now identified two strains of mice, C3H/HeJ and A/J, with profound defects at some stage of the macrophage activation sequence. It is clear from these studies that the genetic basis for cytotoxic defects in A/J and C3H/HeJ mice were different. Further analysis of macrophage activation in these genetic models could provide a system for isolation and characterization of intermediary signals and responsive cells and define mechanisms for genetic control of nonspecific resistance.

### REFERENCES

1. Boraschi, D., and Meltzer, M.S. Cell.Immunol. 45:188, 1979.

2. Boraschi, D., and Meltzer, M.S. J.Immunol. 122:1587, 1979.

3. Boraschi, D., and Meltzer, M.S. J.Immunol. 122:1592, 1979.

4. Boraschi, D., and Meltzer, M.S. J.Immunol., 1980 (in press).

5.  Gordon, S., Unkeless, J.C., and Cohen, Z.A.   J.Exp.Med.
    140:995, 1974.
6.  Hibbs,J.B.,Jr., Taintor, R.R., Chapman, H.A.Jr., and
    Weinberg, J.B.  Science 197:279, 1977.
7.  Meltzer, M.S., Ruco, L.P., Boraschi, D., and Nacy, C.A.
    J.Reticul.Soc. 26:403, 1979.
8.  Mizel, S.B., and Rosenstreich, D.L.   J.Immunol.
    122:2173, 1979.
9.  Nathan, C.F., and Root, R.K.   J.Exp.Med.  146:1648,
    1977.
10. Rietschel, E.Th., and Galanos, C.  Infect.Immun. 15:34,
    1977.
11. Ruco, L.P., and Meltzer, M.S.   J.Immunol.  120:329,
    1978.
12. Ruco, L.P., and Meltzer, M.S.   J.Immunol.  120:1054,
    1978.
13. Ruco, L.P., and Meltzer, M.S.   Cell.Immunol.  41:35,
    1978.
14. Ruco, L.P., and Meltzer, M.S.   J.Immunol.  121:2035,
    1978.
15. Ruco, L.P., Meltzer, M.S., and Rosenstreich, D.L.
    J.Immunol. 121:543, 1978.
16. Russell, S.W., Doe, W.F., and McIntosh, A.T.
    J.Exp.Med. 146:1511, 1977.
17. Watson, J., Largen, M., and McAdam, K.P.W.J.
    J.Exp.Med. 147:39, 1978.

## DISCUSSIONS

Rosenstreich: Meltzer's endotoxin-tolerance data are very interesting, but I wonder whether he might be misinterpreting it. I am not sure that the only defect in a mouse that has been given endotoxin is that it is tolerant to endotoxin. I suspect that there are also a number of other problems - in terms of its reticuloendothelial function.

Meltzer: I agree with Rosenstreich. Macrophages from the endotoxin-tolerant C3H/HeN mice do not develop cytotoxic activity and they behave to BCG like the macrophages from C3H/HeJ mice. Now to go from that observation and to say that there is only a single defect in these mice, I would not want to do. It is just that there are only a limited number of ways one can approach this issue. If we postulate that endotoxin has something to do with macrophage cytotoxicity (a quite unresolved situation), there a minimal number of ways in which one can affect endotoxin responsiveness. One is through the use of genetic models, another through tolerance. In both cases we see the same effect.

Stewart: Does Meltzer think that the defect might be like the sex-linked CBA-LPS defect? Has he looked at that?

Meltzer: That was given on the list of responsive mice. They respond perfectly well to BCG or to C. parvum or to lymphokines in vitro. But I think that macrophages from these mice respond normally to endotoxin. It is the B cells that are defective.

Stewart: But they may not be getting enough signal from the macrophages.

Meltzer: We see no macrophage cytotoxicity defect in them.

Stewart: Another point: because the A/J mice macrophages respond poorly to inflammatory stimuli, could it be that one has different dilutions of resident cells which might not respond, and that one is really focussing on a quantitative difference in numbers of newly elicited cells diluted by resident cells?

Meltzer: We looked into this issue by utilizing peroxidase staining. This method poses technical problems but at least we did not find any differences in numbers of peroxidase-positive cells in these mice. We could adjust our cell concentrations to an equal number of peroxidase-positive mononuclear phagocytes and still see the same defect.

Roder: Does Meltzer think the genetic differences would be overcome by in vitro culture? The reason I ask is that in some collaborative work we have done with Lohman-Matthes, using her bone marrow cultures and then looking at activated macrophage killers, after about a week in culture we could no longer discern any genetic differences between cells of the A/J and other strains.

Meltzer: Well, there are many ways to kill tumor cells and many ways macrophages can kill tumor cells. For example, by bringing in antibody one gets an ADCC-like reaction and there would be no genetic differences at any time. C3H/HeJ, C3H/HeN and A/J mice would all respond perfectly well.

Roder: The studies I referred to dealt with spontaneous killing.

Meltzer: I do not know the answer. I know that it is very hard to compare killing reactions in different systems. When we put the cells in culture for 24 hours we are unable to activate them for killing in our assay system by any of a variety of different ways that we have tried.

Roder: I might mention one further thing concerning the system I referred to. The macrophages from the C3H/HeJ bone marrow, cultured in high concentrations of Con A-supernatant factor (which is like MAF, I suppose), are restored to complete responsiveness. Meltzer's response would probably be that in this situation we have a small contamination with endotoxin, which is always possible.

Meltzer: No, my reply would actually be different from that. As I remember the Lohman-Matthes system, she does not absorb out the mitogenic Con A. In that event, very small amounts of Con A could act like an ADCC reaction and, as we know, there is no defect in ADCC killing.

Cudkowicz: Unlike the C3H/HeJ, the A/J mouse is also deficient in NK activity. Deficient in the sense that the NK activity is low and expecially that it cannot be enhanced by the interferon-inducers - a bit like the SJL mouse. Does Meltzer happen to know whether there is any relationship between the macrophage and NK defects in his $F_1$ mice and the segregting populations?

Meltzer: We have not looked at that. Initially we were very concerned about that question because there was a period of time when others were suggesting that all macrophage cytotoxicity was in fact NK activity. Perhaps the best evidence against this notion is that AKR mice, fully responsive in macrophage cytotoxicity, are as poor in NK activity as the A/J mice. Isn't that so?

Cudkowicz: I did not mean to say that macrophage cytotoxicity is equated with NK activity.

Meltzer: There are actually some good studies showing that the early response to BCG, for example, within the first 2-3 days, may be due to NK activity rather than to macrophages.

Cudkowicz: But you actually do not have the information I requested.

Meltzer: No, we do not.

Participant:  I am especially interested in the genetics of
the A/J hypo-responsiveness.  It would have been interesting
if Meltzer had tested other A independent sublines, long
separated ones, like A/Sn or other A background mice.

Meltzer:  Well, the macrophage cytotoxicity defect was
tested in A/J, A/HeJ and A/HeN;  all three of those were
non-responders.  The A/WySnJ was an intermediate strain.
B10.A/Wy was fully responsive.

# ACTIVATED MACROPHAGES IN NATURAL RESISTANCE TO <u>RICKETTSIA AKARI</u>

Carol A. Nacy, Georgiene Radlick, and Monte S. Meltzer
Division of Communicable Diseases and Immunology
Walter Reed Army Institute of Research
Washington D.C. 20012
and
Laboratory of Immunobiology
National Cancer Institute
National Institutes of Health
Bethesda, Maryland 20205

Mouse peritoneal macrophages are activated for non-specific tumoricidal and microbicidal activities by treatment <u>in vivo</u> with <u>Mycobacterium</u> bovis, strain BCG or <u>Corynebacterium parvum</u> or <u>in vitro</u> with lymphokine-rich supernatants of antigen or mitogen-stimulated leukocytes(3,7,9). Certain strains of mice, however, fail to develop activated tumoricidal macrophages after any of several <u>in vitro</u> or <u>in vivo</u> treatments over a wide range of experimental conditions: (1.) strains with the defective <u>Lps</u> gene (C3H/HeJ, C57BL/10ScN, C57BL/10ScCR), (2.) strains derived from A mice (A/J, A/HeN) and (3.) P/J strain (1). We recently surveyed 15 strains of mice for resistance to the lethal effects of <u>Rickettsia akari</u> infection (Table 1).

<u>Table 1.</u>  Genetic variation in resistance to <u>R. akari.</u>

| RESISTANT | | SUSCEPTIBLE | |
|---|---|---|---|
| AL/N | $(10^{4.8})$ | *A/HeN | $(10^{3.5})$ |
| BALB/c | $(10^{4.3})$ | *A/J | $(10^{2.0})$ |
| CBA/N | $(>10^{5})$ | | |
| C3H/HeN | $(>10^{5})$ | *C3H/HeJ | $(10^{1.5})$ |
| C57BL/6N | $(>10^{5})$ | *C57BL/10ScN | $(10^{2.7})$ |
| C57BL/10J | $(>10^{4.6})$ | *C57BL/10ScCr | $(10^{1.2})$ |
| C57L/N | $(10^{4.6})$ | | |
| DBA/2N | $(>10^{5.3})$ | NZW/N | $(<10^{2.0})$ |
| *P/J | $(10^{4.5})$ | | |

*Mouse strains with defects in macrophage activation for tumor cytotoxicity.
[a]Numbers in parentheses indicate $LD_{50}$ of <u>R. akari</u> in each mouse strain. Resistance was defined as mouse strain in which 50% of animals survived $10^{4}$ rickettsiae challenge.

C3H/HeJ, C57BL/10ScN, C57BL/10ScCR, A/J and A/HeN mice, all
from strains with macrophage cytotoxic defects, were 1,000-
10,000-fold more susceptible than mice from resistant strains.   These data suggested that development of activated
macrophages may be an essential response for host resistance
to R. akari disease.
     The correlation between strain susceptibility to R.
akari infection and defective macrophage function was examined in greater detail.   We have previously shown that
macrophages from mice with regressing R. tsutsugamushi infection were highly activated for both tumoricidal and
rickettsiacidal activities (6).   To ascertain whether a
similar macrophage activation occurred during R. akari infection, we treated mice from six selected strains (C3H/HeN,
C3H/HeJ, C57BL/10J, C57BL/10ScCR, BALB/cN and A/J) with 1000
PFU R. akari intraperitoneally each day for 9 days.   Macrophages were collected from all animals on day 10 and assayed
in vitro for tumoricidal and rickettsiacidal activities
(Figure 1).

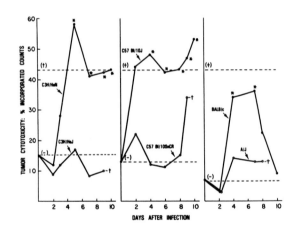

Figure 1.   Macrophages were harvested from mice inoculated
-10 days with R. akari.   Cells were adjusted to 5 x 10⁵
macrophages/culture well, and exposed to $^3$H-thymidine prelabeled tumor mKSA-TU-5 target cells at an effector to
target cell ratio of 10:1.   Tumor cytotoxicity was estimated
by measuring $^3$H-thymidine released into culture supernatants
at 48 hr.   Results are expressed as % total incorporated
counts. (+): % tumor cytotoxicity of macrophages from uninfected resistant mice treated with lymphokines in vitro;
(-): % tumor cytotoxicity of untreated macrophages from uninfected resistant mice; (*): macrophages which were activ-
vated to kill R.akari in vitro.

Macrophages from all resistant mice (C3H/HeN, C57BL/10J and BALB/cN) developed significant levels of both tumor cytotoxicity and rickettsiacidal activity 2-4 days after infection. Macrophages from these resistant mice also developed tumoricidal and rickettsicidal activities after in vitro treatment with lymphokines (Table 2). In contrast, macrophages from susceptible strains of mice (C3H/HeJ, C57BL/10ScCr and A/J) were not activated for tumor cytotoxicity in vivo at any time following inoculation of R. akari. Rickettsiacidal activity of macrophages from these infected mice could not be determined. Since 20-40% of peritoneal macrophages contained intracellular rickettsiae at the time of cell harvest, further analysis of macrophage rickettsiacidal activity in this system was impossible.

Table 2. Rickettsiacidal activity of macrophages from R. akari-infected mice or treated in vitro with lymphokine supernatants[α].

| Mouse strain: | Treatment of macrophages: | | % Rickettsiacidal activity: | |
| | R. akari in vivo: | Lymphokines in vitro: | 1 hr | 24 hr |
|---|---|---|---|---|
| C3H/HeN | + | - | 32 | 74 |
| | - | + | 26 | 69 |
| C57Bl/10J | + | - | 34 | 72 |
| | - | + | 33 | 70 |
| BALB/cN | + | - | 22 | 58 |
| | - | + | 27 | 62 |

[a] Macrophages were harvested from 3 mice infected with rickettsiae 7 days previously and 5 control mice of each strain. Macrophages from rickettsial infected mice were incubated in medium for 4 hr at 37 C in 5% $CO_2$; macrophages from control mice were incubated in medium or 1/10 dilution of lymphokines for 4 h. Cultures were washed, exposed to rickettsiae for 1 hr, and incubated in medium or lymphokines for 18 hr. Samples were removed 1 hr after addition of rickettsiae or at 18 hr and examined microscopically for percent infected macrophages (mφ). Rickettsiacidal activity was determined by:

$$100 \times \frac{\% \text{ infected control } m\phi - \% \text{ infected treated } m\phi}{\% \text{ infected control } m\phi}$$

Table 3. Treatment of macrophages with lymphokines in
vitro: induction of ricketsiacidal activity in macrophages
from resistant and susceptible mouse strains.

| Mouse Strain: | Macrophages treated with lymphokines: | | % Rickettsiacıdal activity at: | |
|---|---|---|---|---|
| | Preinfection | Postinfection | 1 hour | 24 hour |
| C3H/HeN | + | - | 35 | 30 |
| | - | + | 0 | 39 |
| | + | + | 35 | 48 |
| C3H/HeJ | + | - | 0 | 4 |
| | - | + | 0 | 11 |
| | + | + | 0 | 24 |
| C57BL/10J | + | - | 35 | 42 |
| | - | + | 0 | 55 |
| | + | + | 35 | 70 |
| C57BL/10ScCR | + | - | 0 | 7 |
| | - | + | 0 | 20 |
| | + | + | 0 | 26 |
| BALB/cN | + | - | 29 | 37 |
| | - | + | 0 | 70 |
| | + | + | 29 | 78 |
| A/J | + | - | 0 | 15 |
| | - | + | 0 | 8 |
| | + | + | 0 | 14 |

Macrophages were harvested from 4-6 mice of each strain, adjusted to $10^6$ macrophages/ml, and incubated in medium or
lymphokines (1/10 dilution) for 4 hr. Macrophage cultures
were exposed to 5 PFU R. akari for 1 hr, and incubated in
medium or lymphokines for 18 hr. Samples were removed at 1
hr or 18 hr and examined microscopically for percent infected macrophages (mφ). Rickettsiacidal activity was determined
by:

$$100 \times \frac{\text{\% infected control mφ} - \text{\% infected treated mφ}}{\text{\% infected control mφ}}$$

Analysis of mechanisms of microbicidal activity by activated macrophages against R. tsutsugamushi suggested two distinct pathways: an initial decrease in infectivity of rickettsiae for activated cells followed by significant increases in intracellular killing of viable organisms (7). The definition of resistant and susceptible mouse strains to R. akari provided us with a unique opportunity to examine the possible contribution of each antimicrobial pathway to host resistance (Table-3). Lymphokine-treated macrophages from resistant C3H/HeN, C57BL/10J and BALB/cN mice demonstrated both rickettsiacidal effects: rickettsiacidal activity at 1 hour ranged between 30-35%; activity at 24 hours was 30-78%. In contrast, cells from the susceptible mouse strains with macrophage tumoricidal defects (C3H/HeJ, C57BL/10ScCr and A/J) had no initial antimicrobial activity. Moreover, the level of intracellular killing over 24 hours by cells from these mouse strains was 50-90% less than that by cells from resistant strains. Thus, macrophages from susceptible mice exhibit decreased activity in both antimicrobial pathways.

Defects in macrophage rickettsiacidal activity were not limited to cells treated with lymphokines in vitro. Macrophages from BCG-infected C3H/HeJ, C57BL/10ScCR and A/J mice, all from strains susceptible to R. akari infection, showed little or no rickettsicidal activity; cells from resistant BCG-infected C3H/HeN, C57BL/10J or BALB/cN mice were strongly microbicidal and tumoricidal in vitro (Table 4).

Animals infected with BCG show increased nonspecific resistance against a wide variety of microbial pathogens (2,4,8,10). The protective effect of BCG infection against the lethal effects of R. akari was examined in the C3H/HeN-C3H/HeJ strain pair. Mice were inoculated with $10^6$ viable BCG or medium and challenged with graded doses of either R. akari or R. tsutsugamushi. R. tsutsugamushi was included as C3H/HeN and C3H/HeJ mice are equally susceptible to intraperitoneal inoculation of this rickettsial species, but BCG protects only C3H/HeN mice from lethal infection (5) (Table 5). Seventy five percent of C3H/HeN mice treated with BCG survived $10^4$ challenge of R. tsutsugamushi, while all C3H/HeN mice inoculated with R. akari (untreated and BCG-treated) survived infection. C3H/HeJ mice treated with BCG did not survive challenge with R. tsutsugamushi and were protected only minimally from R. akari.

Simultaneous development of macrophage activation for tumor cytotoxicity and for rickettsiacidal activity has been observed over a broad range of experimental conditions both in vivo and in vitro (5,6,7). Analysis of macrophage function in mouse strains susceptible to the lethal effects of

Table 4.    Rickettsiacidal and tumoricidal activities of macrophages from mice treated with M. bovis strain BCG[a].

| Mouse strain | % Rickettsiacidal activity[b] at: | | % Tumor cytotoxicity[c]: |
|---|---|---|---|
| | 1 hour | 24 hour | |
| C3H/HeN | 32 | 89 | 55 |
| C3H/HeJ | 0 | 32 | 11 |
| C57Bl/10J | 35 | 76 | 46 |
| C57Bl/10ScCR | 0 | 28 | 14 |
| BALB/cN | 30 | 72 | 40 |
| A/J | 0 | 8 | 8 |

[a] Mice were inoculated ip with $10^6$ viable BCG 10 days before macrophage (mφ) harvest.

[b] Rickettsiacidal activity was determined by:

$$100 \times \frac{\text{\% infected control mφ} - \text{\% infected treated BCG mφ}}{\text{\% infected control mφ}}$$

[c] Tumor cytotoxicity was estimated by release of $^3$H-thymidine from prelabeled tumor target cells: total incorporated counts were determined by digesting tumor monolayers with SDs and results expressed as percent SDS total counts.

Table 5.    Protective effect of BCG infection against lethal challenge with R. akari and R. tsutsugamushi.

| Mouse strain: | LD$_{50}$ challenge: | R. akari:% survival of mice treated with: | | R. tsutsugamushi:% survival of mice treated with: | |
|---|---|---|---|---|---|
| | | medium | BCG | medium | BCG |
| C3H/HeN | $10^4$ | 100 | 100 | 0 | 75 |
| | $10^3$ | 100 | 100 | 0 | 100 |
| | $10^2$ | 100 | 100 | 0 | 100 |
| | $10^1$ | 100 | 100 | 0 | 100 |
| C3H/HeJ | $10^4$ | 0 | 0 | 0 | 0 |
| | $10^3$ | 0 | 0 | 0 | 0 |
| | $10^2$ | 0 | 0 | 0 | 0 |
| | $10^1$ | 0 | 75 | 0 | 0 |

R. akari infection (C3H/HeJ, C57BL/10ScCR, A/J) suggest that ability of macrophages to respond to immunologic signals for activation is critical for survival. Macrophages from mice with defective tumoricidal capacity also had altered macrophage function for rickettsial killing. However, P/J mice, a strain with macrophage tumoricidal defects phenotypically and genetically distinct from that of C3H/HeJ or A/J mice, were resistant to R. akari infection, while NZW/N mice, a strain with normal macrophage responses for tumor cytotoxicity, were susceptible. In these two instances, tumoricidal and rickettsiacidal activities could be dissociated. Natural resistance to neoplastic diseases and at least some microbial infections may therefore be regulated by different mechanisms, each under separate genetic control.

## REFERENCES

1. Boraschi, D., and Meltzer, M.S. Cell. Immunol. 45: 188, 1979.
2. Clark, I.A., Allison, A.C., and Cox, F.E. Nature 259: 309, 1976.
3. Cleveland, R.P., Meltzer, M.S., and Zbar, B. J. Natl. Cancer Inst. 52:1837, 1974.
4. Maddison, S.E., Chandler, F.W., McDougal, J.S., Slemenda, S.B., and Kagan, I.G. Am.J.Trop.Med.Hyg. 27:966, 1978.
5. Nacy, C.A., Meltzer, M.S., Russell, P.K., and Osterman, J.V. Fed. Proc. 38:1078, 1979.
6. Nacy, C.A., and Osterman, J.V. Infect.Immun. 26:744, 1979.
7. Nacy, C.A., and Meltzer, M.S. J. Immunol. 123:2544, 1979.
8. Ortiz-Ortiz, L., Gonzalez-Mendosa, A., and Lamoyi, E. J.Immunol. 114:1424, 1975.
9. Ruco, L.P., and Meltzer, M.S. J. Immunol. 119:889, 1977.
10. Smrkovski, L.L., and Strickland, G.T. J. Immunol. 121:1257, 1978.

## DISCUSSION

Kirchner: I was wondering about your P strain. Could you elaborate on it?

Nacy: It has a macrophage defect for tumoricidal cytotoxicity which is quite different from that of mice with the LPS defect.

Participant:  What does Nacy find when she adds immune sera
to Rickettsiae before interacting them with macrophages?

Nacy:  This is a question that comes up frequently.  Serum
does something, but it is minimal.  Rickettsiae do not
ordinarily get into macrophages by standard phagocytic
mechanisms.  It is probably a parasite-induced phagocytosis.
If one opsonizes Rickettsiae with antibody, more organisms
can be brought into the cell - but those Rickettsiae which
enter by the phagosome, by Fc-receptor mediated phagocytosis, are then killed.  The killing is, however, at a lower
level of magnitude than the one which is lymphokine-induced.
That, of course, brings up an interesting question;  how
does the macrophage actually kill Rickettsiae which are in
the cytosol, not in a phagocytic vacuole, so that there is
no lysosome-phagosome interaction.

Participant:  Does Nacy have any data pertaining to incidence of spontaneous tumors in any of these mouse strains.
I ask because A mice have high incidence of spontaneous lung
tumors, many of them being invasive - so I suppose that
could be an even more useful model than the methylcholan-
threne-induced sarcoma.  The fibrosarcomas, which are used
too often, are very artificial because mice never develop
them spontaneously.

Nacy:  I do not have any information on the incidence of
spontaneous tumors.

Rosenstreich:  Groves did not make a point of it but, re-
calling his data with the BXH recombinant inbred mice, there
are inbred strains that are unresponsive to endotoxin but
fully resistant to Rickettsia tsutsugamushi.  I wonder how
that observation would correlate with Nacy's hypothesis
about the LPS$^d$ allele, the development of activated macrophages, and the requirement for the resistance to these
organisms.

Nacy:  One thing that has to be kept in mind is that the
Rickettsiae are usually lumped together as obligate intracellular microorganisms.  However, that does not mean that
they necessarily have much in common with each other.  R.
tsutsugamushi is quite a different organism.  Its' cell wall
is different, its' GC content is different, its' DNA-anneal-
ing between strains is very different, and the organism
itself has differential susceptibility to antibiotics and

preferential sites of replication in the cell which R. akari does not have. So there would seem to be some real question about the legitamacy of trying to compare R. tsutsugamushi directly with R. akari. The story about activated macrophages and killing of R. tsutsugamushi is also quite different in vivo when compared with R. akari and this again may be a reflection of the strain differences between the Rickettsiae. In the susceptible animal, the strongest correlation for the macrophage being responsible for resistance to R. tsutsugamushi is the BCG-protection data. One can only protect an animal against lethal R. tsutsugamushi infection if it is capable of responding to BCG by the formation of activated macrophages. When one examines the infection with R. tsutsugamushi in vivo of susceptible animals (C3H/HeN for example), one finds that such mice do develop activated macrophages part way through the course of Rickettsiae infection, and there is a part where the macrophage activation is suppressed. That is a very complex interaction with R. tsutsugamushi whereas, in the case of R. akari, it appears to be much more clear cut. And again this is likely due to strain differences as I said.

Rosenstreich: I cannot help wondering whether under these circumstances Nacy is looking at genetic differences in response to BCG and not so much at genetics of resistance to R. akari.

Nacy: The critical studies for the future will be, of course, to examine the capacity of cells from NZW and P/J mice to kill Rickettsiae in vitro, and compare this with what happens in vivo. I have some preliminary evidence with another system quite similar to Rickettsia, and that is Leishmania. It appears that the P/J strain has a defect for intracellular killing but does not have a defect in the first microbicidal activity that we measure at one hour. This may be the most important aspect in resitance to intracellular parasites.

Rosenstreich: Does R. akari possess an endotoxin?

Nacy: Nobody has looked for endotoxin in R. akari. There is one group of Rickettsiae in which LPS has been demonstrated and that is Coxiella burneti, but this organism is vastly different from either R. akari or R. tsutsugamushi. From this one can only infer that there is indeed a possibility that LPS is present.

# MACROPHAGE INFLAMMATORY RESPONSES IN LISTERIA-RESISTANT AND LISTERIA-SENSITIVE MICE

Mary M. Stevenson, Patricia A.L. Kongshavn
and Emil Skamene

Montreal General Hospital Research Institute
Montreal, Quebec H3G 1A4, Canada

Resistance to infection with <u>Listeria monocytogenes</u> in mice appears to be controlled by a single, dominant, autosomal, non H-2 linked gene (1,2). The genetic advantage of resistant strains (e.g. C57BL/6 or B10.A) when compared with sensitive strains (e.g. A/J) is apparent within 24-48 hrs of infection. In contrast to C57BL/6 mice which show the characteristic response described by Mackaness (3) after a sublethal dose of Listeria, A/J mice are unable to control bacterial proliferation in their livers and spleens following infection with a comparable dose and succumb within 4 days. Studies in our laboratory of the phenotypic expression of the Listeria-resistance gene have shown that the biological advantage of resistant strains is dependent upon the early appearance of a radiosensitive precursor cell of the mononuclear phagocytic system (4). The importance of newly emergent blood monocytes which later become activated with increased microbicidal ability by cellular immune mechanisms was initially described by North (5). Later studies by Mitsayama, Fakeya and their associates (6) have shown that prior to the appearance of activated macrophages in Listeria-infected liver, there is an accumulation of immature, blood-derived monocytes which presumably are inflammatory macrophages. The accumulation of inflammatory cells may be critical in preventing fulminant bacterial growth before the appearance of activated macrophages.

Thus, the cellular basis for different levels of resistance to Listeria may be the <u>production</u> of adequate numbers of mononuclear phagocytes and/or their <u>mobilization</u> to the foci of infection. We have therefore examined these two parameters of macrophage response, namely the macrophage pool size and the degree of the macrophage inflammatory response in Listeria-resistant and sensitive mice.

Resistance to Listeria and the total number of macrophages that could be recovered from peritoneal cavity during the course of infection were determined simultaneously in individual progenitor B10.A, A/J and $F_1$ hybrid and backcross mice. Mice were injected intravenously with a primary dose of $5 \times 10^3$ cfu Listeria and 1 week later with a secondary

dose of 1 x 10$^5$ cfu. Three days later, total cell and differential counts were determined on peritoneal washouts.
Growth of Listeria was determined on corresponding liver and
spleen homogenates.

**Table 1.** Linkage of Peritoneal Macrophage Yield and
Resistance to Listeria of Backcross Mice Derived from A/J
and B10.A Progenitors.

| Mice (n) | Number of peritoneal macrophages x 10$^6$ (mean+range) | Resistance to Listeria log$_{10}$CFU/liver (mean+range) |
|---|---|---|
| A (6) | 0.61 (0.43-0.70) | sensitive 8.26 (8.00-8.5) |
| B10.A (6) | 2.33 (2.01-2.51) | resistant 5.05 (3.62-7.27) |
| F$_1$(AxB10.A) (6) | 2.54 (1.74-3.18) | resistant 5.12 (3.60-7.17) |
| Backcross | | |
| F$_1$ x A | | |
| BC1 | 1.33 | resistant (6.11) |
| BC2 | 1.15 | resistant (7.17) |
| BC3 | 0.74 | sensitive (8.17) |
| BC4 | 2.60 | N.D. |
| BC5 | 0.32 | sensitive (8.30) |
| BC6 | 0.74 | sensitive (8.27) |
| BC7 | 1.84 | resistant (6.86) |
| BC8 | 0.96 | sensitive (8.30) |
| BC9 | 1.38 | resistant (7.20) |
| BC10 | 0.43 | sensitive (8.30) |
| Backcross | | |
| F$_1$ x B10.A | | |
| BC11 | 2.34 | resistant (4.50) |
| BC12 | 2.01 | resistant (5.63) |
| BC13 | 2.91 | resistant (4.83) |
| BC14 | 2.48 | resistant (7.01) |
| BC15 | 2.66 | resistant (6.22) |
| BC16 | 1.54 | resistant (4.35) |
| BC17 | 3.82 | resistant (6.17) |
| BC18 | 2.77 | resistant (7.00) |
| BC19 | 2.87 | resistant (3.90) |
| BC20 | 1.57 | resistant (5.23) |

Listeria-sensitive A/J mice had a mean of $0.61 \times 10^6$ macrophages and more than $1 \times 10^8$ cfu Listeria per liver (Table 1). Listeria-resistant B10.A mice had 4-fold greater numbers of peritoneal macrophages and were at least 100 times more resistant with a mean of $1 \times 10^5$ cfu per liver. $F_1$ hybrid mice likewise had greater numbers of peritoneal macrophages and were resistant to Listeria. Backcross analysis showed that 100% of B10.A x $F_1$ and all the resistant segregants of A/J x $F_1$ backcross had high numbers of macrophages characteristic of resistant B10.A mice. We can conclude, therefore, that host outcome of infection with Listeria is genetically linked to the size of mononuclear phagocyte system.

In order to assess whether, in addition to an augmented pool of macrophages, prompt macrophage inflammatory responses might also contribute to superior anti-listerial ability of the resistant strain, we examined the mobilization of inflammatory cells in vivo following intraperitoneal injection of nonspecific irritants and in vitro response to chemotactic stimuli. The differences in peritoneal cell yields between Listeria-resistant and sensitive strains were magnified following i.p. treatment with thioglycollate. Three days after such treatment, Listeria-resistant B10.A mice had enhanced inflammatory responses in vivo in comparison to Listeria-sensitive A/J mice (Table 2).

Table 2. Peritoneal Macrophage Inflammatory Response in Thioglycollate-Treated Mice

| Mouse Strain | Treatment i.p. | Total Peritoneal Cells x $10^6$ | Total Macrophages x $10^6$ |
|---|---|---|---|
| B10.A | None | $4.1 \pm 0.1$ | $2.4 \pm 0.1$ |
| A/J | None | $3.4 \pm 0.1$ | $1.7 \pm 0.1$ |
| B10.A | Thioglycollate | $28.7 \pm 2.0$ | $20.1 \pm 1.7$ |
| A/J | Thioglycollate | $9.5 \pm 0.6$ | $7.2 \pm 0.5$ |

Enhanced peritoneal macrophage responses were also evident in Listeria-resistant B10.A mice following i.p. injection with other sterile irritants - ConA and PHA (Fig. 1).

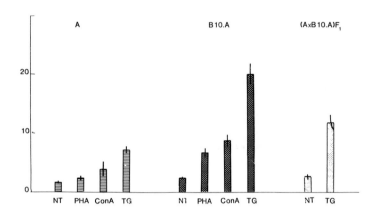

**Figure 1.** Macrophage inflammatory responses to various non-specific stimuli (peritoneal macrophage yield x $10^{-6}$ three days following i.p. injection of 3% thioglycollate (TG), 100 µg Con A, 100 µg PHA). NT = normal untreated mice. Mean of 3 mice per group ± SE.

To further examine the relationship between in vivo inflammatory responses and resistance to Listeria, a mouse strain survey of macrophage inflammatory responses following i.p. treatment with thiglycollate was made. Differences in in vivo inflammatory responses were evident among the strains examined (Table 3). All Listeria-resistant strains exhibited high macrophage inflammatory response in vivo. In contrast, Listeria-sensitive strains had uniformly low macrophage inflammatory responses. C3H/HeJ strain mice which had $LD_{50}$ for Listeria intermediate to resistant and sensitive strains had high inflammatory responses.

Table 3. Resistance to <u>Listeria</u> <u>Monocytogenes</u> and
Peritoneal Macrophage Inflammatory Response:   Strain
Distribution

| Mouse Strain | Resistance to Listeria[a] | Macrophage Inflammatory Response[b] |
|---|---|---|
| C57BL/6J | + | High |
| B10.A | + | High |
| B6.CH.2BA/BY | + | High |
| SJL | + | High |
| DBA/2J | − | Low |
| DBA/1J | − | Low |
| A/J | − | Low |
| C3H/HeJ | ± | High |
| Balb/c | − | Low |

+ $LD_{50}$  $10^5 - 5 \times 10^5$ cfu
− $LD_{50}$  $5 \times 10^3 - 10^4$ cfu
± $LD_{50}$  $3 \times 10^4 - 5 \times 10^4$ cfu

[a]$LD_{50}$ of intravenously-injected Listeria was determined by
Method of Reed and Muench (7).
[b]Numbers of macrophages were calculated from the total and
differential counts performed on samples of peritoneal
exudate cells from 5 to 40 individual mice treated 3 days
previously with thioglycollate.
High > $15 \times 10^6$ macrophages, Low < $10 \times 10^6$ macrophages.

Thioglycollate-induced peritoneal macrophages from
B10.A but not A/J mice also exhibited increased chemotactic
responsiveness <u>in vitro</u> to endotoxin-activated mouse serum
(EAMS) which contains C5a (8).  The enhanced macrophage
chemotactic responsiveness was observed under a wide range
of experimental conditions.  It is of interest to note that
there was no difference in the chemotactic ability of normal
resident peritoneal macrophages from either B10.A or A/J
mice to complement-derived chemotactic factors (Fig. 2).
However, thioglycollate-induced macrophages from A/J mice
were one-third to one-sixth less responsive in comparison to
equal number of similarly induced macrophages from B10.A
mice to various dilutions of EAMS.  The difference was, in

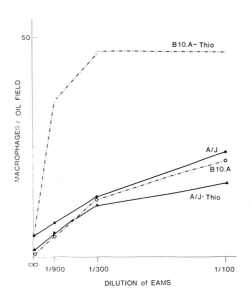

<u>Figure 2.</u>  Chemotaxis of peritoneal macrophages   dose re-
sponse to EAMS.   Peritoneal exudate cells were collected
from untreated mice or mice treated ip with thioglycollate 3
days  previously.    Chemotactic  responses  were  assayed  to
endotoxin-activated mouse serum (EAMS) by standard methods
(9).   Response is expressed as mean number of macrophages
per number of fields shown ± standard error of mean for
triplicate filters.

fact, most obvious at the highest dilution (1/900) of EAMS
tested.    In  addition,  the  difference  in  chemotactic  responsiveness  was  not  related  to  the  time  of  incubation
(Fig. 3).   With macrophages from either strain, there was
accelerated chemotaxis between 0 hr and approximately 3-4
hrs and a plateau in the response by 6 hrs.   In spite of the
similarity in kinetics, macrophages from B10.A mice treated
with thioglycollate were more responsiveness to 1/100 dilution of EAMS at each time point assayed.

        The  cells  responsible  for  the  enhanced  macrophage
chemotactic  responsiveness  were  evident  within  2  days  of
i.p. injection of B10.A mice with thioglycollate and remained evident through 4 days (Fig. 4).   Macrophages from A/J
mice did not show enhanced chemotactic responsiveness

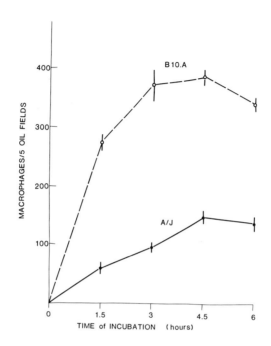

<u>Figure 3.</u>   Kinetics of chemotaxis of thioglycollate-induced
peritoneal   macrophages.    Experimental   conditions   as   per
Figure 2.

through  4  days  post  treatment.    Thioglycollate-induced
peritoneal macrophages from other Listeria-resistant strains
showed both high inflammatory responses <u>in vivo</u> and enhanced
chemotactic  responsiveness  <u>in vitro</u>.    Similarly, Listeria-
sensitive strains which exhibited low inflammatory responses
<u>in vivo</u> did not show enhanced chemotactic responsiveness of
macrophages <u>in vitro</u>.   Thus, the enhanced macrophage inflammatory responses evident in Listeria-resistant mice <u>in vivo</u>
seem to be due both to quantitative differences in macrophage pool and to qualitative differences in responsiveness to
chemotactic stimuli.

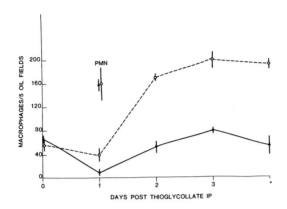

Figure 4. Chemotaxis of peritoneal macrophages (time course following _in vivo_ stimulation with thioglycollate). Experimental conditions as per Figure 2 ●————● A/J mice, o----o B10.A mice.

To examine whether the macrophage inflammatory response is under genetic control similar to host resistance to Listeria, we studied inflammatory responses in (A x B10.A)$F_1$ mice and appropriate backcross populations. $F_1$ hybrid mice showed a high intermediate level of both macrophage inflammatory responses _in vivo_ and chemotactic responses _in vitro_ following treatment with thioglycollate (Table 4).

Table 4. In _Vivo_ and In _Vitro_ Macrophage Inflammatory Responses of (B10.A x A/J)$F_1$ Mice.

| Mouse Strains | Total Macrophages x $10^6$ Mean ± SEM[a] | Macrophages Migrated/ 5 oil fields Mean ± SEM[b] |
|---|---|---|
| B10.A | 22.4 ± 2.82 | 213 ± 11 |
| A/J | 6.0 ± 1.16 | 94 ± 11 |
| (B10.AxA)$F_1$ | 12.5 ± 1.5 | 171 ± 6 |

[a]Mice were injected ip with thioglycollate. Three days later, PC were harvested. Numbers of macrophages were calculated from total and differential counts performed on samples of PC from individual mice. Mean of 6 mice per group ± standard error of the mean.
[b]Chemotactic response of macrophages to EAMS determined by standard methods (9). Mean number of migrated macrophages per 5 oil fields ± standard error of the mean for triplicate filters.

Inflammatory response (<u>in vivo</u>) in individual backcross, $F_1$ and parental mice was then studied and expressed as a percent of the mean response of B10.A mice. The mean macrophage inflammatory response of A/J mice was 37 ± 2%. The upper limit of low macrophage inflammatory responses characteristic of A/J mice was chosen as 63% (μ ± 2SD of A/J response). Using this criteria to distinguish high and low responders 14 of 33 (42%) A/J x $F_1$ backcross mice showed high macrophage inflammatory responses. More than 90% of B10.A x$F_1$ backcross mice exhibited high macrophage inflammatory responses. Analysis of individual hybrid $F_1$ and backcross mice therefore suggested that the trait of enhanced macrophage inflammatory responsiveness is controlled by a single dominant gene thus resembling inheritance of resistance to <u>Listeria monocytogenes</u>.

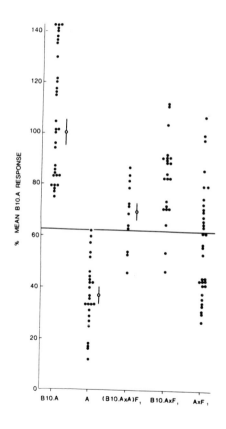

<u>Figure 5.</u>    Macrophage  inflammatory  response:    backcross analysis.

In conclusion, deficiencies in mononuclear phagocyte production by Listeria-sensitive mice (e.g. A/J) are suggested by the finding of low numbers of peritoneal macrophages present in the normal and infected state. This study extends the observation that the degree of peritoneal blood monocytosis is significantly higher in the infected Listeria-resistant B10.A than in the sensitive A/J strain mice (10). In addition, intraperitoneal injection of Listeria-resistant mice with sterile irritants resulted in 2-3 fold increases in macrophage yields in comparison to Listeria-sensitive mice. This quantitative difference in inflammatory responsiveness in vivo was paralleled by qualitative differences in chemotactic responsiveness in vitro. Thus, Listeria-sensitive A/J mice have defects in mononuclear phagocyte mobilization as assessed by in vivo and in vitro macrophage inflammatory responses. There was a strong correlation between resistance to Listeria monocytogenes and macrophage inflammatory responsiveness in vivo. Backcross analysis showed that the macrophage inflammatory response is genetically controlled by a single autosomal dominant gene. It will be of interest to determine if this gene is linked to the gene(s) controlling resistance to Listeria.

## REFERENCES

1. Cheers, C., and Mckenzie, I.F.C. Infect.Immun. 19:763, 1978.
2. Skamene, E., Kongshavn, P.A.L., and Sachs, D.H. J.Infect.Dis. 139:228, 1979.
3. Mackaness, G.B. J.Exp.Med. 116:381, 1962.
4. Sadarangani, C., Skamene, E., and Kongshavn, P.A.L. Infect.Immun. 28:381, 1980.
5. North, R.J. J.Exp.Med. 132:521, 1970.
6. Mitsuyama, M., Jakeya, K., Nomoto, K., and Shemotori, S. J.Gen.Micro. 106:165, 1979.
7. Reed, L.J., and Muench, H. Am.J.Hyg. 27:493, 1938.
8. Snyderman, R., Pike, M.C., McCurley, D., and Long, L. Infect.Immun. 11:488, 1975.
9. Boetcher, D.A., and Meltzer, M.S. J.Natl.Cancer Inst. 54:795, 1975.
10. Kongshavn, P.A.L., Sadarangani, C., and Skamene, E. 1980 (this volume).

# THE BEIGE (CHEDIAK-HIGASHI SYNDROME) MOUSE AS A MODEL FOR MACROPHAGE FUNCTION STUDIES

Page S. Morahan, Stephen S. Morse
and Keith H. Mahoney

Department of Microbiology
Medical College of Virginia
Virginia Commonwealth University
Richmond, Virginia 23298

Macrophages are important cells in host defense and regulatory processes, but the mechanisms involved in these functions are still being elucidated. A naturally occurring macrophage deficiency would be helpful for assessing the significance of macrophage functions. Although "macrophage-less" mutants are unknown, abnormalities of phagocyte function occur in the Chediak-Higashi syndrome (CH). CH might therefore serve as a useful model for defining certain macrophage functions. Since the disease includes lysosomal deficiencies, it would also be useful for defining the role of lysosomes in macrophage function.

CH is a rare autosomal recessive genetic disease characterized by pigmentary dilution and the presence of giant granules (abnormal lysosomes) in several cell types, including leukocytes (9). The condition has been described in humans, mink, mice, and other species. The mouse CH homologue, known as beige (bg), was first identified in the C57BL/6J line at Jackson (10,12). At present, two independently arising beige mutations are known in the C57BL/6J mouse; both are phenotypically identical (4). The beige mutation has also been observed in the C3H/HeJ mouse. Most research has been done with the C57BL/6J $bg^J/bg^J$ mutant.

Increased susceptibility to infections or neoplasia has been reported in CH. In humans, CH is associated with a lymphoma-like condition known as the accelerated phase (3). Increased susceptibility to pyogenic bacterial infections has been reported in both humans (23) and the beige mouse (12). Granulocytes have been the most studied cell in CH, and various abnormalities have been reported. CH granulocytes show a delay in bactericidal activity (23), which may be involved in the increased susceptibility that these patients exhibit to bacterial infection. The delay in killing of phagocytized bacteria appears to be correlated with a delay in fusion of the phagosome with lysosomes (20). Other functional abnormalities reported include defective chemotaxis in vitro (6).

Table 1.  Phagocytic Cell Abnormalities Reported in the
Beige Mouse

|  | Abnormality | Reference |
|---|---|---|
| **Histochemical** | | |
| Lysosomes; peroxidase granules (G, M)* | Giant granules | 1,12 |
| Lysosomes in bone marrow precursor cells (G, M) | Abnormal (large, self-fusion) | 16 |
| Concanavalin A capping (G) | Abnormal | 18 |
| Granulocyte neutral protease | Reduced or absent | 21 |
| **Functional** | | |
| Chemotaxis (G, M) | Reduced in vitro | 6 |
| Exudate formation in vivo (G, M) | Normal | 14,21 |
| NK cell activity | Reduced or absent | 19 |
| Macrophage tumor cell cytolysis and cytostasis | Delayed | 14 |
| Microbicidal activity against: | | |
|   Staphylococcus aureus | Delayed | 6 |
|   Group D Streptococci | Delayed | 6 |
| **Susceptibility to infection** | | |
| Experimental infection with Candida albicans, Streptococcus pneumoniae, Klebsiella pneumoniae, Staphylococcus aureus, or Escherichia coli | Increased susceptibility and mortality rates | 5 |
| Natural susceptibility reported increased to | | |
|   Eye and lung infections | | 12 |
|   Periodontal disease | | 11 |
|   Spontaneous pneumonitis (beige--satin double mutant) | | 10 |

*Cell type: G = Granulocyte; M = Macrophage or monocyte

Although mononuclear phagocytic cells have not been well studied, our results indicate that this cell lineage also possesses the characteristic abnormalities of CH. Both monocytes and promonocytes are abnormal (16). Table 1 summarizes the phagocyte abnormalities described in the beige mouse. Mononuclear phagocytes, like neutrophils in the beige mouse, possess the characteristic giant lysosomes, visible by acridine orange fluorescence. Peripheral blood counts are normal in the beige mouse, and both granulocytes and monocytes contain giant peroxidase-positive granules.

Treatment of mice with Corynebacterium parvum (Propion-ibacterium acnes) (70 mg/kg administered intraperitoneally 5-7 days before macrophage collection) is widely used to elicit macrophages which possess increased function. The numbers of peritoneal cells and proportion of macrophages are also increased by this treatment. A splenomegaly occurs which is related to the macrophage activation. In our laboratory, C. parvum caused comparable increases in both peritoneal cell yields and spleen weights in beige and C57BL/6J +/+ (control) mice (Table 2).

Table 2. Characteristics of Peritoneal Cells (PC) from the Beige Mouse

| Mouse | C. parvum | PC per mouse (X $10^{-6}$) | Percent macrophages[a] | %Fc rosette[b] | %C3b phagocytosis[b] |
|-------|-----------|------------------------------|-------------------------|-----------------|------------------------|
| Beige | - | $1.6 \pm 0.4$ | $23.1 \pm 2.4$ | $70.8 \pm 12.6$ | <5 |
| Control | - | $2.5 \pm 0.2$ | $24.9 \pm 2.5$ | $69.0 \pm 12.4$ | <5 |
| Beige | + | $3.0 \pm 0.6$ | $44.6 \pm 4.0$ | $85.1 \pm 7.4$ | $66.6 \pm 2.9$ |
| Control | + | $3.5 \pm 0.8$ | $46.7 \pm 4.0$ | $94.3 \pm 2.3$ | $67.1 \pm 4.2$ |

[a] Macrophages by acridine orange fluorescence
[b] Rosettes and phagocytosis of the adherent peritoneal macrophages

Spleen weights increased from a mean of 80.0 mg in untreated control mice to 284.4 mg after C. parvum. In the beige mouse, spleen weight increase from 99.7 to 319.1 mg. representing an increased of 3-3.5 fold in each case. The increases in peritoneal cell yield and percent macrophages from approximately 25% macrophages in untreated animals to about 47% after C. parvum) were also comparable in beige and control mice. Finally, macrophage response to Brewer's thioglycollate broth was similar in beige and control animals. These observations indicate that the beige reticuloendothelial system marshals a normal macrophage response after an eliciting stimulus. Previous reports have indicated that a normal granulocyte response also occurs (13,21).

Although macrophages from the beige mouse possess the morphologic hallmarks of CH (such as abnormal lysosomes), surface markers of the beige macrophage appeared relatively normal. Capping with Concanavalin A has been reported to be abnormal in macrophages of the beige mouse (17). We have studied macrophage surface receptors for the Fc portion of the IgG molecule and for the complement component C3b, which are also often used to enumerate macrophages. Macrophage phagocytosis can also be mediated by Fc or C3b receptors, with C3b receptor-mediated phagocytosis often used a criterion of macrophage activation (2). Resident beige and control macrophages showed comparable Fc and C3b surface receptor binding (Table 2). In addition, C. parvum macrophages from beige and control mice demonstrated comparable C3b-mediated phagocytosis.

The macrophages of the beige mouse therefore possess the characteristic lysosomal abnormalities and demonstrate abnormal capping with ConA (suggesting abnormalities in cytoskeleton). However, the beige mouse mobilizes a normal macrophage inflammatory response to stimuli tested. Moreover, although there may be some abnormalities in macrophage surface structure and cytoskeleton, these do not affect all surface receptors and do not markedly alter phagocytosis.

The normal C3b receptor mediated phagocytosis of C. parvum elicited macrophages suggests that macrophages from the beige mouse appear capable of normal activation. Activated macrophages mediate a number of host defense functions, including tumor cell cytolysis and cytostasis (8) and antiviral activities (15). We have investigated the antitumor activity of C. parvum elicited beige macrophages. Lysosomes have been implicated in macrophage antitumor activity (7). The beige mouse, with its lysosomal deficiency, could be used to define the role of lysosomal function.

Using Lewis lung carcinoma as the target cell, cytolysis (by $^3$H-T$^{dR}$ release) and cytostasis (by inhibition of $^{125}$IUdR uptake) were at normal levels at the end of the 72-hr assays. However, the kinetics of these antitumor activities were altered in the beige mouse, showing a delay of approximately 6-12 hours in expression. Thus, by 6 hour C. parvum control macrophages inhibited $^{125}$IUdR uptake in the tumor cells (cytostasis assay) by 86.3%, while beige macrophages inhibited the target cells by only 49.7% (p<0.05). The differences were even more pronounced at earlier times. However, by 24 hours, there was virtually no difference between the beige and control activity. In tumor cell cytotoxicity assays, similar results were observed. Although beige and control C. parvum elicited macrophages showed approximately equal cytolytic activity at 48 hours, there were striking differences at earlier times. At 12 hours, the beige macrophages had less than one third the activity of control cells.

These delays in macrophage antitumor function are similar to the delays observed in granulocyte bactericidal activity (23). At present, it is unknown whether similar mechanisms are involved in these activities. An anbormality in macrophage function should also be evident in vivo, if not masked by compensatory increases in other host defense systems. Macrophages appear to be consistently involved in immunomodulator induced resistance to the Lewis lung carcinoma which is syngeneic in C57BL/6 mice. Therefore, growth of Lewis lung carcinoma injected in foot pad was measured in controls and beige mice. There was no significant difference in tumor volume or mean survival time. In a typical experiment we observed mean survival times of 27.9 (± 1.5) days for control mice and 28.0 (± 1.2) days for beige. The role of macrophages is being further assessed by immunomodulator treatment of the Lewis lung carcinoma in the two mouse strains. In experiments with the B16 melanoma, which is another metastasizing solid tumor, the beige mouse has shown markedly decreased resistance as compared to the +/+ mouse to intravenous tumor inoculation but less difference with subcutaneous inoculation. These data suggest that impaired macrophage or NK cell function in the beige mouse may be more pronounced in the peritoneum and spleen than peripherally (N. Hanna, personal communication). Reports of virus-like particles in leukocytes of CH patients in the lymphoproliferative accelerated phase (22) suggest that there may be abnormal responses to some viruses. Macrophage antiviral activity is currently being defined. Only limited data are available on response of the beige mouse to virus challenge and on antiviral activity of beige mouse macrophages.

It is not yet known whether the delayed expression of macrophage in vitro antitumor activity is related to the lysosomal abnormalities of the beige mouse; further studies with the beige mouse may help to elucidate the early step in macrophage expression. Moreover, recent reports (19) have demonstrated that the beige is deficient in natural killer (NK) cell function. The beige mouse would therefore be an ideal animal for defining the roles of NK cells and for distinguishing macrophage- and NK-mediated defenses.

ACKNOWLEDGEMENT

This work was supported by Grant CA24686 and by Postdoctoral Fellowship CA 06332 (S.S.M.) from the National Cancer Institute, DHEW, Grant AI 70863 from the National Institutes of Health, DHEW, and Grant IN-105C from the American Cancer Society.

REFERENCES

1.   Bennett, J.M., Blume, R.S., and Wolff, S.M.  J.Lab.-
     Clin.Med. 73:235, 1969.
2.   Bianco, C., and Edelson, P.J.  In Molecular Basis of
     Cell-Cell Interaction. (Birth Defectrs vol. 14, No.2).
     R.A. Lerner (ed). New York: Alan R. Liss, p119, 1978.
3.   Blume, R.S., and Wolff, S.M.  Medicine (Balt.) 51:247,
     1972.
4.   Brandt, E.J., and Swank, R.T.  Amer.J.Pathol. 82:573,
     1976.
5.   Elin, R.J., Edelin, J.B., and Wolff, S.M.  Infect.-
     Immun. 10:88, 1974.
6.   Gallin, J.I., Bujak, J.S., Patten, E., and Wolff, S.M.
     Blood 43:201, 1974.
7.   Hibbs, J.B.,Jr.  Science 184:468, 1974.
8.   Kaplan, A.M., Brown, J., Collins, J.M., Morahan, P.S.,
     and Snodgrass, M.J.  J.Immunol. 119:1738, 1978.
9.   Klebanoff, S.J., and Clark, R.A.  In The Neutrophil.
     S.J. Klebanoff and R.A. Clark (eds).  New York:
     Elsevier/North-Holland, p735, 1979.
10.  Lane, P.W., and Murphy, E.D.  Genetics 72:451, 1972.
11.  Lavine, W.S., Page, R.C., and Padgett, G.A.
     J.Periodont 47:621, 1976.
12.  Lutzner, M.A., Lowrie, C.T., and Jordon, H.W.  J.Hered.
     58:299, 1967.
13.  McGarry, M.P., Brandt, E.J., and Swank, R.T.  Amer.J.-
     Pathol. 85:685, 1976.
14.  Mahoney, K.H., Morse, S.S., and Morahan, P.S.  In
     Current Chemotherapy and Infectious Disease.  J.D.
     Nelson, C. Grassi, and R.W. Sarber (eds).  Washington
     DC: American Society for Microbiology, 1980 (in press).
15.  Morahan, P.S., Morse, S.S., and McGeorge, M.B.  J.Gen.-
     Virol. 46:291, 1980.
16.  Oliver, C., and Essner, E.  Lab.Invest. 32:17, 1975.
17.  Oliver, J.M., and Berlin, R.D.  In Immunobiology of the
     Macrophage.  D.S. Nelson (ed).  New York: Academic
     Press, p259, 1976.

18.  Oliver, J.M., Zurier, R.B., and Berlin, R.D.  Nature
     253:471, 1975.
19.  Roder, J., and Duwe, A.  Nature 278:451, 1979.
20.  Root, R.K., Rosenthal, A.S., and Balestra, D.J.
     J.Clin.Invest. 51:649, 1972.
21.  Vassalli, J.D., Granelli-Piperno, A., Griscelli, C.,
     and Reich, E.  J. Exp.Med. 147:1285, 1978.
22.  White, J.G.  Cancer 19:877, 1966.
23.  Wolff, S.M., Dale, D.C., Clark, R.A., Root, R.K., and
     Kimball, H.R.  Ann.Intern.Med. 76:293, 1972.

## DISCUSSION

Collins:  Morahan gave a list of organisms to which there
was an increased susceptibility.  Most of these are extracellular parasites or at least involve polymorphonuclear re-
spones.  Has she any information on how the beige mice behave against certified intracellular parasites such as M.
tuberculosis.  There is a great deal of difference in the
susceptibility of the C57BL mouse against M. tuberculosis
infection (BCG included) and many other inbred strains of
mice and I wonder whether in fact these beige mice are perhaps one step further advanced in their susceptibility.

Morahan:  I have no idea.  They handle C. parvum fine, but
these are killed organisms.  We have not seen any differences which might be related to LPS.  But that again is not
exactly related to BCG infection.

Burton:  My comment is about the growth of Lewis lung tumor
in beige mice.  We have been studying the C57BL and beige
mice with alloantisera directed against NK alloantigens.
There clearly seem to be at least two types of NK cells in
mice, one type being preferentially directed against lymphomas, the other preferentially, but not exclusively, directed
against non-lymphomatous tissues.  We would have predicted
that tumor induction in beige mice would not be much different than what is usual for the solid tumors, but quite
different in the case of the leukemias and lymphomas.  The
same thing would probably apply to transplantation studies.

Morahan:  I think this is an important observation and that
is my feeling also.

Burton:  It would be interesting to see whether the Lewis
lung tumor in fact is a target for the natural killer

directed against the non-lymphomatous tissues rather than for the cell that kills the lymphoma.

Morahan: I think that would indeed be interesting.

Kiessling: Did you use the in vivo line of B16 melanoma?

Morahan: We have used both the in vivo and the in vitro lines. There was no difference.

Kiessling: There is a paper in press by Talmage et al. that, when they used the in vitro line of B16 melanoma, they saw more rapid growth of tumor in beige mice as compared to heterozygous littermates.

Morahan: Right. I think some of the differences may involve the route of inoculation of the tumor and so forth, i.e., whether it is inoculated intravenously in which case it goes directly to the lung, or by looking at spontaneous metastasis.

# DEFECTIVE Fc-MEDIATED PHAGOCYTOSIS BY LPS-HYPORESPONSIVE (Lps^d) C3H/HeJ MACROPHAGES: CORRECTION BY AGENTS THAT ELEVATE INTRACELLULAR CYCLIC AMP

Stefanie N. Vogel, Lynda L. Weedon, Joost J. Oppenheim and David L. Rosenstreich[1]

Laboratory of Microbiology and Immunology
National Institute of Dental Research
National Institutes of Health
Bethesda, Maryland
and
[1]The Albert Einstein College of Medicine
Departments of Medicine, Microbiology and Immunology
New York, N.Y.

Endotoxin, the lipopolysaccharide (LPS) derived from many Gram negative organisms, can induce profound immunological alterations resulting in lethality and tumor necrosis, as well as a number of other clinically important manifestations (reviewed in 1). Sometime between 1961 and 1965, a spontaneous mutation occurred in the C3H/He mouse strain, resulting in the endotoxin-resistant C3H/HeJ substrain (5). Studies of this mouse mutant have revealed that the gene controlling LPS responsiveness (Lps) is located on the 4th chromosome (8). This gene has since been shown to control macrophage (Mφ) sensitivity to LPS, the ability of Mφ to become activated, and resistance to infection with Salmonella typhimurium (reviewed in 7). We have recently demonstrated that thioglycollate-induced peritoneal Mφ derived from LPS-hyporesponsive (Lps^d) C3H/HeJ mice lose, over a 48 hour culture period, the capacity to bind and phagocytose IgG-coated, sheep erythrocytes (EA). In contrast, fully LPS-responsive (Lps^n) C3H/HeN mice exhibit a progressive increase in phagocytic ability with time in culture (6). Since Fc-receptor expression is felt to be a reflection of the differentiation state of the Mφ, the inability of C3H/HeJ Mφ to maintain their Fc-binding capacity in vitro may reflect a broader defect in Mφ differentiation. Support for this hypothesis stems from our recent findings that a lymphokine-rich culture supernatant derived from Concanavalin A-stimulated spleen cells (CS), which has the capacity to activate Mφ to a microbicidal state in vitro (4), also reverses the phagocytic defect in C3H/HeJ Mφ cultures (Table 1).

Table 1. Phagocytosis of IgG-coated sheep erythrocytes (EA)
by C3H/HeN and C3H/HeJ Mφ

| | $^{51}$Cr-EA (cpm) Ingested after 48 Hr Culture | |
| --- | --- | --- |
| | C3H/HeN (Lps$^n$) | C3H/HeJ (Lps$^d$) |
| + 0 | 50,462 ± 1667 | 21,108 ± 194 |
| + CS (5%) | 46,486 ± 1888 | 47,276 ± 1914 |

Taken from (6).

The mechanisms leading to the expression of macrophage
membrane markers during differentiation, such as Fc receptors, have not been well delineated. However, dibutyryl
cyclic adenosine monophosphate (DBcAMP) has been shown <u>in
vitro</u> to induce the expression of membrane markers in both B
and T lymphocytes derived from C3H/HeJ mice (2). Additionally, Muschel et al. (3) demonstrated that DBcAMP increased
the number of phagocytic Mφ in nonphagocytic mutant Mφ cell
lines. Therefore, we examined the effects of DBcAMP on the
induction of Fc receptor capacity in C3H/HeN and C3H/HeJ Mφ.
As seen with CS-treated C3H/HeJ cultures (6), DBcAMP increased the capacity of C3H/HeJ Mφ to bind EA (Table 2).

Table 2. Effect of DBcAMP on EA binding capacity of C3H/HeJ
Mφ cultured 48 hr.

| | $^{51}$Cr-EA (cpm) Bound[*] |
| --- | --- |
| + 0 | 1,740 ± 485 |
| + DBcAMP ($10^{-4}$M) | 9,918 ± 353 |

[*]Binding experiments were carried out in the presence of 1.5
X $10^{-3}$M iodoacetic acid to inhibit Fc-mediated phagocytosis.

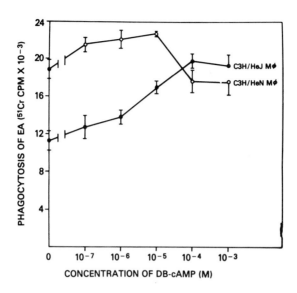

**Figure 1.**

Furthermore, Figure 1 demonstrates that DBcAMP not only reverses the binding defect in C3H/HeJ Mφ cultures, but also restores phagocytosis to the level of C3H/HeN Mφ cultures.

8-Bromo-cAMP was also capable of enhancing Fc-mediated phagocytosis in C3H/HeJ Mφ cultures, but neither butyric acid nor DBcGMP (tested from $10^{-3}$ M to $10^{-8}$ M) were active (Table 3). These data implicate the cAMP moiety as the active agent in the enhancement of EA ingestion by C3H/HeJ Mφ.

Table 3. Agents containing the cAMP moiety enhance
Fc-mediated phagocytosis in C3H/HeJ Mφ cultures

|  | $^{51}$Cr-EA (cpm) Ingested |
|---|---|
| + 0 | 4,352 ± 960 |
| + DBcAMP ($10^{-4}$ M) | 8,916 ± 17 |
| + 8-Br-cAMP ($10^{-4}$ M) | 8,317 ± 250 |
| + Butyric acid ($10^{-4}$ M) | 4,492 ± 1433 |
| + DBcGMP ($10^{-4}$ M) | 4,988 ± 619 |

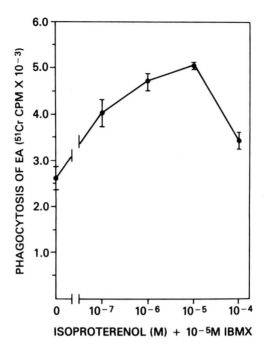

<u>Figure 2.</u>

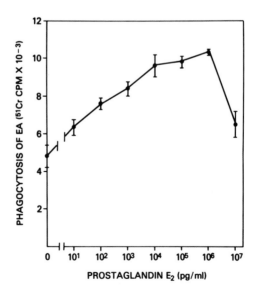

<u>Figure 3.</u>

Treatment of C3H/HeJ Mφ with cAMP agonists also corrected the phagocytic defect in a dose dependent fashion.  The
β-adrenergic agonist, isoproterenol, in the presence of the
phosophodiesterase inhibitor, isobutylmethylxanthine (IBMX),
and prostaglandin $E_2$ ($PGE_2$) increased the ingestion of EA by
C3H/HeJ Mφ cultures (Figures 2 and 3).  These data support
the hypothesis that the expression of Fc-receptors by macrophages can be mediated by agents which increase the intracellular levels of cAMP.

Since $PGE_2$ is an important Mφ product, in addition to
being a potent cAMP agonist, we examined whether the CS-induced increase in Fc-mediated phagocytosis was due to the
presence of $PGE_2$ in the CS or due to CS-induced production
of $PGE_2$ by C3H/HeJ Mφ.  The presence of indomethacin, a
potent inhibitor of $PGE_2$ production, during the production
of CS, failed to alter its ability to enhance phagocytosis
of EA by C3H/HeJ Mφ did not inhibit the increase in Fc-receptor capacity (Table 4).  Thus, CS enhances EA phagocytosis independently of $PGE_2$.

Table 4.   Indomethacin does not inhibit CS-enhancement of
           C3H/HeJ Mφ Fc-mediated phagocytosis.

|  | $^{51}$Cr-EA (cpm) Ingested |
| --- | --- |
| + 0 | 9099 ± 1127 |
| + CS (5%) | 22,668 ± 3956 |
| + Indomethacin (1 ug/ml) | 9659 ± 1315 |
| + Indomethacin + CS | 23,249 ± 1760 |

48 hr cultures

We next analyzed whether CS treatment of C3H/HeJ Mφ
cultures resulted in an increase in intracellular cAMP.
Table 5 demonstrates that CS-treatment of C3H/HeJ Mφ results
in a small but significant overall increase in intracellular
cAMP of approximately 60%.

Table 5.  Effect of CS on intracellular cAMP levels in 48
hr C3H/HeJ Mφ cultures.

Intracellular cAMP/2 X $10^6$ Mφ (pM/culture)

|         | Expt.1 | Expt.2 | Expt.3 | Expt.4 | $\overline{X}$ |
|---------|--------|--------|--------|--------|------|
| +0      | 0.514  | 0.520  | 0.181  | 0.368  | 0.396 |
| + CS (5%) | 0.861 | 0.898 | 0.294  | 0.469  | 0.631 |

## CONCLUSIONS

Thioglycollate-induced C3H/HeJ Mφ exhibit a differentiation defect expressed by an inability to maintain their
Fc-receptor binding and phagocytic capacity in vitro.  In
contrast, C3H/HeN Mφ exhibit a marked enhancement of Fc-
mediated phagocytosis with time in culture.  Treatment of
C3H/HeJ Mφ with a lymphokine-rich, Con A stimulated, spleen
cell culture supernatant (CS) corrects the C3H/HeJ phagocytic defect.

Additionally, DBcSMP, 8-Br-cAMP, as well as several intracellular cAMP agonists, also corrected the phagocytic
defect of C3H/HeJ Mφ.  As seen with CS-treatment, DBcAMP
enhanced both EA binding and phagocytosis by the C3H/HeJ Mφ.
These data suggest that the defective C3H/HeJ Mφ differentiation can be corrected by treatments which increase levels
of intracellular cAMP.  CS-stimulation of C3H/HeJ Mφ cultures also induced an increase in intracellular cAMP.  This
raises the possibility that correction of the C3H/HeJ differentiation defect by CS may act through a mechanism involving a cAMP signal.

It is highly likely that the C3H/HeJ differentiation
defect is another manifestation of the C3H/HeJ gene defect,
Lps[d].  Additional evidence supporting this hypothesis is
that Mφ derived from C57BL/10ScN (Lps[d]), but not C57BL/
10ScSn (Lps[n]) mice, also exhibited the same phagocytic
defect which was correctable by CS-treatment.

Our working hypothesis is that the differentiation
defect in C3H/HeJ Mφ is secondary to the inability of Mφ
precursor cells to respond to LPS or to LPS-induced differentiation factors.  The data presented in this report demonstrate that cAMP can act as a differentiation signal for
these macrophages.  However, direct evidence for a role for
cAMP in modulating LPS-hyporesponsiveness remains to be
obtained.

## REFERENCES

1.   Berry, L.J.   Crit.Rev.Toxicol. 5:239, 1977.
2.   Koenig, S., Hoffmann, M.K., and Thomas, L.   J.Immunol. 118:1910, 1977.
3.   Muschel, R.J., Rosen, N., Rosen, O.M., and Bloom, B.R. J.Immunol. 119:1813, 1977.
4.   Nogueira, N., and Cohn, Z.A.   J.Exp.Med. 148:288, 1978.
5.   Sultzer, B.   Infect.Immun. 5:107, 1972.
6.   Vogel, S.N., and Rosenstreich, D.L.   J.Immunol. 123:- 2842, 1979.
7.   Vogel, S.N., Weinblatt, A.C., and Rosenstreich, D.L. In Immunologic Defects in Laboratory Animals.   M.E. Gershwin and B. Merchant (eds). New York: Plenum Press, 1980 (in press).
8.   Watson, J., Kelly, K., Largen, M., and Taylor, B.A. J.Immunol. 120:422, 1978.

# GENETIC CONTROL OF MACROPHAGE DIFFERENTIATION AND FUNCTION

## Chairman's Summary

### Peter Ralph

Memorial Sloan-Kettering Cancer Center
New York, N.Y.

In focussing on genetic resistance to specific diseases, preceding sessions of this conference generally dealt with whole animal experiments, mostly with multigene and complicated environmental interactions. The critical role of the macrophage and the cellular and molecular levels of genetic defects surfaced from time to time. Controversy continued concerning the essential participation of macrophages in natural resistance to viruses (HSV-2),as opposed to the concept that a variety of cell types, including macrophages, exhibit resistance in the appropriate strains of mice (MHV-3, and influenza virus in hepatocytes).

This session was concerned with the generation, recruitment, activation and cytotoxic mechanisms of macrophages as critically important components of host resistance.

## GENERATION OF MONOCYTES AND MACROPHAGES

There are mouse strain differences in numbers of peritoneal exudate macrophage colony forming cells (M-CFC) and size of colonies. In chimera experiments between A/J and B10.A, low numbers of M-CFC was determined by the B10.A genotype while Listeria resistance was associated with the host environment. These CFC results were obtained with a L cell source of colony stimulating factor (CSF) that contained an inhibitor preferentially acting on B/6 and B10.A. Purified CSF gave similar numbers of CFC in the different strains. The possibility of strain differences in endogenous inhibitors that have been found in peritoneal fluids is being further explored (Stewart et al.).

A water-soluble monocytosis-promoting activity (MPA) can be derived from Listeria. MPA did not have a direct CSF-like effect on bone marrow precursors in vitro, but did induce production of a monocytosis-promoting serum factor. MPA was active in several strains of mice including B10.A, but failed to induce appreciable monocytosis in A/J mice.

C3H/HeJ mice are LPS-unresponsive in contrast to C3HeB-/FeJ mice with respect to generation of macrophages. HeJ mice have reduced CSF levels and splenic pluripotent CFC and G,M-CFC in response to endotoxin. Using pregnant mouse uterus extract (PMUE) as a source of CSF, normal HeJ mice had elevated levels of M-CFC in bone marrow, spleen, peripheral blood and especially peritoneal exudate when compared with FeJ. Spleen, marrow and peritoneal leukocytosis followed different kinetics in the two strains after LPS i.p., presumably reflecting differences in their handling of endotoxin (MacVitie et al.).

## MACROPHAGE RESISTANCE TO INFECTION AND MALIGNANCY

BCG-activated or lymphokine (LK)-treated macrophages from mouse strains developing tumoricidal capacity (C3H/HeN, C57BL/6N) kill a fraction of Rickettsia akari or Leishmania tropica at an early stage of in vitro infection (1 hr) and the majority of organisms within 24 hr. Tumoricidal-deficient strains (HeJ, B10/ScCR, A/J, etc.) are $10^3$-$10^4$ fold more susceptible to R. akari infection. Their macrophages fail to kill parasites early and are anergic at 24 hr. Strain A/J macrophages apparently could not be stimulated by any treatment to kill L. tropica. P/J was an exceptional strain, deficient in tumoricidal macrophages, but resistant to R. akari and able to kill both parasites in vitro. This strain fails to produce a 50,000 molecular weight LK responsible for tumoricidal activity, but does produce analogous LK that stimulates macrophage parasiticidal activity. P/J macrophages can be stimulated by the proper LK, from other strains, to kill tumor targets. HeJ and B/10ScCR macrophages respond to the non-50,000 LKs by killing parasites within 24 hr but do not show a normal LK of response to 50,000 MW. Genetic control at the level of host activating mechanisms and at the level of macrophage responsiveness to activation are evident in these experiments (Nacy et al.).

The concept was introduced of a time-dependent, irreversible series of steps to primed and then cytotoxic macrophages. A/J, C3H/HeJ, P/J and a few other mouse strains do not develop typical tumoricidal macrophages after i.p. injection of BCG or other strong stimuli. The HeJ mouse has at least two genetic defects. One is the well characterized unresponsiveness to LPS seen in fibroblasts, lymphocytes and macrophages. The second abnormality is hyporesponsiveness of macrophages to activation by a variety of agents unrelated to endotoxin. This effect is unrelated to inflammatory response (number of exudate macrophages, degree of chemotaxis, phagocytosis, peroxidase staining) or ability of BCG-primed spleen cells to make tumoricidal LK upon secondary antigen (PPD) stimulation in culture. Several mouse strains on the A background (but not B10.A) have macrophages manifesting a similar defect in activation (Meltzer et al.). As with the LPS-unresponsive strains, such strains require strong stimuli both in vivo and in vitro to develop tumoricidal capacity. This defect is also associated with failure to kill Rickettsia and Leishmania, although exceptions are noted (P/J,NZW).The possibility that the "activated macrophage" gene is different from the LPS gene comes from the finding that C3Heb/FeJ mice have normal tumoricidal activity but are susceptible to Salmonella typhimurium. It may be necessary to ascertain whether another gene, such as Ity, has "crept" into this strain for confirmation of a multilocus defect in the region of the Lps gene in C3H/HeJ.

Ruco described a number of unsuccessful in vivo experiments designed to bring C3H/HeJ mice up to the level of other mouse strains in developing activated tumoricidal macrophages. These included multiple i.p. injections of BCG, Con A, LPS, LK, etc. LK free of extrinsic inflammatory agents apparently does not activate responsive mouse strains in vivo either. It is important to develop in vitro models of exudation, such as "priming", and better ways to analyze cellular and molecular events leading to inflammatory responses.

In the case of strain A/J (susceptible) and B10.A (resistant) mice infected with Listeria, fewer inflammatory macrophages induced by Con A, PHA or thioglycollate with lower chemotactic response are seen in the susceptible strain (Stevenson et al.). It was proposed that these two-fold differences in numbers could be responsible for successful outcome of infection by Listeria in the competition between host defenses and bacterial multiplication and invasiveness. Suggestions in the workshop to inject infected A/J mice with syngeneic resident or early and late exudate macrophages were considered as an approach to test this hypothesis.

With the discovery that they lack NK cell activity and are less resistant to some transplantable leukemias, the beige (bg) mutation in C56BL/6 mice has become important for the study of host resistance. Beige macrophages manifest the same morphologic abnormality as granulocytes, namely giant cytoplasmic granules. However, macrophage surface receptors, phagocytosis, % peroxidase positive and numbers of cells in exudates are normal. Cytostatic and cytotoxic effects of beige macrophages against Lewis lung tumor targets are delayed early in incubation, but attain normal levels by 12 - 24 hr cocultivation. Lewis lung tumor growth and mean survival times were similar in bg/bg and +/+ control mice (Morahan). This result is consistent with the demonstration that the beige mutation affects $NK_L$ active on lymphomas, but not the $NK_S$ subset preferentially killing solid tumors.

### MOLECULAR MECHANISMS OF MACROPHAGE EFFECTOR FUNCTIONS

Thioglycollate-induced peritoneal macrophages from C3H-/HeJ mice lose the capacity to bind and phagocytose antibody-coated RBC in the course of 2 days in culture. In contrast, LPS-responsive HeN macrophages show an increase in these activities during culture. LK, cAMP derivatives, and agents that increase cytoplasmic cAMP levels correct the HeJ defect. The culture medium may contain substances stimulating normal cells to which HeJ macrophages cannot respond. These results suggest that LK maintains HeJ functions in vitro by acting through a cAMP signal (Vogel et al.).

Con A-induced exudate macrophages that are tumoricidal pinocytose more than thioglycollate-induced macrophages, but phagocytose fewer antibody-coated RBC. Two variants of the J774.2 cell line deficient in RBC ingestion had reduced pinocytic ability, and further study of mutants is proceeding (Norin).

In assessing the tumoricidal capacity of eight macrophage-related cell lines, three immature lines proved inactive whereas the other lines showed varying degrees of spontaneous toxicity and killing enhanced by LPS, NK, tumor promoter phorbol myristate, and antibody to targets. The differences in killing of six tumor targets tested suggests diverse mechanisms of toxicity and perhaps the operation of several sublines of macrophages. Two variants of J774 line deficient in superoxide anion production maintained tumoricidal capacity induced by several agents (Ralph et al.). Development of macrophage lines lacking other postulated toxic mechanisms should prove helpful in analyzing resistance to parasitic, bacterial and viral infections as well as resistance to malignancy.

# INDEX